Urodynamics, Neurourology and Pelvic Floor Dysfunctions

Series Editor

Enrico Finazzi Agrò
Tor Vergata University
Urology Department
Rome, Italy

The aim of the book series is to highlight new knowledge on physiopathology, diagnosis and treatment in the fields of pelvic floor dysfunctions, incontinence and neurourology for specialists (urologists, gynecologists, neurologists, pediatricians, physiatrists), nurses, physiotherapists and institutions such as universities and hospitals.

More information about this series at http://www.springer.com/series/13503

Giovanni Mosiello • Giulio Del Popolo
Jian Guo Wen • Mario De Gennaro
Editors

Clinical Urodynamics in Childhood and Adolescence

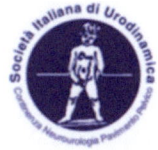

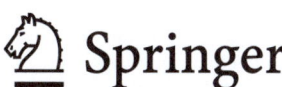

Editors
Giovanni Mosiello
Pediatric NeuroUrology Research and Clinic
Bambino Gesù Pediatric Hospital
Rome, Italy

Giulio Del Popolo
Neurourology Department
Careggi Hospital
Florence, Italy

Jian Guo Wen
Pediatric Urodynamic Center
First Affiliated Hospital of Zhengzhou University
Zhengzhou, China

Mario De Gennaro
Urology Unit
Bambino Gesù Pediatric Hospital
Rome, Italy

Pediatric Surgery and Urology
First Affiliated Hospital of Xinxiang Medical University
Xinxiang, China

ISSN 2510-4047 ISSN 2510-4055 (electronic)
Urodynamics, Neurourology and Pelvic Floor Dysfunctions
ISBN 978-3-030-13252-1 ISBN 978-3-319-42193-3 (eBook)
https://doi.org/10.1007/978-3-319-42193-3

© Springer International Publishing AG, part of Springer Nature 2018
Softcover re-print of the Hardcover 1st edition 2018
This work is subject to copyright. All rights are reserved by the Publisher, whether the whole or part of the material is concerned, specifically the rights of translation, reprinting, reuse of illustrations, recitation, broadcasting, reproduction on microfilms or in any other physical way, and transmission or information storage and retrieval, electronic adaptation, computer software, or by similar or dissimilar methodology now known or hereafter developed.
The use of general descriptive names, registered names, trademarks, service marks, etc. in this publication does not imply, even in the absence of a specific statement, that such names are exempt from the relevant protective laws and regulations and therefore free for general use.
The publisher, the authors and the editors are safe to assume that the advice and information in this book are believed to be true and accurate at the date of publication. Neither the publisher nor the authors or the editors give a warranty, express or implied, with respect to the material contained herein or for any errors or omissions that may have been made. The publisher remains neutral with regard to jurisdictional claims in published maps and institutional affiliations.

Printed on acid-free paper

This Springer imprint is published by the registered company Springer International Publishing AG part of Springer Nature
The registered company address is: Gewerbestrasse 11, 6330 Cham, Switzerland

Series Editor's Preface

As President of the Italian Society of Urodynamics, I am very proud to present this new book in our series: *Clinical Urodynamics in Childhood and Adolescence*.

When our Society defined this project with Springer, we had exactly the idea to offer to clinicians, and all health care providers, some practical books to use in their daily clinical practice.

The readers will be able to find three different parts: diagnostic tests, pathologies, and management, stressing the value of urodynamics that is sometimes confused with a minor part of urological practice, not considering the value to represent the functional part of urology.

All the authors are recognized experts of bladder and bowel, or in pediatric or in adult people, in some cases in both, because involved in transitional care project. All of them are valuable and active in different scientific societies. Furthermore, the majority of them are members of the International Continence Society and the International Children Continence Society.

I would like to thank all of them for their valuable contribution. A special thanks to the editors Giulio, Jian, Mario, and last but not least to Giovanni Mosiello for involving all of us in this book and for his perseverance and his efforts to publish it.

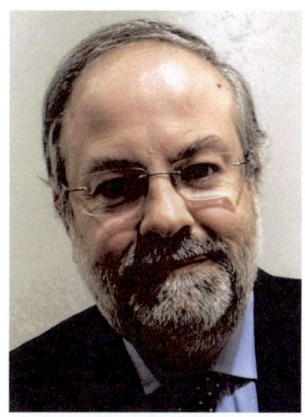

Enrico Finazzi Agrò
Rome, Italy

Foreword

Pediatric urodynamics has always been a challenging field, for both the referring doctors and those who are performing the studies. This special population of children and adolescent patients usually suffers from complex or complicated lower urinary tract dysfunction. Other pathologies such as congenital anomalies, high-grade vesico-ureteral reflux, and outlet obstructions can add to the difficulty of urodynamic studies.

The International Continence Society (ICS) is very pleased with this textbook, which discusses clinical urodynamics in this patient population to shed light on the typical indications and critical technical aspects relevant to this age group. I am proud of Giovanni Mosiello, who is Chairman of the ICS Children and Young Adults Committee, for authoring this valuable book. I expect that it will serve as a valuable reference for those who are interested in urodynamics performance and knowledge.

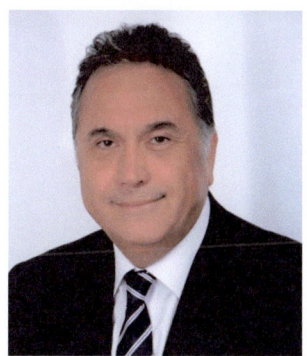

Sherif Mourad
ICS General Secretary
Cairo, Egypt

Preface

Pediatric urology often involves reconstruction of congenital malformations, which requires specialized surgical skills. Many patients with these congenital malformations commonly experience continence dysfunction. For this reason, reconstructive surgery must be performed while keeping function in mind. Thus, a pediatric urologist must be a functional urologist, with knowledge of the long-term effects of pathologies and the treatment performed. A pediatric urologist must be able to distinguish between functional incontinence (which is very common in childhood) and incontinence related to neurogenic or anatomic causes.

Many pathologies that are surgically treated in childhood may still have lifelong effects, such as incontinence. In all of these situations, it is important to understand the possible future effects of any treatments performed in childhood. For this reason, we decided to publish the first book on clinical urodynamics in children and young adults.

We offer a special thanks to all friends who agreed to participate in the writing of this book by sharing their great experiences.

On behalf of the other editors—Giulio De Popolo, Mario De Gennaro and Jian Guo Wen—we hope you enjoy.

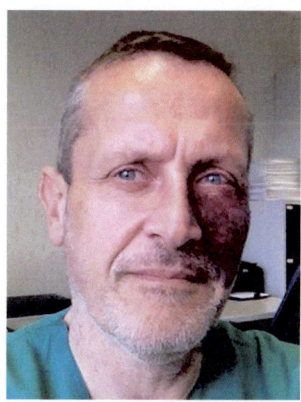

Giovanni Mosiello
Rome, Italy

Contents

Part I Diagnostic Evaluation

1. **Anatomy and Neurophysiology of the Lower Urinary Tract and Pelvic Floor** 3
   Lotte Kaasgaard Jakobsen, Jens Christian Djurhuus, and L. Henning Olsen

2. **Clinical Evaluation: History Taking and Urological, Gynaecological and Neurological Evaluation** 11
   Cevdet Kaya and Christian Radmayr

3. **Diagnostic Scores, Questionnaires and Quality-of-Life Measures in Paediatric Continence** 21
   Wendy F. Bower

4. **Diaries** 29
   Ana Ludy Lopes Mendes, Ilaria Jansen, and Giovanni Mosiello

5. **Ultrasound and MRI** 37
   J.M. Nijman

6. **Endoscopy** 45
   Murat Ucar, Selcuk Keskin, and Selcuk Yucel

7. **Noninvasive Urodynamics and Flowmetry in Children, Adolescents, and Young Adults** 63
   Mario Patricolo

8. **Cystometry, Pressure Flow Study and Urethral Pressure Measurement** 73
   Jian Guo Wen

9. **Videourodynamic in Children** 95
   Valerio Iacovelli, Giuseppe Farullo, Andrea Turbanti, and Enrico Finazzi Agrò

10. **The Neurophysiological Testing** 101
    Giorgio Selvaggio and Roberto Cordella

11	Diagnostic Tests for Defecation Disorders 109
	Peter Christensen

Part II Pathological Conditions

12	Lower Urinary Tract Dysfunction in Children and Young Adults: An Introduction... 117
	Tryggve Nevéus

13	Neurogenic Bladder: Myelomeningocele, Occult Spina Bifida, and Tethered Cord 127
	Pieter Dik, Laetitia M.O. de Kort, and Paul W. Veenboer

14	Spinal Cord Injury and Iatrogenic Lesions 143
	Giulio Del Popolo and Elena Tur

15	Cerebral Palsy and Other Encephalopathies..................... 153
	Stuart Bauer

16	Urinary Incontinence in Children and Adolescents with Mental and Physical Disabilities: Comorbidities and Barriers 165
	Mario Patricolo and June Rogers

17	Monosymptomatic Enuresis.................................. 175
	Eliane Garcez da Fonseca

18	Nonmonosymptomatic Nocturnal Enuresis 189
	Kwang Myung Kim

19	Overactive Bladder... 193
	Lorenzo Masieri, Chiara Cini, and Maria Taverna

20	Daytime Lower Urinary Tract Conditions 205
	Marleen van den Heijkant

21	Congenital and Iatrogenic Incontinence: Ectopic Ureter, Ureterocele, and Urogenital Sinus.............................. 213
	Keara N. DeCotiis, Liza M. Aguiar, and Anthony A. Caldamone

22	Bladder Exstrophy 225
	Alan Dickson

23	Posterior Urethral Valves.................................... 237
	Mario De Gennaro, Maria Luisa Capitanucci, Giovanni Mosiello, and Antonio Zaccara

24	Hypospadia and Urethral Stricture............................. 251
	Carlos Arturo Levi D'Ancona, Juliano Cesar Moro, and Caio Cesar Citatini de Campos

Part III Therapies

25 Cognitive Behavioral Therapy on the Basis of Urotherapy 261
   Anka J. Nieuwhof-Leppink and M.A.W. Vijverberg

26 Pelvic Floor Rehabilitation and Biofeedback 277
   Sandro Danilo Sandri

27 Pharmacological Therapy 297
   John Weaver and Paul Austin

28 Sacral Neuromodulation in Children 303
   Ilaria Jansen, Ana Ludy Lopes Mendes, Francesco Cappellano,
   Mario De Gennaro, and Giovanni Mosiello

29 Bowel Dysfunction Management 313
   Giuseppe Masnata, Valeria Manca, Laura Chia, and Francesca Esu

**30 Percutaneous Tibial Nerve Stimulation (PTNS)
   and Transcutaneous Electrical Nerve Stimulation (TENS)** 319
   Maria Luisa Capitanucci, Giovanni Mosiello,
   and Mario De Gennaro

31 Botulinum Toxin, Endoscopy, and Mini-Invasive Treatment 327
   Giovanni Palleschi, Antonio Luigi Pastore, Davide Moschese,
   and Antonio Carbone

32 Laparoscopic Procedures 337
   Rafał Chrzan

33 Open Surgery for Incontinence 349
   Tom P.V.M. de Jong and Aart J. Klijn

Index 371

Contributors

Enrico Finazzi Agrò Department of Experimental Medicine and Surgery, Urology Division, Tor Vergata University of Rome, Rome, Italy

Liza M. Aguiar, M.D. Division of Pediatric Urology, Hasbro Children's Hospital, Warren Alpert School of Medicine, Brown University, Providence, RI, USA

Paul Austin, M.D. Division of Urologic Surgery, St. Louis Children's Hospital, Washington University School, St. Louis, USA

Stuart Bauer, M.D. Department of Urology, Boston Children's Hospital, Boston, MA, USA

Wendy F. Bower, FACP,PhD,Dip EpiBio,BAppSc(PT) Division of Medicine and Community Care, Melbourne Health, Melbourne, VIC, Australia

Anthony A. Caldamone, M.D. Division of Pediatric Urology, Hasbro Children's Hospital, Warren Alpert School of Medicine, Brown University, Providence, RI, USA

Caio Cesar Citatini de Campos Division of Urology, Universidade Estadual de Campinas—UNICAMP, Campinas, São Paulo, Brazil

Maria Luisa Capitanucci, M.D. Division of Urology, Surgery for Continence and Urodynamics, Bambino Gesù Children Hospital, Rome, Italy

Francesco Cappellano Department of Urologist, Nation Hospital, Abu Dhabi, UAE

Department of Neuro-Urology, Verona University, Verona, Italy

Antonio Carbone Faculty of Pharmacy and Medicine, Department of Medico-Surgical Sciences and Biotechnologies, Sapienza University of Rome, Latina, Italy

ICOT Hospital—Uroresearch Association, Latina, Italy

Laura Chia Pediatric Urology Unit and Spina Bifida Center, Brotzu Hospital, Cagliari, Italy

Peter Christensen Pelvic Floor Unit, Department of Surgery, Aarhus University Hospital, Aarhus, Denmark

Rafał Chrzan Department of Pediatric Urology, Children's University Hospital, Jagiellonian University Medical College, Krakow, Poland

Chiara Cini Division of Pediatric Urology, Meyer Pediatric Hospital, Florence, Italy

Roberto Cordella, M.Sc., Ph.D. Department of Neurosurgery, Fondazione IRCCS Istituto Neurologico "Carlo Besta", Milan, Italy

Carlos Arturo Levi D'Ancona Division of Urology, Universidade Estadual de Campinas—UNICAMP, Campinas, São Paulo, Brazil

Keara N. DeCotiis, M.D. Division of Pediatric Urology, Hasbro Children's Hospital, Warren Alpert School of Medicine, Brown University, Providence, RI, USA

Alan Dickson Consultant Paediatric Urologist, Royal Manchester Childrens Hospital, Stony Littleton, Bath, UK

Pieter Dik Department of Pediatric Urology, Wilhelmina Children's Hospital, Utrecht, The Netherlands

Jens Christian Djurhuus Department of Clinical Medicine, Aarhus University, Aarhus, Denmark

Giuseppe Farullo Department of Experimental Medicine and Surgery, Urology Division, Tor Vergata University of Rome, Rome, Italy

Francesca Esu Pediatric Urology Unit and Spina Bifida Center, Brotzu Hospital, Cagliari, Italy

Eliane Garcez da Fonseca The University of the State of Rio de Janeiro, Souza Marques Medical School, Rio de Janeiro, RJ, Brazil

Mario De Gennaro Urology, Robotic Surgery and Urodynamic Unit—Department of Surgery, Children's Hospital Bambino Gesù, Rome, Italy

Marleen van den Heijkant, F.E.B.U., F.E.A.P.U. Department of Urology, UZ Leuven, Gasthuisberg, Leuven, Belgium

L. Henning Olsen Department of Clinical Medicine, Department of Urology, Section of Pediatric Urology, Aarhus University Hospital, Aarhus, Denmark

Valerio Iacovelli Department of Experimental Medicine and Surgery, Urology Division, Tor Vergata University of Rome, Rome, Italy

Lotte Kaasgaard Jakobsen Department of Clinical Medicine, Department of Urology, Section of Pediatric Urology, Aarhus University Hospital, Aarhus, Denmark

Ilaria Jansen Department of Urology, AMC, Amsterdam, Netherlands

Department of Biomedical Engineering and Physics, AMC, Amsterdam, Netherlands

Tom P.V.M. de Jong Department of Pediatric Urology, University Children's Hospitals UMC Utrecht and AMC Amsterdam, Utrecht, The Netherlands

Cevdet Kaya, M.D. Department of Urology, School of Medicine, Marmara University, Istanbul, Turkey

Selcuk Keskin, M.D. Department of Urology, Acıbadem University School of Medicine, İstanbul, Turkey

Kwang Myung Kim, M.D. Department of Pediatric Urology, Seoul National University Children's Hospital, Seoul, Republic of Korea

Aart J. Klijn Department of Pediatric Urology, University Children's Hospitals UMC Utrecht and AMC Amsterdam, Utrecht, The Netherlands

Laetitia M.O. de Kort Department of Urology, University Medical Center Utrecht, Utrecht, The Netherlands

Ana Ludy Lopes Mendes Division of Urology, Surgery for Continence and Neuro-Urology, Bambino Gesù Pediatric Hospital, Rome, Italy

Valeria Manca Pediatric Urology Unit and Spina Bifida Center, Brotzu Hospital, Cagliari, Italy

Lorenzo Masieri Division of Pediatric Urology, Meyer Pediatric Hospital, Florence, Italy

Giuseppe Masnata Pediatric Urology Unit and Spina Bifida Center, Brotzu Hospital, Cagliari, Italy

Juliano Cesar Moro Division of Urology, Universidade Estadual de Campinas—UNICAMP, Campinas, São Paulo, Brazil

Davide Moschese Faculty of Pharmacy and Medicine, Department of Medico-Surgical Sciences and Biotechnologies, Sapienza University of Rome, Latina, Italy

Giovanni Mosiello, M.D. Pediatric NeuroUrology Research and Clinic, Bambino Gesù Pediatric Hospital, Rome, Italy

Tryggve Nevéus, M.D., Ph.D. Uppsala University Children's Hospital, Uppsala, Sweden

Anka J. Nieuwhof-Leppink Pediatric Psychology and Social Work, Wilhelmina's Children Hospital, University Medical Center Utrecht, Utrecht, The Netherlands

J.M. Nijman Department of Urology and Pediatric Urology, University Medical Center, Groningen, The Netherlands

Giovanni Palleschi Faculty of Pharmacy and Medicine, Department of Medico-Surgical Sciences and Biotechnologies, Sapienza University of Rome, Latina, Italy

ICOT Hospital—Uroresearch Association, Latina, Italy

Antonio Luigi Pastore Faculty of Pharmacy and Medicine, Department of Medico-Surgical Sciences and Biotechnologies, Sapienza University of Rome, Latina, Italy

ICOT Hospital—Uroresearch Association, Latina, Italy

Mario Patricolo Al Noor Hospital, Abu Dhabi, UAE

Giulio Del Popolo Neuro-Urology and Spinal Unit, Careggi University Hospital, Florence, Italy

Christian Radmayr, M.D. Department of Urology, School of Medicine, Innsbruck University, Innsbruck, Austria

June Rogers Manchester Disabled Living, Manchester, UK

Sandro Danilo Sandri Department of Urology and Spinal Unit, Hospital of Legnano, Legnano, Italy

Department of Urology and Spinal Unit, Hospital of Magenta, Milan, Italy

Giorgio Selvaggio, M.D. Department of Pediatric Surgery, Children's Hospital "V.Buzzi", Milan, Italy

Maria Taverna Division of Pediatric Urology, Meyer Pediatric Hospital, Florence, Italy

Elena Tur Neuro-Urology and Spinal Unit, Careggi University Hospital, Florence, Italy

Andrea Turbanti Department of Experimental Medicine and Surgery, Urology Division, Tor Vergata University of Rome, Rome, Italy

Murat Ucar, M.D. Department of Urology Section of Pediatric Urology, Saglik Bilimleri University Tepecik Training and Research Hospital, İzmir, Turkey

Paul W. Veenboer Department of Urology, University Medical Center Utrecht, Utrecht, The Netherlands

M.A.W. Vijverberg Pediatric Psychology and Social Work, Wilhelmina's Children Hospital, University Medical Center Utrecht, Utrecht, The Netherlands

John Weaver, M.D. Division of Urologic Surgery, St. Louis Children Hospital, Washington University School, St. Louis, MO, USA

Jian Guo Wen Pediatric Urodynamic Center, First Affiliated Hospital of Zhengzhou University, Zhengzhou, China

Pediatric Surgery and Urology, First Affiliated Hospital of Xinxiang Medical University, Xinxiang, China

Selcuk Yucel, M.D. Department of Urology, Acıbadem University School of Medicine, İstanbul, Turkey

Antonio Zaccara Division of Urology, Surgery for Continence and Urodynamics, Bambino Gesù Children Hospital, Rome, Italy

Part I
Diagnostic Evaluation

Anatomy and Neurophysiology of the Lower Urinary Tract and Pelvic Floor

Lotte Kaasgaard Jakobsen, Jens Christian Djurhuus, and L. Henning Olsen

1.1 Bladder

The urinary tract undergoes a very dynamic development during foetal life. Emerging from the metanephros, the human kidney begins to produce urine at 10–12 weeks of gestation [1, 2]. At this time the bladder is a cylindrical tube of cuboidal cells in a single layer. During the second trimester, 4–5 cell layers develop, forming a low compliant 'bladder' at the 21st week of gestation [3–5]. The foetal bladder handles a relatively large amount of fluid, draining to the amniotic cavity with a subsequent oral reuptake by the foetus. The salt and water homeostasis, however, is cleared by the placenta and eventually by the mother's kidneys [6]. Any deviation from this cycle may lead to a more or less pathological consequence for the foetus. In the beginning the lower urinary tract is a conduit with coordinated peristalsis propulsing the urine through the urethra, as is the case with the upper urinary tract. After the formation of the external sphincter, the lower urinary tract develops graduate filling and emptying, and the bladder wall properties change. From being a coordinated peristaltic conduit, the bladder becomes an organ with chaotic micromotions in the bladder wall.

L.K. Jakobsen (✉) • L. Henning Olsen
Department of Clinical Medicine, Department of Urology, Section of Pediatric Urology, Aarhus University Hospital, Aarhus, Denmark
e-mail: lottekj@clin.au.dk

J.C. Djurhuus
Department of Clinical Medicine, Aarhus University, Aarhus, Denmark

© Springer International Publishing AG, part of Springer Nature 2018
G. Mosiello et al. (eds.), *Clinical Urodynamics in Childhood and Adolescence*, Urodynamics, Neurourology and Pelvic Floor Dysfunctions,
https://doi.org/10.1007/978-3-319-42193-3_1

1.2   Urethra, Sphincter and Pelvic Floor

The external rhabdosphincter is crucial for continence. In male foetuses a common sphincter urethrae primordium can be found already at the ninth week of gestation. However, the final horseshoe-shaped rhabdosphincter is not seen until late in gestation [7–9]. Its musculature primarily consists of type-1 slow twitch fibres as a marked contrast to the rest of the pelvic floor which predominantly is type-2 fast-twitch fibres. Together with the external anal sphincter and the ischiocavernosus and bulbocavernosus muscles, the urethral sphincter has been shown to be controlled from the Onuf's nucleus at level S1–S2, situated in the front horn as two separate densities, one innervating the external urethral sphincter and ischiocavernosus and the other one the external anal sphincter and bulbocavernosus. This nucleus has a very high density of serotonin and norepinephrine receptors.

The external striated sphincter not only deviates in muscular characteristics from the surrounding pelvic floor; it is also, from an investigational and diagnostic point of view, difficult to monitor. It is mainly lying in front of the urethra, almost as a horseshoe. Therefore, when it is claimed that sphincter electromyography has been obtained, it is usually a misinterpretation. One has to settle with monitoring pelvic floor activity which gives a far more lenient investigational situation because one can use perianal surface electrodes instead of the more invasive needle electrodes.

The rest of the pelvic floor, which as mentioned consists of musculature with fast-twitch fibres, supports the urethra and acts as a guarding reflex elicitor and resistance in increased musculature during coughing and Valsalva.

The innervation and the properties of the external sphincter may, in the future, have significant clinical importance since it has been shown that OAB symptoms can be elicited through lack of stability of the urethra.

1.3   Voiding

Knowledge pertaining to the normal development of voiding function is crucial to the understanding of normal voiding and distinguishing it from abnormal voiding function. Evolution of voiding function begins in the first trimester of pregnancy and continues throughout childhood and adolescence [10–17]. Major developments are apparent such as the development of continence; others are more subtle. The simultaneous development of the neurogenic voiding reflex pathway has been shown as early as the 17th week of gestation by immunohistochemistry of autonomic innervated detrusor muscle bundles, while the adrenergic nerve supply was not seen before the 30th week of gestation [18]. In 1995 Yeung et al. showed that voiding in the neonatal period was not a mere autonomic reflex but also involved immature cortical mechanisms [19].

The voiding frequency undergoes a very dynamic development from foetal life to adolescence.

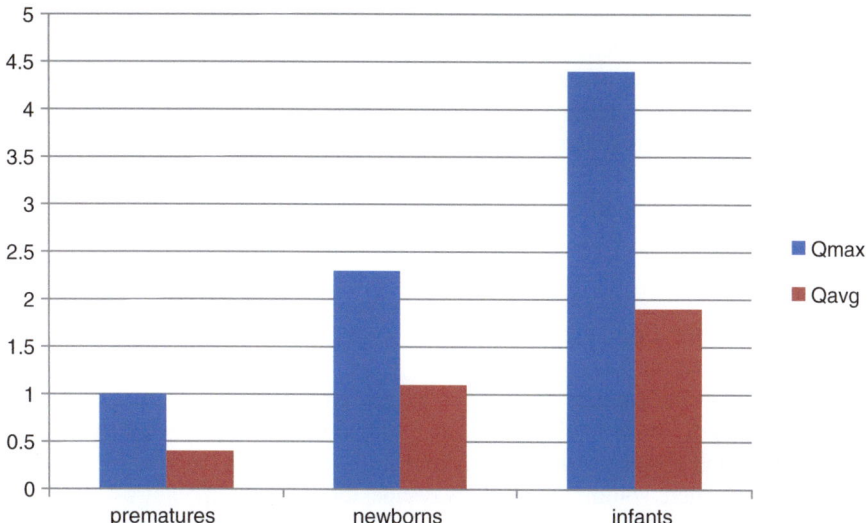

Fig. 1.1 Development of average (Q_{avg}) and maximum (Q_{max}) (mL/sec) flow rate with time

In the last trimester, there is a frequent rhythmic filling and emptying of the bladder at a rate of up to 30 sequences per 24 h.

During infancy the voiding frequency decreases to approximately one third with a further decrease towards stability from age 7, where more than seven voidings a day and less than three are considered abnormal. Conversely the flow rate increases with age (Fig. 1.1).

A normal voiding is described as a bell-shaped flow curve leading to a complete emptying of the bladder. The physiologic background consists of a relaxation of the bladder neck elicited via NO release, an introduction of urine into the proximal part of the urethra causing stimulation of mechano- and chemoreceptors, leading to stimulation of a detrusor contraction which overcomes the resistance of the external sphincter, and then the voiding is in progress. This pattern is considered to be the normal, but voidings both in children and in normal adult volunteers have been shown to be far more versatile, with several configurations including the bell shaped. Schmidt et al. showed that voiding shows a rather low degree of consistency in normal young men [20]. Lu et al. have confirmed the same both using natural fill overnight ambulatory urodynamics and artificial filling conventional urodynamics in children with OAB [21]. In the early stages of postnatal life into infancy and childhood, several interesting observations have been made. Flow curves with plateau shaped can be seen in prematures and newborns, while the spike-dome configuration is displayed in newborns and infants [22–24]. These patterns seem to be transient, while staccato and interrupted flow continues to occur in older children. The predominant flow curve shape in kindergarten and school children seems to be the bell and tower pattern [12, 14, 25, 26]. However, Bower et al. found in flow studies of 96 healthy 5–14-year-old children staccato-shaped flow curves in 30% of all initial voids [17]. They describe this surprising finding which is not in accordance with other studies, but had no plausible explanation [12, 14, 25]. Mattsson et al. showed that the number of staccato or interrupted voidings, seen in 16% of the children during an initial voiding, decreased to less than 3% in the subsequent voiding, while this fraction was stable in the observations of Bower et al. who recorded on average 4.4 micturitions per child [17, 27].

Consequently normality and abnormality of voiding seem far from fully elucidated.

1.4 Bladder Capacity

Estimating bladder capacity in children is not only relevant when determining whether or not the voided volume is within normal range but also when evaluating the need for, and frequency of, intermittent catheterization. In the investigative setting, the estimated volume is used to decide the amount of contrast used for MCUG. Bladder capacity obviously varies depending on age and weight of the child, but also depending on the filling media, the rate of filling and the presence of a urethral or suprapubic catheter.

The bladder has a paradox reaction to filling. The faster it is filled, the more it can accommodate [28], a factor which has to be taken into consideration when urodynamics are to be analysed. The relationship between filling and volume is even more complicated since it seems as if the change in filling rate results in even more volume changes during the day having a maximum during night.

Following these variations there are different measures of bladder capacity, according to the situation. The expected maximum voided volume, being the term for capacity recommended by the ICCS [29, 30], can be calculated by the following formula: *Estimated bladder capacity = 30 mL × (age + 1)*, which is a modification from the original formula (*Bladder capacity (ounces) = age + 2 years*), presented by Koff in 1983 [31] and later validated in other studies [32]. Several alternative formulas have been proposed, most of them based on cystometric data. Fairhurst et al. proposed two formulas based on either L1–L3 distance on X-ray or weight (*Estimated bladder capacity (mL) = (7 × weight in kg) + 1,2*) which offer a more accurate estimate in younger infants [33], an important supplement to Koff's version, which is applicable for children aged 4–12 years.

How to measure the actual bladder capacity in a relevant way can also be debated. When using the bladder diary, voided volumes and maximum voided volume (earlier referred to as functional bladder capacity) are obtained from a physiological setting with natural filling of the bladder. Alternative terms for bladder capacity are cystometric bladder capacity (recorded at first sensation) and maximum cystometric capacity (recorded when voiding commences), both obtained during urodynamic investigation, with a catheter in the bladder filling the bladder at a faster rate and with another medium, than under physiological conditions, inevitably affecting the measurements.

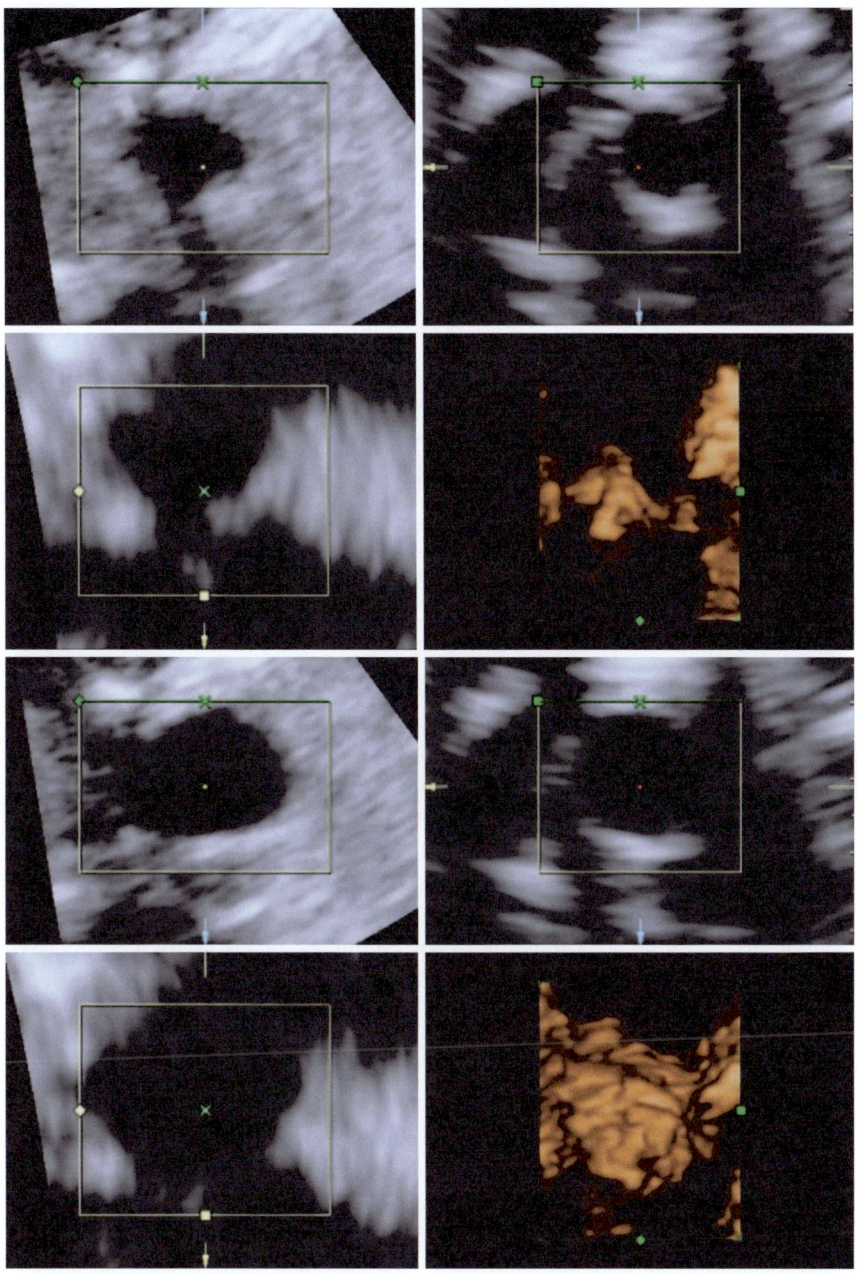

Fig. 1.2 Voiding in third trimester obtained by way of 3-D ultrasound. A bladder volume of appr. 4 mL is reduced to appr. 1 mL during the voiding

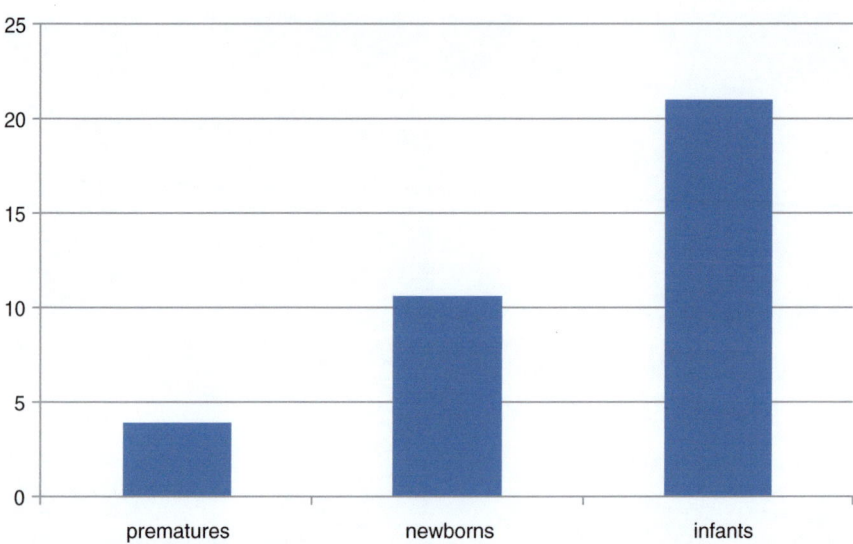

Fig. 1.3 Development of voided volume with age (mL (median)) assessed by transit-time ultrasound flow measurement [21–23]. The voided volume is smaller than the estimated bladder capacity indicating incomplete bladder emptying [10]

The 4-h observation period gives insight into both voided volume and post-void residual urine. While diapers are weighed after each voiding, the concomitant residual urine is assessed by transabdominal ultrasound [34]. The sum gives an estimate of bladder capacity. In prematures Sillen et al. found a bladder capacity of 12 mL at 32 weeks of gestation [35, 36]. Gladh et al. estimated the bladder capacity of 2-week-old newborns to 48 mL, while Bachelard found a bladder capacity of only 20 mL in 3-month-old infants [13, 37]. Bachelard et al.'s subjects were the asymptomatic siblings of infants with vesicoureteral reflux studied by invasive cystometry. The indwelling urethral catheter may therefore well explain some of these discrepancies. A later study from the same institution reported a median bladder capacity of 52 mL at 8 months of age [38]. It is evident that the aforementioned studies report large inter- and intraindividual variation with regard to the bladder volume that initiates voiding, voided volume and post-void residual urine. The influence of frequent manipulation of diapers, ink indicators and transabdominal ultrasound in these studies has undoubtedly affected outcomes [39]. The ICCS definition of estimated bladder capacity (EBC), originally proposed by Hjälmås and Koff, seems therefore reasonable to go by in the clinical setting [29–31, 40]. However, it is worth remembering that prematures, newborns at term and infants void at varying degrees of EBC which again limits the value of an absolute EBC (Figs. 1.2 and 1.3). The voided volume does not seem to influence the flow curve pattern [24].

References

1. Cuckow PM, Nyirady P, Winyard PJ. Normal and abnormal development of the urogenital tract. Prenat Diagn. 2001;21:908–16.
2. Chevalier RL. Chronic partial ureteral obstruction and the developing kidney. Pediatr Radiol. 2008;38(Suppl 1):S35–40.
3. Newman J, Antonakopoulos GN. The fine structure of the human fetal urinary bladder. Development and maturation. A light, transmission and scanning electron microscopic study. J Anat. 1989;166:135–50.
4. Coplen DE, Macarak EJ, Levin RM. Developmental changes in normal fetal bovine whole bladder physiology. JURO. 1994;151:1391–5.
5. Dean GE, Cargill RS, Macarak E, Snyder HM, Duckett JW, Levin R. Active and passive compliance of the fetal bovine bladder. JURO. 1997;158:1094–9.
6. Rabinowitz R, Peters MT, Vyas S, Campbell S, Nicolaides KH. Measurement of fetal urine production in normal pregnancy by real-time ultrasonography. Am J Obstet Gynecol. 1989;161:1264–6.
7. Sebe P, Schwentner C, Oswald J, Radmayr C, Bartsch G, Fritsch H. Fetal development of striated and smooth muscle sphincters of the male urethra from a common primordium and modifications due to the development of the prostate: an anatomic and histologic study. Prostate. 2005;62:388–93.
8. Ludwikowski B, Oesch Hayward I, Brenner E, Fritsch H. The development of the external urethral sphincter in humans. BJU Int. 2001;87:565–8.
9. Kokoua A, Homsy Y, Lavigne JF, Williot P, Corcos J, Laberge I, Michaud J. Maturation of the external urinary sphincter: a comparative histotopographic study in humans. JURO. 1993;150:617–22.
10. Holmdahl G, Hanson E, Hanson M, Hellström AL, Sillén U, Sölsnes E. Four-hour voiding observation in young boys with posterior urethral valves. JURO. 1998;160:1477–81.
11. Jansson UB, Hanson M, Hanson E, Hellström AL, Sillén U. Voiding pattern in healthy children 0 to 3 years old: a longitudinal study. JURO. 2000;164:2050–4.
12. Jensen KM, Nielsen KK, Jensen H, Pedersen OS, Krarup T. Urinary flow studies in normal kindergarten--and schoolchildren. Scand J Urol Nephrol. 1983;17:11–21.
13. Gladh G, Persson D, Mattsson S, Lindström S. Voiding pattern in healthy newborns. Neurourol Urodyn. 2000;19:177–84.
14. Mattsson S, Spångberg A. Urinary flow in healthy schoolchildren. Neurourol Urodyn. 1994;13:281–96.
15. Mattsson S, Spångberg A. Flow rate nomograms in 7- to 16-year-old healthy children. Neurourol Urodyn. 1994;13:267–80.
16. Mattsson SH. Voiding frequency, volumes and intervals in healthy schoolchildren. Scand J Urol Nephrol. 1994;28:1–11.
17. Bower WF, Kwok B, Yeung CK. Variability in normative urine flow rates. JURO. 2004;171:2657–9.
18. Jen PY, Dixon JS, Gosling JA. Immunohistochemical localization of neuromarkers and neuropeptides in human fetal and neonatal urinary bladder. Br J Urol. 1995;75:230–5.
19. Yeung CK, Godley ML, Ho CK, Ransley PG, Duffy PG, Chen CN, Li AK. Some new insights into bladder function in infancy. Br J Urol. 1995;76:235–40.
20. Schmidt F, Jørgensen TM, Djurhuus JC. Twenty-four-hour ambulatory urodynamics in healthy young men. Scand J Urol Nephrol Suppl. 2004;38:75–83.
21. Lu YT, Jakobsen LK, Djurhuus JC, Bjerrum SN, Wen JG, Olsen LH. What is a representative voiding pattern in children with lower urinary tract symptoms? Lack of consistent findings in ambulatory and conventional urodynamic tests. J Pediatr Urol. 2016;12(3):154.e1–7.
22. Olsen LH, Grothe I, Rawashdeh YF, Jørgensen TM. Urinary flow patterns in premature males. J Urol. 2010;183:2347–52.

23. Olsen LH, Grothe I, Rawashdeh YF, Jørgensen TM. Urinary flow patterns of healthy newborn males. J Urol. 2009;181:1857–61.
24. Olsen LH, Grothe I, Rawashdeh YF, Jørgensen TM. Urinary flow patterns in first year of life. J Urol. 2010;183:694–8.
25. Chang S-J, Yang SSD. Inter-observer and intra-observer agreement on interpretation of uroflowmetry curves of kindergarten children. J Pediatr Urol. 2008;4:422–7.
26. Gutierrez Segura C. Urine flow in childhood: a study of flow chart parameters based on 1,361 uroflowmetry tests. JURO. 1997;157:1426–8.
27. Gladh G, Mattsson S, Lindström S. Anogenital electrical stimulation as treatment of urge incontinence in children. BJU Int. 2001;87:366–71.
28. Sørensen SS, Nielsen JB, Nørgaard JP, Knudsen LM, Djurhuus JC. Changes in bladder volumes with repetition of water cystometry. Urol Res. 1984;12:205–8.
29. Nevéus T, Gontard von A, Hoebeke P, et al. The standardization of terminology of lower urinary tract function in children and adolescents: report from the standardisation Committee of the International Children's continence society. JURO. 2006;176:314–24.
30. Austin PF, Bauer SB, Bower W, et al. The standardization of terminology of lower urinary tract function in children and adolescents: update report from the standardization committee of the international Children's continence society. Neurourol Urodyn. 2015;35(4):471–81. https://doi.org/10.1002/nau.22751.
31. Koff SA. Estimating bladder capacity in children. Urology. 1983;21:248.
32. Rittig S, Kamperis K, Siggaard C, Hagstroem S, Djurhuus JC. Age related nocturnal urine volume and maximum voided volume in healthy children: reappraisal of international Children's continence society definitions. J Urol. 2010;183:1561–7.
33. Fairhurst JJ, Rubin CM, Hyde I, Freeman NV, Williams JD. Bladder capacity in infants. J Pediatr Surg. 1991;26:55–7.
34. Holmdahl G, Hanson E, Hanson M, Hellström AL, Hjälmås K, Sillén U. Four-hour voiding observation in healthy infants. JURO. 1996;156:1809–12.
35. Sillén U, Sölsnes E, Hellström AL, Sandberg K. The voiding pattern of healthy preterm neonates. JURO. 2000;163:278–81.
36. Sillén U. Bladder function in healthy neonates and its development during infancy. JURO. 2001;166:2376–81.
37. Bachelard M, Sillén U, Hansson S, Hermansson G, Jodal U, Jacobsson B. Urodynamic pattern in asymptomatic infants: siblings of children with vesicoureteral reflux. JURO. 1999;162:1733–7. discussion 1737–8.
38. Jansson UB, Hanson M, Sillén U, Hellström AL. Voiding pattern and acquisition of bladder control from birth to age 6 years–a longitudinal study. JURO. 2005;174:289–93.
39. de Groat WC. Central neural control of the lower urinary tract. Ciba Found Symp. 1990;151:27–44. discussion 44–56.
40. Hjälmås K. Micturition in infants and children with normal lower urinary tract. A urodynamic study. Scand J Urol Nephrol Suppl. 1976;37:1–106.

Clinical Evaluation: History Taking and Urological, Gynaecological and Neurological Evaluation

2

Cevdet Kaya and Christian Radmayr

2.1 Introduction

Paediatric urology practice encompasses a spectrum of disorders from complex congenital anomalies to more routine but important problems such as voiding dysfunction (LUTD) in a school-aged child. The evaluation process of a child with LUTD should begin with a good history consisting of perinatal issues, developmental milestones, current mental status, scholastic performance, nature of toilet training, bladder and bowel emptying patterns and frequency, timing and severity of incontinent episodes. The second important step is the physical examination, a careful inspection of the lower spine to identify possible cutaneous manifestations of an occult spinal dysraphism and/or sacral agenesis, an assessment of the lower extremity function and an examination of the external genitalia, respectively.

The development of lower urinary tract function requires maturation of the neural system. The process of having control over the bladder and sphincter function is complex, and therefore highly susceptible for the development of various types of dysfunction [1]. While the normal bladder function is usually gained during the second year of life, the child becomes able to express a need to void, initiate a void and inhibit micturition if needed during the third and fourth year of life. Eventually, a healthy school child voids less than seven times per day, and most of them empty their bladders completely. The overactive bladder with normal micturition, dysfunctional voiding with staccato pattern and detrusor underactivity with significant residual urine comprise the main clinical patterns of LUTD in children. In response to the uninhibited contractions during toilet training, many children learn to contract

---

C. Kaya, M.D.
Department of Urology, School of Medicine, Marmara University, Istanbul, Turkey

C. Radmayr, M.D. (✉)
Department of Urology, School of Medicine, Innsbruck University, Innsbruck, Austria
e-mail: christian.radmayr@i-med.ac.at

© Springer International Publishing AG, part of Springer Nature 2018
G. Mosiello et al. (eds.), *Clinical Urodynamics in Childhood and Adolescence*, Urodynamics, Neurourology and Pelvic Floor Dysfunctions,
https://doi.org/10.1007/978-3-319-42193-3_2

their sphincters to avoid wetting, and many of these can develop a form of urge syndrome as they learn to overcome the urge and voiding by sphincter contractions and different holding manoeuvers like squatting.

Giggle incontinence is characterized by large-volume voiding that occurs while laughing and no voiding symptoms between these episodes. On the other hand, vaginal voiding is more likely to occur in obese girls and characterized as incontinence when standing up after voiding because of temporarily trapped urine in the vagina.

The neurologic causes of lower urinary tract dysfunction originate from a group of spinal abnormalities. The open spinal canal lesions, meningomyelocele, are obvious on inspection of the back, whereas closed lesions consists of lipomeningocele, lipoma of the cauda equina, diastematomyelia or thickened filum terminale. Sacral agenesis, another form of spinal dysraphism, is more difficult to detect because lower extremity function and sensation are normal, with the only clues being a low gluteal cleft and flattened buttocks. Acquired neurologic causes include central nervous system abnormalities, such as cerebral palsy and spinal cord injury [2–4].

Many children with LUTD require urodynamics studies (UDS) to determine whether their lower urinary tract symptoms (LUTS) are neurologic or functional in origin [3].

2.2 Role of a Paediatric Urologist in the Evaluation of a Child with LUTD

The spectrum of LUTD in children comprises a wide variety of disorders. The assessment of the child with LUTS has to involve ruling out any underlying neurologic or anatomic abnormality. LUTD in children with spinal dysraphism may be present from birth in those with open neural tube defects or later in life in those with closed neural tube defects and a tethered cord syndrome [5]. Therefore, the monitoring of the child throughout the clinical course of spinal dysraphism is very important for the prevention of progressive deterioration of upper urinary tract function. Children with closed spinal dysraphisms may explicit themselves with signs and symptoms much more insidious in nature, with the exception of the cutaneous markers that may be associated with at least half of the cases [6–8]. Because clinically significant symptoms are usually the result of abnormalities caused by spinal cord tethering, the diagnosis generally relies on the history and monitoring of lower urinary tract symptoms to assess changes in voiding patterns compared to the baseline urological findings. A long-term follow-up study in children after myelomeningocele repair demonstrated the importance of regular follow-up of urinary tract function, since some children, particularly younger ones, were at higher risk of secondary tethered cord and subsequent upper urinary tract deterioration [9, 10]. Children with spinal dysraphism were reported to have abnormal baseline urodynamic studies in most of them with open defects and more than half of them with closed defects [11, 12].

The presence of lower urinary tract symptoms is well correlated with preoperative UDS results and eventual voiding patterns. All these factors imply the importance of good acquisition of history taking from the parents or children. UDS, combined with a multidisciplinary approach under the guidance of paediatric urologists, provide a reliable way to evaluate the lower urinary tract function in these children.

2.3 The Evaluation of a Child with LUTD: History Taking

The history should focus on the identification of children with neurologic or anatomic causes of their symptoms and then distinguish the various forms of voiding dysfunction. It is important to identify the person who is able to give the detailed history and to clarify the relationship to the child. The child should feel that they are the primary interest of the interaction, and regardless of the age, the paediatric urologist has to concentrate on the child and to communicate in a way to develop a trusting relationship. The role of the paediatric urologist is to determine what key questions are necessary to formulate the most accurate description of the patient's genitourinary condition. The child or the parents should be questioned about possible associated genitourinary symptoms including flank or abdominal pain, haematuria, dysuria, frequency, any previous urologic surgery and scrotal pain or swelling. The past medical history should include information about the prenatal history of the child and pregnancy period of the mother, including any disease and/or treatment the mother was exposed to. The family history can be also very significant for various paediatric urologic conditions like vesicoureteral reflux, urinary tract infections, genital malformations and voiding dysfunction. Since family characteristics often play a significant role in progression of LUTD, issues about siblings, any loss of a family member, parental separation or divorce and family move may give additional clues [13–16].

In children with LUTD related to spinal cord injury or myelomeningocele, eliciting a diagnostic history is not really a challenging condition. However, children with no obvious neurologic abnormality can sometimes be challenging even in experienced hands. Important parameters to be elucidated include voiding schedule and symptoms such as urgency, frequency, timing of incontinence episodes, squatting, postponement or holding manoeuvers [14].

Components of a detailed history include maternal medical issues, perinatal history, developmental milestones, scholastic performance, behavioural history, toilet training history, patterns of voiding and bowel movements, history of UTI and family history of voiding dysfunction. In the evaluation of LUTD, the use of a detailed 2–3-day voiding diary is often helpful to identify the frequency of voiding, the voided volumes, the presence or absence of incontinence and the timing of incontinent episodes. Using this bladder diary, the child's functional bladder capacity may also be assessed as the largest voided volume. Volume of the morning micturition represents night-time bladder capacity. This record is usually kept during the weekend to make it easier for patients and parents. When filled in properly, it also provides valuable information on fluid intake which is sometimes useful in distinguishing idiopathic urinary frequency from polyuria. Additionally, many parents and children are unaware of LUTD on routine questioning, and symptoms may not be apparent. It is a useful tool to help identify those who may warrant further studies, as well as in the follow-up during any kind of treatment. Whenever possible, the diary should be the responsibility of the child and part of the motivational process to ensure that the child takes an active role in the treatment [15, 17].

Many efforts have been made to develop methods to quantify or grade voiding symptoms in children. The dysfunctional voiding scoring system (DVSS), one of the symptom scores frequently used, was developed to serve as an objective instrument for grading of voiding behaviours in children [18]. Such instruments can contribute to diagnose and manage voiding dysfunction. Voiding symptoms, such as hesitancy, straining and weak or intermittent stream, should also be recorded [19, 20]. Defecation frequency, constipation and soiling, should also be documented and become an integrated part of a proper voiding diary. A defecation diary includes frequency, soiling and stool consistency based on the Bristol Stool Form scale [21]. Stool habits with regard to interval, size and consistency should be investigated. A stool and diet diary can be used for any child with daytime voiding disorder if the history indicates bowel-related problems. It provides information on drinking of small amounts of water during the day and large amounts of alternative liquids, such as soft drinks and juices. Dietary information including fluid intake and caffeine consumption are further important parameters [16, 22].

Maternal prenatal and perinatal histories consisting of prematurity, Apgar scores, systemic infection and respiratory distress are very critical steps to evaluate the child with lower urinary dysfunction. Newborns with constant dribbling or signs of overflow incontinence may have undergone a traumatic delivery with the possibility of hyperextension injury to the cervical spinal cord. Infants of diabetic mothers have an increased risk of neural tube defects. The details of the developmental milestones of the child are important steps to understand the lower urinary tract function. A complete history always includes mental medical issues such as a history of attention deficit hyperactivity disorder, ability to stay focused, educational performance at school, behavioural patterns and gross and fine-motor coordination of the child.

Another important aspect is to consider the posture of the child while voiding. Young girls often slump while sitting on the toilet without an upright posture or spread their legs apart inadequately. Some children may exhibit leg crossing, squatting on the floor or sitting on the edge of a chair to compress their pelvic floor. These posturing manoeuvers represent compensatory responses to overcome bladder spasms, and the perineal pressure inhibits bladder contraction through the sacral reflex arc [23]. Documentation of urinary tract infection may suggest urinary stasis or incomplete emptying. Many children with LUTD experience symptoms consistent with cystitis, such as dysuria, urinary frequency and suprapubic pain or discomfort related to voiding, although urine culture is sterile. These children may have findings of leukocyturia, haematuria and amorphous debris that reflect chronic inflammation and irritation in response to urinary stasis.

2.4 Physical Examination

A comprehensive physical examination is mandatory with particular emphasis on the genitourinary system including the abdomen and external genitalia, neurological examination for lower extremity strength and sensation, deep tendon reflexes, gait, fine-motor coordination, perineal/anal sensation, rectal tone, and bulbocavernosus and anal reflex. Urological examination includes inspection of meatus, skin excoriation or irritation in the scrotum, faecal staining on underpants and perianal staining. The abdominal examination includes inspection and palpation in all four quadrants for abdominal wall tension, masses, rigidity, guarding or tenderness and the presence of umbilical hernias. The evaluation of the flanks looks for enlarged kidneys, enlarged bladder or masses. In case of severe constipation, the sigmoid colon may be palpable in the left lower quadrant. In infants, large amounts of gas may be present within the gastrointestinal tract.

Musculoskeletal examination consists of spinal abnormalities such as tufts of hair, haemangiomas, masses, scoliosis and lower extremity abnormalities. On physical examination, attention has to be paid to the back and lower spine for cutaneous manifestations of possible occult spinal dysraphism and/or sacral agenesis including sacral malformation, lipoma, hairy patches, dermal vascular malformation, dermal sinus tract and asymmetry of the gluteal crease [14–16].

2.4.1 Neurological Examination

A detailed neurological examination is significant for a correct diagnosis [24]. LUTD is reported as one of the main discomforts in cases of occult spinal dysraphism, together with pain, foot deformity, gait disturbance, progressive scoliosis, bowel dysfunction and other neurological deficits [25]. A paediatric urologist needs to ask for symptoms such as back lump, skin appendage, urinary incontinence, foot deformity, leg weakness, imperforate anus and scoliosis. A careful neurological examination should include an assessment of strength, sensation and coordination of all extremities. Any central cutaneous abnormalities overlying the spine, such as a sacral dimple, gluteal cleft, lipoma or hair tuft, should prompt further investigation to rule out occult spinal cord anomalies such as tethered cord, diastematomyelia and other lumbosacral defects.

Spinal cord injury often leads to severe neurological dysfunction and disability in addition to the development of a neurogenic bladder with the risk of renal failure. Examination can rule out the level of the injury including the status of sensation, tendon reflex, muscular tension and pathologic reflex of lower extremities, sensation of perineum and autonomic contraction of anus. Accurate evaluation and subsequent management represent the keys to reduce complications. Unfortunately the type of voiding dysfunction cannot be assumed based on the site of spine injury. Precise evaluation is dependent on the timely and dynamic examination of urodynamics. It is a fact that the type and status of a neurogenic bladder cannot be predicted according to the level of a spinal cord injury [26–28].

A detailed physical examination is a critical step in the evaluation of spinal dysraphism. Meningomyelocele represents an extreme form of myelodysplasia, in which the dysplastic neural tissue leads to neurogenic bladder dysfunction. Occult spinal dysraphism causes bladder dysfunction by an abnormal caudal fixation of the conus medullaris which results in neuronal damage due to kinking and stretching of the blood supply to the spinal cord.

Neurological examination is normal in most of the children with non-neurogenic dysfunction, but careful examination is required to exclude those who may require further neurologic evaluation. Lesions such as an asymmetric gluteal fold, hairy patch, dermovascular malformation or lipomatous abnormality of the sacral region should prompt further imaging for occult spinal dysraphism. Radiographic visualization is as important as functional assessment of the lower urinary tract in characterizing and managing these conditions. In addition, on careful inspection of the legs, one may note a high arched foot or feet, hammer toes or claw toes, a discrepancy in muscle size, and shortness and decreased strength in one leg compared with the other. The absence of perineal sensation and the finding of back pain and secondary incontinence are common symptoms in older children and adolescents. New-onset urinary incontinence, changes in voiding patterns or recurrent urinary tract infections may represent clinically significant symptoms which are usually the result of pathologies or abnormalities causing spinal cord tethering [29–33].

Occasionally, in some patients without an obvious back lesion, delayed traction on the spinal cord can cause urinary or lower extremity symptoms or back pain after puberty. When these children are evaluated during their neonatal period or early infancy, they have a perfectly normal neurourologic examination.

Spina bifida cystica and occulta present with a wide spectrum of urodynamic abnormalities including upper and lower neuron types of bladder and urethral dysfunction [24, 34, 35]. The anocutaneous reflex is mediated through S2–S4 spinal neurological level. It consists of an immediate and transient contraction of the external anal sphincter when the perineal skin is pricked or pinched. The absence of this sacrally mediated anal reflex implies that a person would be unable to develop such urethral sphincter spasm. Therefore, assessment of the anocutaneous reflex provides a promising non-invasive clinical tool to quantify the risk of upper tract damage [36, 37].

2.4.2 Urological Examination

The detection of an abdominal mass may be the first sign of a distended bladder, a multicystic dysplastic kidney, a hydronephrotic kidney or a tumour, respectively. The palpation of the abdomen is advised to be initially soft, gentle and superficial and progresses to a more deliberate, deeper palpation. Any renal pathology is the source of up to two-thirds of neonatal abdominal masses. The cystic abdominal masses may include hydronephrosis, multicystic dysplastic kidneys, hydrometrocolpos and intestinal duplication, and the solid ones may include neuroblastoma, congenital mesoblastic nephroma, hepatoblastoma and teratoma.

The external genitalia should be examined to exclude any obvious anatomic malformations. It includes gentle retraction of the foreskin for signs of phimosis and inspection of the meatus for stenosis, epispadias and hypospadias. A hidden penis should be differentiated from the rare but more serious micropenis.

The inguinal canal should be inspected on each side for signs of asymmetry or mass, undescended testis, hernia or hydrocele. The scrotum needs to be palpated with special attention to the testicles, the epididymis and the vas deferens. Scrotal masses can be transilluminated to determine if the component is primarily fluid, such as a tense hydrocele, a varicocele or solid like a testicular tumour. The consistency and approximate size of the testes should be noted, as well as the stage of sexual development. A child with acute scrotal pain must be presumed to have spermatic cord torsion regardless of age until proven otherwise. A digital rectal examination should be reserved for special circumstances, such as urinary retention or for the assessment of the neurologically impaired child, or in cases of severe constipation. It is best performed using a well-lubricated, gloved, small finger [15, 16].

2.4.3 Gynaecological Examination

Gynaecologic examination should be conducted in the supine position with the legs in a frog-like position, asking the patient to perform Valsalva's manoeuver to inspect the introitus. After observing the external genital appearance, the labia majora should be firmly, but not tightly, grasped between the thumb and index finger and pulled outwards and upwards, allowing full assessment of the open introitus, distal vaginal canal and urethral meatus. The vaginal introitus should be examined for pooling of urine or irritation. If there is continuous incontinence, examination of the introitus for an ectopic ureteral orifice should be performed. If a child has chronic irritation of the genitalia and perineum, skin changes or labial hypertrophy may be observed [38]. Examination of the female genitalia may identify primary epispadias, a urogenital sinus anomaly, fused labia minora and imperforate hymen. The labial adhesions may contribute to retrograde filling of the vagina while voiding and subsequent dribbling when the girl stands up from the toilet. While it is important to consider the diagnosis of labial adhesions in girls with postvoid dribbling, this phenomenon can also occur in the absence of labial adhesions. In the case of congenital short urethra, continuous urinary leakage is detected and the urethral meatus is typically both, wide and patulous. Isolated lesions that are not associated with anorectal or cloacal anomalies sometimes present with urinary incontinence, due to either neuropathic bladder resulting from an associated spinal anomaly or to a form of urogenital sinus anomaly associated with an incompetent sphincteric mechanism. All urogenital sinus anomalies are characterized by a single vulval orifice that resembles neither vagina nor urethra.

The clitoris should be examined for evidence of hypertrophy that may be suggestive of a disorder of sexual differentiation. Additionally any introital masses should be examined for site of origin, laterality, symmetry and signs of infection or irritation. Placing a small feeding tube into the urethral meatus is recommended to help distinguish between an asymmetrical prolapsed ureterocele or the circular oedema and congestion associated with urethral prolapse. In older girls an imperforate hymen generally appears as a midline, bulging pearly white membrane and may result in hydrometrocolpos and a lower abdominal mass. The palpation of the vaginal wall and cervix and bimanual examination of the uterus with a small speculum completes the examination in older girls. Another common and important symptom is vaginal discharge, which can be associated with vaginal voiding and is particularly common in girls who hold urine and subsequently dribble urine into the vagina. Vaginal bleeding in the prepubertal may result from foreign bodies in the vagina. One should always consider the possibility of sexual abuse, and careful attention has to be paid to possible signs and symptoms that require further workup. Labial fusion may be associated with congenital adrenal hyperplasia, gonadal dysgenesis or cloaca. Further imaging with contrast medium may be indicated in cases where the urethra cannot be distinguished from the vaginal orifice and a urogenital sinus is suspected. An ectopic ureteric orifice is hardly evident on gross inspection, although in some affected individuals urine can be seen leaking from the introitus. To avoid distress in older girls and adolescents, it is generally recommended to carry out the examination under sedation or anaesthesia [16, 39–41].

2.5 Less Common Conditions Affecting Lower Urinary Tract Function

Anorectal anomalies comprise a spectrum of congenital malformations in which the anus fails to open normally on to the perineum. Because some of these children with congenital anorectal malformations suffer from severe LUTD in addition to other urologic manifestations such as vesicoureteral reflux, appropriate investigation of the urinary tract is necessary to lower the risk of subsequent renal damage. In females the most severe expression is cloacal malformation, in which the rectum, urethra and vagina join to form a single confluent channel draining by a common opening on the perineum. Coexisting anomalies comprise vesicoureteric reflux, undescended testes, bifid scrotum, hypospadias and vaginal and uterine duplications occurring in approximately two-thirds of patients with anorectal malformations. Initial evaluation in the neonatal period should include a careful inspection of the perineum looking for a fistulous site from the bowel, an examination of the upper and lower extremities and an assessment of the spine and spinal cord. Many of these children have associated intraspinal pathology, carrying a risk of tethered cord syndrome and, in turn, urological, neurological and orthopaedic complications. Bladder dysfunction may be the result of a congenital neuropathy associated with a coexisting spinal anomaly, or it may represent neurological damage acquired during surgical repair of the anorectal malformation [15, 42, 43].

Cerebral palsy is a nonprogressive injury of the brain occurring in the perinatal period that results in a neuromuscular disability, or cerebral dysfunction. Affected children are found to have delayed gross motor development, abnormal fine-motor performance, altered muscle tone and exaggerated deep tendon reflexes. About one-fourth of affected children are reported to have persistent urinary incontinence.

UDS in children with cerebral palsy is reserved for those who appear to be trainable and do not seem to be hampered too much by their physical impairment and have not achieved continence till late childhood or early puberty [44, 45].

References

1. Hinman F, Baumann FW. Vesical and ureteral damage from voiding dysfunction in boys without neurologic or obstructive disease. J Urol. 1973;109:727.
2. Piatt JH Jr. Treatment of myelomeningocele: a review of outcomes and continuing neurosurgical considerations among adults. A review. J Neurosurg Pediatr. 2010;6:515–25.
3. Abrahamsson K, Olsson I, Sillen U. Urodynamic findings in children with myelomeningocele after untethering of the spinal cord. J Urol. 2007;177:331–4.
4. Kaplan KM, Spivak JM, Bendo JA. Embryology of the spine and associated congenital abnormalities. Spine J. 2005;5:564–76.
5. Sutherland RS, Mevorach RA, Baskin LS, Kogan BA. Spinal dysraphism in children: an overview and an approach to prevent complications. Urology. 1995;46:294–304.
6. Ackerman LL, Menezes AH. Spinal congenital dermal sinuses: a 30-year experience. Pediatrics. 2003;112:641–7.
7. Assaad A, Mansy A, Kotb M, Hafez M. Spinal dysraphism: experience with 250 cases operated upon. Child Nerv Syst. 1989;5:324–9.
8. Guggisberg D, Hadj-Rabia S, Viney C, Bodemer C, Brunelle F, Zerah M, et al. Skin markers of occult spinal dysraphism in children: a review of 54 cases. Arch Dermatol. 2004;140:1109–15.
9. Tamaki N, Shirataki K, Kojima N, Shouse Y, Matsumoto S. Tethered cord syndrome of delayed onset following repair of myelomeningocele. J Neurosurg. 1988;69:393–8.
10. Tarcan T, Bauer S, Olmedo E, Khoshbin S, Kelly M, Darbey M. Long-term followup of newborns with myelodysplasia and normal urodynamic findings: is followup necessary? J Urol. 2001;165:564–7.
11. Macejko AM, Cheng EY, Yerkes EB, Meyer T, Bowman RM, Kaplan WE. Clinical urological outcomes following primary tethered cord release in children younger than 3 years. J Urol. 2007;178:1738–43.
12. Maher CO, Bauer SB, Goumnerova L, Proctor MR, Madsen JR, Scott RM. Urological outcome following multiple repeat spinal cord untethering operations. J Neurosurg Pediatr. 2009;4:275–9.
13. Kaplan WE. Urodynamics of upper and lower urinary tract. In: Docimo SG, editor. Kelalis-King-Belman textbook of clinical pediatric urology. London: Informa healthcare; 2007. p. 747–64.
14. Sillén U, Hellström AL. Pragmatic approach to the evaluation and management of non-neuropathic daytime voiding disorders. In: Gearhart JP, Rink RC, Mouriquand PDE, editors. Pediatric urology. Philadelphia: Saunders Elsevier; 2010. p. 366–79.
15. Wilcox DT. The urinary tract in anorectal malformations, multisystem disorders and syndromes. In: Thomas DFM, Duffy PG, Rickwood AMK, editors. Essentials of pediatric urology. London: Informa healthcare; 2008. p. 189–98.
16. Canning DA, Lambert SM. Evaluation of the pediatric urology patient. In: Wein AJ, editor. Campbell-Walsh urology. Philadelphia: Elsevier Saunders; 2012. p. 3067–84.
17. Bauer SB, Nijman RJ, Drzewiecki BA, Sillen U, Hoebeke P. International Children's continence society standardization report on urodynamic studies of the lower urinary tract in children. Neurourol Urodyn. 2015;34:640–7.
18. Farhat W, Bägli DJ, Capolicchio G, O'Reilly S, Merguerian PA, Khoury A, McLorie GA. The dysfunctional voiding scoring system: quantitative standardization of dysfunctional voiding symptoms in children. J Urol. 2000;164:1011–5.
19. Greydanus DE, Torres AD, O'Donnel DM, Feinberg AN. Enuresis: current concepts. Indian J Pediatr. 1999;66:425–38.

20. Agarwal SK, Bagli DJ. Neurogenic bladder. Indian J Pediatr. 1997;64:313–26.
21. Heaton KW, Radvan J, Cripps H, Mountford RA, Braddon FE, Hughes AO. Defecation frequency and timing, and stool form in the general population: a prospective study. Gut. 1992;33(6):818–24.
22. Combs AJ, Van Batavia JP, Chan J, Glassberg KI. Dysfunctional elimination syndromes: how closely linked are constipation and encopresis with specific lower urinary tract conditions? J Urol. 2013;190(3):1015–20.
23. Roth EB, Austin PF. Evaluation and treatment of Nonmonosymptomatic enuresis. Pediatr Rev. 2014;35(10):430–8.
24. Kaplan WE, McClone DG, Richards I. The urological manifestations of the tethered spinal cord. J Urol. 1988;140:1285–8.
25. Kumar R, Singhal N, Gupta M, Kapoor R, Mahapatra AK. Evaluation of clinic-urodynamic outcome of bladder dysfunction after surgery in children with spinal dysraphism. Acta Neurochir. 2008;150:129–37.
26. Ku JH. The management of of neurogenic bladder and quality of life in spinal cord injury. BJU Int. 2006;98(4):739–45.
27. Samson G, Cardenas DD. Neurogenic bladder in spinal cord injury. Phys Med Rehabil Clin N Am. 2007;18(2):255–74.
28. Moslavac S, Dzidic I, Kejla Z. Neurogenic detrusor overactivity: comparison between complete and incomplete spinal cord injury patients. Neurourol Urodyn. 2008;27(6):504–6.
29. Feldman AS, Bauer S. Diagnosis and management of dysfunctional voiding. Cur Opin Pediatr. 2006;18:139–47.
30. Bauer SB. Special considerations of the overactive bladder in children. Urology. 2002;60(suppl 5A):43–8.
31. Schulman SL. Voiding dysfunction in children. Urol Clin N Am. 2004;31:481–90.
32. Keating MA, Rink R, Bauer SB, et al. Neuro-urologic implications in changing approach in management of occult spinal lesions. J Urol. 1988;140:1299.
33. Anderson FM. Occult spinal dysraphism. Pediatrics. 1975;55:826–35.
34. Kang H, Wang K, Kim SK, Cho BK. Prognostic factors affecting urologic outcome after untethering surgery for lumbosacral lipoma. Childs Nerv Syst. 2006;22:1111–21.
35. Amarante MA, Shrensel JA, Tomei KL, Carmel PW, Gandhi CD. Management of urological dysfunction in pediatric patients with spinal dysraphism: review of the literature. Neurosurg Focus. 2012;33(4):1–9.
36. Marshall DF, Boston VE. Does the absence of anal reflexes guarantee a safe bladder in children with spina bifida? Eur J Paediatr Surg. 2001;11(Suppl I):S21–3.
37. Sakakibara R, Hattori T, Uchiyama T, Kamura K, Yamanishi T. Uroneurological assessment of spina bifida cystic and occulta. Neurourol Urodyn. 2003;22:328–34.
38. Neveus T, Eggert P, Evans J, International Children's Continence Society, et al. Evaluation of and treatment for monosymptomatic enuresis: a standardization document from the international Children's continence society. J Urol. 2010;183(2):441–7.
39. Redman JF. Conservative management of urethral prolapse in female children. Urology. 1982;19(5):505–6.
40. Powell DM, Newman KD, Randolph J. A proposed classification of vaginal anomalies and their surgical correction. J Pediatr Surg. 1995;30(2):271–275; discussion 275–6.
41. Soyer T, Aydemir E, Atmaca E. Paraurethral cysts in female newborns: role of maternal estrogens. J Pediatr Adolesc Gynecol. 2007;20(4):249–51.
42. Peña A. Anorectal malformations. Semin Pediatr Surg. 1995;4:35–47.
43. Peña A, Levitt MA. Anorectal malformations: experience with the posterior sagittal approach. In: Stringer MD, Oldham KT, Mouriquand PDE, editors. Pediatric surgery and urology: long-term outcomes. 2nd ed. Cambridge: Cambridge University Press; 2006. p. 401–15.
44. Silva JA, Alvares RA, Barboza AL, Monteiro RT. Lower urinary tract dysfunction in children with cerebral palsy. Neurourol Urodyn. 2009;28(8):959–63.
45. Richardson I, Palmer LS. Clinical and urodynamic spectrum of bladder function in cerebral palsy. J Urol. 2009;182(4 Suppl):1945–8.

Diagnostic Scores, Questionnaires and Quality-of-Life Measures in Paediatric Continence

Wendy F. Bower

3.1 Introduction

The process of providing clinical care to a child or adolescent with continence issues is essentially about targeting the patient's concerns whilst balancing medical care. In the case of children, it is equally about impacting what matters to the family. Aspects of lower urinary tract dysfunction (LUTD) that bother the child do not necessarily correlate with the severity of incontinence and commonly differ from issues of concern to the patient or caregiver. Engaging the child or young person in identifying their needs at the outset of treatment is associated with improved quality of interactions and higher levels of satisfaction [1] that in turn predict better treatment compliance [2–4]. Patient goal-setting has been well described; the process identifies patient expectations and treatment outcomes that are most significant to each individual [5]. Some authors describe the patient and family's view of care provided as an indicator of quality and health system performance [6–8].

Routine intervention that prioritizes the child and targets their concerns improves their journey through the healthcare system. Children will usually answer unambiguous questions truthfully; when pertinent or goal-oriented issues are raised, the patient's voice can typically be heard. Efficacy can be evaluated and outcomes of care become transparent. In order for specific results or effects to be demonstrable, measurement must capture what matters. If we want to hear the continence details from the child or young person, and understand and quantify current bladder and bowel function, enquiry must be carefully framed. Self-report of bladder and bowel variables is notoriously unreliable, largely due to recall bias, downplaying, catastrophizing or anxiety about the problem. An understanding of the extent of symptoms, and their impact, can rarely be derived from verbal or proxy report.

W.F. Bower, FACP,PhD,Dip EpiBio,BAppSc(PT)
Division of Medicine and Community Care, Melbourne Health, Melbourne, VIC, Australia
e-mail: wendy.bower@mh.org.au

Table 3.1 Potential pitfalls of new metrics

Problematic characteristic	Limitation to clinical usefulness
Unvalidated tool	• May not measure what it is meant to • May not have been tested in specific patient populations
No reliability data reported	• Data obtained may not be stable over time • Unknown whether it will reproduce responses when administered by different clinicians
No proven sensitivity	• The measure has not been shown to change with improvement in patient condition
Unacceptable to patients	• Too long/complicated/repetitive/difficult to understand • Uses age-inappropriate language • Not developed for different cultural groups • Too cumbersome to repeat after treatment
Not relevant to your patients	• Doesn't appear to measure what is important to them • Gender/age/education/economic status bias
Complex scoring ± challenging interpretation	• Difficult to obtain immediate feedback to discuss with patient • Time consuming to use

A robust clinical measurement tool will quantify baseline variables and track changes in patients over time. Table 3.1 summarizes some of the pitfalls to avoid when choosing a metric to capture clinical variables. These basic epidemiological hazards are particularly relevant in emerging clinical areas, such as paediatric LUTD, where clinical research and many of the metrics used are relatively recent.

3.2 LUTD Measures

A worthwhile continence measurement tool will use easily collected information to identify the presence or absence of signs and symptoms, allow classification and quantify the severity of dysfunction. Symptom scores provide structured non-invasive evaluation and are helpful for diagnosing non-neurogenic symptoms. When repeated over time, they should indicate resolution or stasis of symptoms. In summary, symptom scoring systems "have been devised to confirm diagnosis of lower urinary tract dysfunction, classify its severity, and serve as a monitoring instrument to determine response to treatment" [9]. One study showed no greater diagnostic benefit conferred by the addition of a behavioural comorbidity score and ultrasound measures to a symptom score [10]. The limitations of LUTD symptom scores are that they are restricted in content and may not reflect real-world functioning or cultural response to symptoms.

The first reported tool, the pediatric lower urinary tract scoring system, was composed of items used in the International Reflux Study. Items were then modified and two subsequent symptom scores developed, the Dysfunctional Voiding Scoring System (DVSS) [11] and the Wetting and Functional Voiding Disorder Score [12]. The first is child-completed, whilst the latter uses the parent as a proxy. The scores establish the presence and severity of urinary urge, urge leak, nocturnal enuresis, frequency of voiding and any disordered mechanics of emptying. The DVSS was first described in 2000 and has been translated into Korean [13], Chinese [14], Japanese [15] and Brazilian Portuguese [16]. It has been shown to be specific to voiding disorders in children [11] and sensitive to resolution of vesicoureteric reflux [17] and compliance with treatment recommendations [18].

It is known that the presence of clinically relevant behaviours can be associated with poor treatment compliance. Two measures exist to assist the continence clinician in identifying whether a child has behavioural traits that may negatively impact treatment outcomes. The more comprehensive of the two measures is the Child Behaviour Checklist (CBCL) [19]. Designed by a psychologist for children aged 6–18 years, this questionnaire is used to quantify behavioural and emotional functioning, social problems and competencies and to identify if the child manifests clinically significant problems. The measure can generate scores from the child themselves, their parents or a third party. Although often used as a research and screening tool, the Achenbach CBCL is complex and time-consuming to score. To provide a clinical screening tool for non-psychologist continence clinicians, the Short Screening Instrument for Psychological Problems in Enuresis (SSIPPE) was developed [20]. A discrimination process was used on items from both the CBCL and the Disruptive Behaviour Disorders Rating Scale, and the short tool was validated for emotional, attention and hyperactivity/impulsivity problems. Clinicians in continence clinics can thus screen for behavioural issues that warrant closer investigation and psychological management prior to implementing therapy for LUTD.

Aside from summary scores, there are reliable measures of symptoms that capture variables useful in diagnosis and as outcome measures. Urgency can be quantified using the Urge Visual Analogue Scale [21], severity of incontinence (i.e. wetness) tracked with the Dry Pie [21] and voiding mechanics screened with uroflowmetry. If the child is prepared adequately and the environment is comfortable and safe, the initial uroflowmetry is likely to be indicative of traits identified on subsequent voids [22].

Bladder diaries are the backbone of evaluating paediatric continence issues. Careful explanation of the optimal completion strategy will improve the quality of data that can be derived from the bladder diary. Documented voids and fluid intake should be compared to the routine and habits of individual children on school days. Some bladder diaries include time and place descriptions of incontinence episodes, which is helpful information for the clinician. Clearly bladder diaries cannot measure voiding pressure nor estimate efficiency of emptying. It is, however, possible to make assumptions about urge syndrome, infrequent voiding, extraordinary urinary frequency and poor hydration from information on the bladder diary. A less well-known bladder diary is the 14-night enuresis record, in which the child documents wet and dry nights. Table 3.2 summarizes other variables that can be derived from this enuresis record.

An understanding of the impact of bladder issues on the child and their family cannot readily be gained from symptom scores; instead health-related quality of life (QoL) should be assessed. Although generic paediatric QoL measures exist, there are few

Table 3.2 Information that can be derived from a 14-night nocturnal enuresis diary

- Time of sleep and duration
- Whether enuresis/other alarm used
- Any medication taken
- Any parental lifting during the night
- Number of wet nights
- Approximate time of enuresis episode
- Any arousal during enuresis episode
- Spontaneous arousal to void on dry nights
- Change in weight of diaper after wet night
- Size of first morning void
- Total overnight urine production
- Using alongside bladder diary: day to night ratio of urine production

disease-specific tools for use in children with bladder or bowel dysfunction (BBD). The earliest tool was the PinQ (paediatric incontinence quality of life), a cross-cultural two-factor measure shown to be valid and reliable in the target population [23]. The measure has been translated into a number of languages and used in clinical trials to measure QoL as a secondary endpoint and marker of treatment efficacy.

The paediatric enuresis module to assess quality of life (PEMQOL) has also been designed for use in clinical practice and research and to monitor the impact of enuresis on the child and family [24]. A German version of the short form was found to be poor for the child impact scale, where reliability coefficients have been reported from 0.54 to 0.78, although acceptable for measuring family impact of enuresis [24, 25].

3.3 Bowel Dysfunction Measures

Children presenting for help with bowel dysfunction commonly disclose the symptom of faecal incontinence. On questioning there may be evidence suggestive of constipation or defaecation dysfunction. A two-week bowel diary completed prospectively by the child and family will clarify frequency of both bowel actions and faecal incontinence episodes. Additional information that can be derived from this measure includes stool shape and consistency, whether the stool was spontaneous or prompted, any straining, bleeding or pain whilst passing the stool and episodes of stool refusal or failure to attend to call to stool. The Bristol Stool Form Scale, commonly used in paediatric bowel evaluation to describe faeces, is often included on bowel diaries [26]. Whilst constipation can be suspected when a rectal ultrasound diameter of ≥ 30 mm is noted [27], diagnosis of childhood functional constipation requires scoring according to the Rome III criteria (http://www.romecriteria.org). Similar criteria have been described for faecal incontinence (FI). Table 3.3 describes these diagnostic benchmarks.

Quality of life is known to be impaired in children with faecal incontinence [28] and to be more compromised in children with bowel dysfunction compared to those

3 Metrics in Paediatric Evaluation

Table 3.3 Rome III diagnostic criteria

Functional constipation
Two or more of the following over the preceding 2 months in a child with a developmental age of at least 4 years and insufficient diagnostic criteria for irritable bowel syndrome:
• Two or fewer defecations in the toilet per week
• At least one episode of faecal incontinence per week
• History of retentive posturing or excessive volitional stool retention
• History of painful or hard bowel movements
• Presence of a large faecal mass in the rectum
• History of large diameter stools that may block the toilet
Non-retentive faecal incontinence
Must include all of the following over the preceding 2 months in a child with a developmental age of at least 4 years:
• Defaecation in inappropriate places at least once per month
• No evidence of faecal retention
• No evidence of inflammatory, metabolic or neoplastic processes

with bladder symptoms [29]. One valid and reliable instrument quantifying the impact on well-being of issues related to faecal incontinence in children is the Faecal Incontinence Quality of Life Scale [30, 33]. Another such tool is the Virginia Faecal Incontinence–Constipation apperception Test which has demonstrated sensitivity to symptom improvement post-therapy [31].

3.4 Outcome of Clinical Care

Treatment efficacy in childhood BBD can be evaluated by resolution of signs and symptoms. From a clinician perspective, the signs of interest relate to safe pressure within the urinary tract. This requires evidence of synergic voiding patterns, normal detrusor wall thickness, resolution of vesicoureteric reflux and minimal post-void residual volumes. Improvement for patients and their families relates to their needs, goals and motivation for seeking help. Symptoms communicate improved function and will include number and severity of incontinence episodes, severity of urge incidents, intervals between urinary tract infections and number of wet nights. Less commonly in paediatric care, the number of pads used each day may be compared.

Baseline documentation will allow change during intervention and up to final status to be observed. Treatment success or failure is measured by many of the same tools used to evaluate and monitor the problem in the first instance—voiding and bowel diaries, flow rate recording, post-void residual urine measurement and recurrence of urinary tract infection. The International Children's Continence Society has defined different levels of response to intervention by the proportion of reduction in specific symptoms rather than by grouping of children into responders and non-responders [32]. No response is described as 0–49% drop, partial response 50–89%, response ≥90% and full response 100% symptom reduction. Complete success implies no relapse within 2 years after treatment cessation, that is, no more than 1 symptom/month.

3.5 Summary

In a child-centred care model, clinical practice is tailored to address the needs of the patient and their family. Nonetheless, clinical outcome does not equate to how the child feels. Efficacy of treatment must be demonstrated with robust measurement of signs and symptoms, along with improvement in continence-specific quality of life.

References

1. Jackson JL, Chamberlin J, Kroenke K. Predictors of patient satisfaction. Soc Sci Med. 2001;52(4):609–20.
2. Fitzpatrick R. Surveys of patients satisfaction: I–important general considerations. BMJ. 1991;302(6781):887–9.
3. Linn LS, Greenfield S. Patient suffering and patient satisfaction among the chronically ill. Med Care. 1982;20(4):425–31.
4. Weisman CS, Nathanson CA. Professional satisfaction and client outcomes. A comparative organizational analysis. Med Care. 1985;23(10):1179–92.
5. Williams KS, Perry S, Brittain KR, The Leicestershire MRC Incontinence Study Team. Patient goal setting in continence care: a useful assessment tool? Clin Eff Nurs. 2001;5:10–7.
6. Hall JA, Dornan MC. What patients like about their medical care and how often they are asked: a meta-analysis of the satisfaction literature. Soc Sci Med. 1988;27(9):935–9.
7. Lochman JE. Factors related to patients' satisfaction with their medical care. J Community Health. 1983;9(2):91–109.
8. Pascoe GC. Patient satisfaction in primary health care: a literature review and analysis. Eval Program Plann. 1983;6(3-4):185–210.
9. Wallis MC, Khoury AE. Symptom score for lower urinary tract dysfunction in pediatric urology. Curr Urol Rep. 2006;7(2):136–42.
10. Hooman N, Hallaji F, Mostafavi SH, Mohsenifar S, Otukesh H, Moradi-Lakeh M. Correlation between lower urinary tract scoring system, behavior check list, and bladder Sonography in children with lower urinary tract symptoms. Korean J Urol. 2011;52(3):210–5.
11. Farhat W, Bägli DJ, Capolicchio G, O'Reilly S, Merguerian PA, Khoury A, McLorie GA. The dysfunctional voiding scoring system: quantitative standardization of dysfunctional voiding symptoms in children. J Urol. 2000;164(3 Pt 2):1011–5.
12. Akbal C, Genc Y, Burgu B, Ozden E, Tekgul S. Dysfunctional voiding and incontinence scoring system: quantitative evaluation of incontinence symptoms in pediatric population. J Urol. 2005;173(3):969–73.
13. Lee HE, Farhat W, Park K. Translation and linguistic validation of the Korean version of the dysfunctional voiding symptom score. J Korean Med Sci. 2014;29(3):400–4.
14. Chang SJ, Chen TH, Su CC, Yang SS. Exploratory factory analysis and predicted probabilities of a Chinese version of dysfunctional voiding symptom score (DVSS) questionnaire. Neurourol Urodyn. 2012;31(8):1247–51.
15. Imamura M, Usui T, Johnin K, Yoshimura K, Farhat W, Kanematsu A, Ogawa O. Cross-cultural validated adaptation of dysfunctional voiding symptom score (DVSS) to Japanese language and cognitive linguistics in questionnaire for pediatric patients. Nihon Hinyokika Gakkai Zasshi. 2014;105(3):112–21.
16. Calado AA, Araujo EM, Barroso U Jr, Netto JM, Filho MZ, Macedo A Jr, Bagli D, Farhat W. Cross-cultural adaptation of the dysfunctional voiding score symptom (DVSS) questionnaire for Brazilian children. Int Braz J Urol. 2010;36(4):458–63.
17. Upadhyay J, Bolduc S, Bagli DJ, McLorie GA, Khoury AE, Farhat W. Use of the dysfunctional voiding symptom score to predict resolution of vesicoureteral reflux in children with voiding dysfunction. J Urol. 2003;169(5):1842–6.

18. Farhat W, McLorie GA, O'Reilly S, Khoury A, Bägli DJ. Reliability of the pediatric dysfunctional voiding symptom score in monitoring response to behavioral modification. Can J Urol. 2001;8(6):1401–5.
19. Achenbach TM, Ruffle TM. The child behavior checklist and related forms for assessing behavioral/emotional problems and competencies. Pediatric Review. 2000;21(8):265–71.
20. Van Hoecke E, Baeyens D, Vanden Bossche H, Hoebeke P, Vande Walle J. Early detection of psychological problems in a population of children with enuresis: construction and validation of the short screening instrument for psychological problems in enuresis. J Urol. 2007;178(6):2611–5.
21. Bower WF, Moore KH, Adams RD. A novel clinical evaluation of childhood incontinence and urinary. J Urol. 2001;166(6):2411–5.
22. Bower WF, Kwok B, Yeung CK. Variability in normative urine flow rates. J Urol. 2004;171(6 Pt 2):2657–9.
23. Bower WF, Sit FK, Bluyssen N, Wong EM, Yeung CK. PinQ: a valid, reliable and reproducible quality-of-life measure in children with bladder dysfunction. J Pediatr Urol. 2006;2(3):185–9.
24. Landgraf JM. Precision and sensitivity of the short-form pediatric enuresis module to assess quality of life (PEMQOL). J Pediatr Urol. 2007;3(2):109–17.
25. Bachmann C, Ackmann C, Janhsen E, Steuber C, Bachmann H, Lehr D. Clinical evaluation of the short-form pediatric enuresis module to assess quality of life. Neurourol Urodyn. 2010;29(8):1397–402.
26. Lewis SJ, Keaton KW. Stool form scale as a useful guide to intestinal transit time. Scand J Gastroenterology. 1997;32(9):920–4.
27. Joensson IM, Siggaard C, Rittig S, Hagstroem S, Djurhuus JC. Transabdominal ultrasound of rectum as a diagnostic tool in childhood constipation. J Urol. 2008;179(5):1997–2002.
28. Bai Y, Yuan Z, Wang W, Zhao Y, Wang H, Wang W. Quality of life for children with faecal incontinence after surgically corrected anorectal malformation. J Paed Surg. 2000;35(3):462–4.
29. Bower WF. Self-reported effect of childhood incontinence on quality of life. J Wound Ostomy Continence Nurs. 2008;35(6):617–21.
30. Rockwood TH, Church JM, Fleshman JW, Kane RL, Mavrantonis C, Thorson AG, Wexner SD, Bliss D, Lowry AC. Fecal incontinence quality of life scale: quality of life instrument for patients with fecal incontinence. Dis Colon Rectum. 2000;43(1):9–16.
31. Cox DJ, Ritterband LM, Quillian W, Kovatchev B, Morris JB, Sutphen JL, Borrowitz SM. Assessment of behavioural mechanisms maintaining faecal incontinence: Virginia Faecal incontinence-constipation apperception test. J Pediatr Psychol. 2003;28:375–82.
32. Austin PF, Bauer SB, Bower W, Chase J, Franco I, Hoebeke P, Rittig S, Vande Walle J, von Gontard A, Wright A, Yang SS, Nevéus T. The standardization of terminology of lower urinary tract function in children and adolescents: update report from the standardization Committee of the International Children's continence society. J Urol. 2014;191(6):1863–5.
33. Filho HS, Mastroti RA, Klug WA. Quality-of-life assessment in children with fecal incontinence. Dis Colon Rectum. 2015;58(4):463–8.

Diaries

4

Ana Ludy Lopes Mendes, Ilaria Jansen, and Giovanni Mosiello

4.1 Introduction

The bladder function of young children is different from that of adults. In fact during the first years of life, there is still a progressive development of the micturition, from the initial indiscriminate way of voiding to a conscious and voluntary adult way. During growth, the functional storage capacity of the bladder increases, the voluntary micturition control matures and the ability to control the initiation and inhibition of the micturition through the sphincter-bladder unit starts [1].

The increase in bladder capacity during growth is a crucial step in the development of the bladder function and for urinary continence.

According to the international children continence society (ICCS), the recording of voiding symptoms at home under normal conditions is crucial for the assessment of lower urinary tract (LUT) function in childhood, and it is relevant after attainment of bladder control of age 5 years [2].

The assessment of lower urinary tract symptoms (LUTS) in children should be detailed and must include consistent and structured medical history and physical examination; and for assessment of the voiding diary, enough time must be taken [2, 3].

The International Continence Society (ICS) has proposed three main forms to record the micturition events: the *micturition time chart* that records only

A.L. Lopes Mendes (✉)
Division of Urology, Surgery for Continence and Neuro-Urology,
Bambino Gesù Pediatric Hospital, Rome, Italy
e-mail: olalu@hotmail.it

I. Jansen
Department of Urology, AMC, Amsterdam, Netherlands

Department of Biomedical Engineering and Physics, AMC, Amsterdam, Netherlands

G. Mosiello
Pediatric NeuroUrology Research and Clinic, Bambino Gesù Pediatric Hospital, Rome, Italy

© Springer International Publishing AG, part of Springer Nature 2018
G. Mosiello et al. (eds.), *Clinical Urodynamics in Childhood and Adolescence*,
Urodynamics, Neurourology and Pelvic Floor Dysfunctions,
https://doi.org/10.1007/978-3-319-42193-3_4

micturition times for at least 24 h, the *frequency volume chart (FVC)* that sets the time and the volume of each micturition and the *bladder diary* that registers the time and the volume of each micturition, incontinence episodes, pad usage and other information such as fluid intake, degree of urgency and urine loss [4].

In the paediatric population, bladder diaries or FVC are routinely used in clinical practice and provide a non-invasive method to evaluate children with LUTS.

4.2 Voiding and Bowel Diaries

Voiding diaries are a part of the diagnostic tools and play an important role in children with micturition problems. However, they always need to be accompanied by the assessment of patients' medical history, physical examination and often other questionnaires. The medial history generally starts at the perinatal or prenatal period and often regards eventual foetal distress, anoxia, birth trauma, oligohydramnios or prenatal hydronephrosis. Information regarding toilet training and the presence of incontinence, urge or age in which continence appeared is important to assess [3]. Other questions, such as holding manoeuvres, post-micturition dribble and urinary retention, should be addressed as well, together with previous surgery or urinary tract infections.

The most common voiding diaries used in clinical practice include properly filled out records of the daily fluid intake, the total voided volume and frequency in 24 h, given information about the mean voided volume, lowest and largest voided volume in 24 h, the distribution of urinary volume during day and night and episodes of urgency and leakage.

Concerning paediatric storage symptoms, it has been proved that voiding frequency is variable and it is mostly influenced by age, as well as by diuresis and fluid intake and in lesser terms the bladder capacity [5–7]. An increased frequency is considered when the child has a micturition frequency of ≥ 8 per day and a decreased daytime micturition frequency when the frequency is ≤ 3 a day [7].

Incontinence occurs when involuntary leakage of urine is seen, and continued incontinence, daytime incontinence, intermittent incontinence and enuresis have to be considered [7].

With a bladder diary it is also important to understand the increase or the decrease of the nocturnal bladder capacity elemental to diagnose nocturnal polyuria. Nocturnal polyuria is considered when the nocturnal urine production exceeds 130% of the expected bladder capacity (EBC) for age. The current formula to calculate the EBC in children is (30 x [age in years +1] ml. EBC is advised to be applicable in children between 4 and 12 years old [2, 7].

In literature, the ideal minimal time for completing the bladder diary is controversial. In adults, several studies have been performed investigating the optimal duration of the voiding diary without reaching an agreement. For the paediatric population, the 2016 ICCS report states that the complete bladder diary (Fig. 4.1) consists of a seven-night recording of incontinence episodes and night-time urinary measurements to evaluate enuresis and a 48 hour daytime frequency and volume chart (not necessarily recorded on 2 consecutive days) to evaluate the LUTD [7].

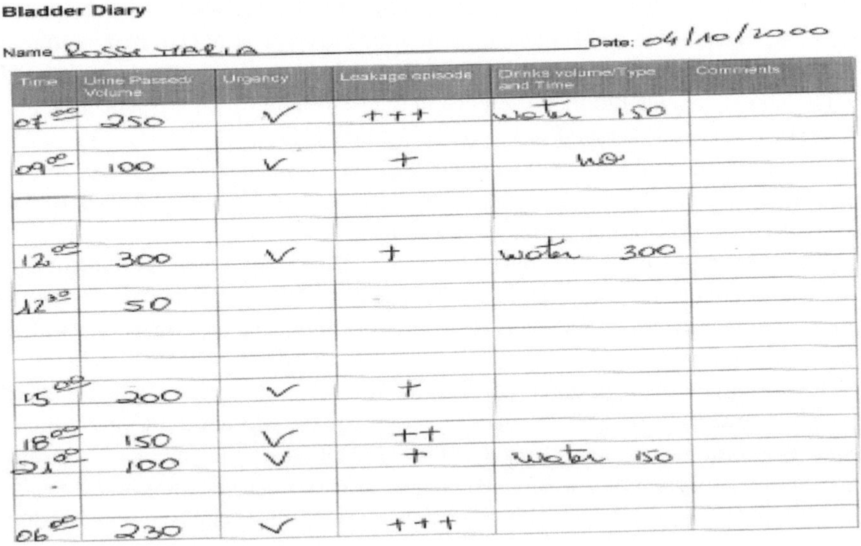

Bladder Diary

Name: Rossi Italia   Date: 04/10/2000

Time	Urine Passed/ Volume	Urgency	Leakage episode	Drinks volume/Type and Time	Comments
07:00	250	✓	+++	water 150	
09:00	100	✓	+	no	
12:00	300	✓	+	water 300	
12:30	50				
15:00	200	✓	+		
18:00	150	✓	++		
21:00	100	✓	+	water 150	
06:00	230	✓	+++		

Fig. 4.1 Example of paediatric bladder diary

In the adult population, according to literature, a voiding diary is recommended to be recorded for at least 3 or more days [8, 9]. In the EAU guidelines for non-neurogenic male LUTS, the recommendation is to use the FVC or a bladder diary to assess male LUTS with a storage component or nocturia but without any mentioning about how longer has to be filled [10–12]. Some studies for the adult population stated that the time has to be long enough to avoid sampling errors and short enough to avoid non-compliance [13].

Schick et al. analysed women with LUTS and compared various variables of the FVC for 1 up to 6 days and studied the reliability and compliance for each recorded parameter each day during 7 days. While days 1, 2 and 3 presented a different results from the total 7 days diary, the rest, day 3 (4, 5 and 6), were comparable, and they concluded that a 4 day diary gives accurate clinical information [14].

In literature there has been a lack of studies regarding bladder diaries for children.

A study comparing a 3-day versus a 2-day voiding diary in children showed that regarding urinary frequency, the 3-day diary had an agreement of 83.4% compared to the 2-day diary, but the average number of urinations was greater in the 2-day bladder diary. No statistical difference regarding the voided volume was seen. Their conclusion was that a 2-day diary gives comparable result and stated that when using the 2-day diary, a false-negative rate of 16% for frequency can be expected and a 2-day diary is sufficient to evaluate bladder capacity and fluid intake in children [15].

The international consensus of the ICCS for the management of enuresis recommends a *daytime diary* (has to be taken ideally during holidays or weekends), used to assess the child's bladder capacity. The measurement of maximum voided volume (excluding the first morning void) needs to be done for at least 3–4 days

[16, 17]. However, is also recommended a *bedwetting diary*, that has to be completed for seven consecutive days/nights, to access the presence of nocturnal polyuria; in this case, to calculate the night-time urinary production, the first morning voided volume must be added to the difference in diaper weight. In case of nocturia, it is recommended to add the night-time voided volume [16].

In children from 5 years old with incontinence, the pad test, the assessment of urine loss by repeating measurements of the weight of the absorptive pads placed in the underwear, is also important to be recorded [7].

There is an important relationship between bladder and bowel dysfunction. In fact, the genitourinary tract and the gastrointestinal tract share the same embryological origin, aspects of innervation and pelvic location, and they both pass through the levator ani muscle.

It is seen that after treatment of constipation, 66% of children with increased PVR had also an improvement in bladder emptying [18]. Moreover, in 1997, another study demonstrated an improvement of 89% of daytime wetting and a 63% resolution of night-time wetting with prevention of urinary tract infection [19]. For this reason, bowel diaries are helpful to evaluate and monitor children with voiding problems.

According to the ICCS, regarding this close relationship between bladder and bowel function described above, the bowel diary is required in association with bladder diary to rule out the bladder bowel dysfunction and to manage the functional constipation in children with LUTS. The Bristol stool scale is a useful tool in children, and constipation is stated when type 1 or 2 stool is present [20], but the most common diagnostic criterion used for constipations is the Rome-III criteria [7].

4.3   Why Do We Use Voiding Diary in Paediatric Population

Dysfunction of the lower urinary tract in children is common and can be related to detrusor and sphincter disorders, structural abnormalities (acquired or congenital) and other conditions, such us giggle incontinence or the Hinman syndrome [2]. However, according to the ICCS, a child with intact neurological system with dysfunctional voiding habitually contracts the urethra sphincter or pelvic floor during voiding [7].

In children the most common conditions for which diaries are useful are, enuresis and LUTS, including bladder bowel dysfunction.

The first non-invasive step to understand the micturition mechanism together with the medical history and questionnaires in paediatric population is through the compilation and the analysis of voiding and bowel diaries.

In studies of children presented with wetting problems, it was demonstrated that 32% of them had dysfunctional voiding [21]. Considering that dysfunctional voiding is often overlooked by families, the child and family education regarding the correct bladder and bowel management through timed voiding, adequate fluid intake during daytime, correct dietary advices (such as avoiding a high protein diet or salt in the evening), correct position to void, hygiene and remembering to void before bedtime is an important tool for the clinical practice to start the management of bedwetting [22, 23].

In the management of enuresis, the consensus of ICCS proposed to provide families of a child with no apparent symptoms of non-monosymptomatic enuresis (NMNE) with bladder diaries the completion also before the second appointment (evidence level 3 grade B) [16]. It has been shown that the nocturnal urine output in many enuretic children is exceeding the bladder capacity during sleep at night [24].

In this way a bladder diary should help to distinguish between monosymptomatic enuresis and NMNE, giving important information about the bladder capacity and the nocturnal urine production.

4.4 Limitations of Bladder Diary in Children

With a bladder diary, it is impossible to obtain the PVR, being the biggest limitation of its diagnostic function.

The evaluation of the bladder before and after voiding should demonstrate residual urine, which is an important diagnostic parameter.

To be reliable, the PVR must be obtained immediately, within <5 min after voiding. Based on an Taiwanese study, the 2016 ICCS terminology stated that for children of 4–6 years old, abnormal PVR is considered when a single PVR >30 mL or 21% of the bladder capacity, where the BC is determined as voided volume + PVR expressed as percent of the expected bladder capacity. For children of 7–18 years old, a single PVR >20 mL or 15% BC or repetitive PVR > 10 mL or 6% BC is considered significant [2, 7].

This is why without PVR, the voiding diary is lacking.

Another limitation of completing the voiding diary is the parents', caregivers' or child's motivation. When some errors and mistakes during registration are identified, or changes on fluid intake are made, it will influence the clinical evaluation.

In conclusion, a diary is an important tool to evaluate voiding symptoms and bowel habits and help clinicians in better diagnostic and therapeutic approach. It is important to combine the voiding diaries with bowel diaries to obtain the best knowledge of bladder bowel dysfunction and other voiding disturbances.

References

1. Yeung CK. The normal infant bladder. Scand J Urol Nephrol Suppl. 1995;173:19–23. PubMed PMID: 8719561.
2. Neveus T, von Gontard A, Hoebeke P, Hjalmas K, Bauer S, Bower W, et al. The standardization of terminology of lower urinary tract function in children and adolescents: report from the standardisation Committee of the International Children's continence society. J Urol. 2006;176(1):314–24. PubMed PMID: 16753432.
3. Hoebeke P, Bower W, Combs A, De Jong T, Yang S. Diagnostic evaluation of children with daytime incontinence. J Urol. 2010;183(2):699–703. PubMed PMID: 20022025.

4. Abrams P, Cardozo L, Fall M, Griffiths D, Rosier P, Ulmsten U, et al. The standardisation of terminology of lower urinary tract function: report from the standardisation sub-committee of the international continence society. Neurourol Urodyn. 2002;21(2):167–78. PubMed PMID: 11857671.
5. Bower WF, Moore KH, Adams RD, Shepherd RB. Frequency-volume chart data from incontinent children. Br J Urol. 1997;80(4):658–62. PubMed PMID: 9352709.
6. Mahler B, Hagstroem S, Rittig N, Mikkelsen MM, Rittig S, Djurhuus JC. The impact of daytime diuresis on voiding frequency and incontinence classification in children. J Urol. 2008;179(6):2384–8. PubMed PMID: 18433779.
7. Austin PF, Bauer SB, Bower W, Chase J, Franco I, Hoebeke P, et al. The standardization of terminology of lower urinary tract function in children and adolescents: update report from the standardization committee of the international Children's continence society. Neurourol Urodyn. 2016;35(4):471–81. PubMed PMID: 25772695.
8. Yap TL, Cromwell DC, Emberton M. A systematic review of the reliability of frequency-volume charts in urological research and its implications for the optimum chart duration. BJU Int. 2007;99(1):9–16. PubMed PMID: 16956355.
9. Homma Y, Ando T, Yoshida M, Kageyama S, Takei M, Kimoto K, et al. Voiding and incontinence frequencies: variability of diary data and required diary length. Neurourol Urodyn. 2002;21(3):204–9. PubMed PMID: 11948713.
10. Cornu JN, Abrams P, Chapple CR, Dmochowski RR, Lemack GE, Michel MC, et al. A contemporary assessment of nocturia: definition, epidemiology, pathophysiology, and management--a systematic review and meta-analysis. Eur Urol. 2012;62(5):877–90. PubMed PMID: 22840350.
11. Weiss JP, Bosch JL, Drake M, Dmochowski RR, Hashim H, Hijaz A, et al. Nocturia think tank: focus on nocturnal polyuria: ICI-RS 2011. Neurourol Urodyn. 2012;31(3):330–9. PubMed PMID: 22415907.
12. Gratzke C, Bachmann A, Descazeaud A, Drake MJ, Madersbacher S, Mamoulakis C, et al. EAU guidelines on the assessment of non-neurogenic male lower urinary tract symptoms including benign prostatic obstruction. Eur Urol. 2015;67(6):1099–109. PubMed PMID: 25613154.
13. Bright E, Drake MJ, Abrams P. Urinary diaries: evidence for the development and validation of diary content, format, and duration. Neurourol Urodyn. 2011;30(3):348–52. PubMed PMID: 21284023.
14. Schick E, Jolivet-Tremblay M, Dupont C, Bertrand PE, Tessier J. Frequency-volume chart: the minimum number of days required to obtain reliable results. Neurourol Urodyn. 2003;22(2):92–6. PubMed PMID: 12579624.
15. Lopes I, Veiga ML, Braga AA, Brasil CA, Hoffmann A, Barroso U Jr. A two-day bladder diary for children: is it enough? J Pediatr Urol. 2015;11(6):348 e1–4. PubMed PMID: 26386888.
16. Vande Walle J, Rittig S, Bauer S, Eggert P, Marschall-Kehrel D, Tekgul S, et al. Practical consensus guidelines for the management of enuresis. Eur J Pediatr. 2012;171(6):971–83. PubMed PMID: 22362256. Pubmed Central PMCID: 3357467.
17. Hansen MN, Rittig S, Siggaard C, Kamperis K, Hvistendahl G, Schaumburg HL, et al. Intra-individual variability in nighttime urine production and functional bladder capacity estimated by home recordings in patients with nocturnal enuresis. J Urol. 2001;166(6):2452–5. PubMed PMID: 11696810.
18. Dohil R, Roberts E, Jones KV, Jenkins HR. Constipation and reversible urinary tract abnormalities. Arch Dis Child. 1994;70(1):56–7. PubMed PMID: 8110010. Pubmed Central PMCID: 1029685.
19. Loening-Baucke V. Urinary incontinence and urinary tract infection and their resolution with treatment of chronic constipation of childhood. Pediatrics. 1997;100(2 Pt 1):228–32. PubMed PMID: 9240804.
20. Heaton KW, Radvan J, Cripps H, Mountford RA, Braddon FE, Hughes AO. Defecation frequency and timing, and stool form in the general population: a prospective study. Gut. 1992;33(6):818–24. PubMed PMID: 1624166. Pubmed Central PMCID: 1379343.

21. Hoebeke P, Van Laecke E, Van Camp C, Raes A, Van De Walle J. One thousand video-urodynamic studies in children with non-neurogenic bladder sphincter dysfunction. BJU Int. 2001;87(6):575–80. PubMed PMID: 11298061.
22. Hjalmas K, Arnold T, Bower W, Caione P, Chiozza LM, von Gontard A, et al. Nocturnal enuresis: an international evidence based management strategy. J Urol. 2004;171(6 Pt 2):2545–61. PubMed PMID: 15118418.
23. Vande Walle J, Vande Walle C, Van Sintjan P, De Guchtenaere A, Raes A, Donckerwolcke R, et al. Nocturnal polyuria is related to 24-hour diuresis and osmotic excretion in an enuresis population referred to a tertiary center. J Urol. 2007;178(6):2630–4. PubMed PMID: 17945292.
24. Hjalmas K. Pathophysiology and impact of nocturnal enuresis. Acta Paediatr. 1997;86(9):919–22. PubMed PMID: 9343267.

Ultrasound and MRI

J.M. Nijman

5.1 Introduction

In most children suffering from urinary incontinence, additional imaging studies are not necessary. Children with enuresis most often have no structural abnormalities of the urinary tract, and an extensive history, physical examination, as well as bladder and bowel diary will be adequate for making the diagnosis and starting subsequent treatment.

In children with daytime symptoms, the same is true, but determining post-void residual urine following flowmetry using ultrasound may be helpful. When these children also have urinary tract infections, especially when accompanied with fever, additional imaging studies are required. In this chapter the different indications for ultrasound as well as MRI will be discussed. When looking at the literature hardly any studies have looked at the impact these studies have on treatment outcome. Looking at the level of evidence, most studies would classify at best as "good clinical practice" and "expert opinion."

In children born with complex abnormalities of the urinary tract such as bladder exstrophy, anorectal malformations, and spina bifida, the emphasis of imaging mostly has been on the preservation of the upper urinary tract. Specific studies in these abnormalities on the pelvic floor anatomy and neural innervation are beginning to emerge but are not part of routine investigations yet.

J.M. Nijman
Department of Urology and Pediatric Urology, University Medical Center,
Groningen, The Netherlands
e-mail: j.m.nijman@umcg.nl

5.2 Ultrasound Imaging

The most common use of US in children with urinary incontinence is for determining post-void residual urine in the bladder, usually in combination with flowmetry. It is however also extremely helpful to determine if the bladder is filled adequately before starting with the flowmetry. Many children will tell you that they can void, but it is important to have the flow performed when an adequate volume can be voided. Using the voiding diary as a guide to what volume the child will normally void at home can save a lot of frustration. In daily practice, the "Bladderscan" is most often used: they are easy to operate and are not only used in the urology departments but in most hospitals in recovery rooms to measure bladder volume postoperatively to avoid urinary retention following surgery. Each study must be repeated several times to make sure that the measurements are accurate [1]. Most bladder scans are accurate between 20 and 300 ml, but with smaller and larger volumes, the range of measuring variations increases. The software used for the calculation of bladder volume is based on the assumption that the bladder represents a sphere: but in many instances, this is not entirely true.

In case a more accurate determination of bladder volume is necessary, a formal ultrasound study can be done [2, 3]. In Fig. 5.1 the bladder is imaged in two directions: the width, length, and height are measured, and a formula is used to automatically generate the volume (also based on the assumption that the bladder is more or less spherical). The outcomes are operator dependent: to become more experienced, it is advised to use the ultrasound probe during, e.g., urodynamic investigations for some time. The volume infused into the bladder is known, and also at the end of the study when the bladder is emptied, the volume is known.

Some US machines use also a quick method using only one (transverse) view: drawing a circle over the bladder will provide a rough estimate of bladder volume (this method is less adequate than the one described above).

Bladder wall thickness can also be measured using US; this can be useful especially in the neurogenic bladder or trabeculated bladders (Fig. 5.2). Children with detrusor overactivity may show an increase in bladder wall thickness. In order to obtain reproducible results, the bladder needs to be filled at least >50% of normal voided volumes.

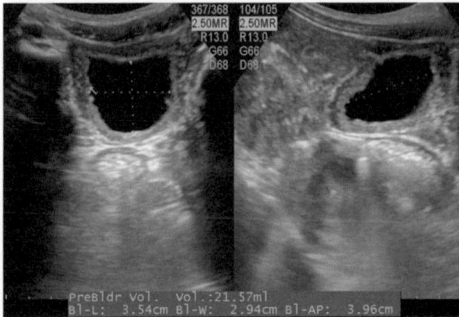 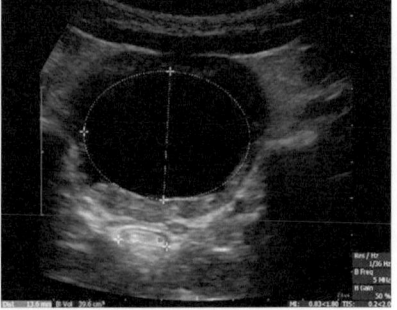

Fig. 5.1 Determination of bladder volume by ultrasound. Two planes are needed to determine width, height, and length to calculate bladder volume. The figure on the right shows a simplified method to estimate volume using a single image

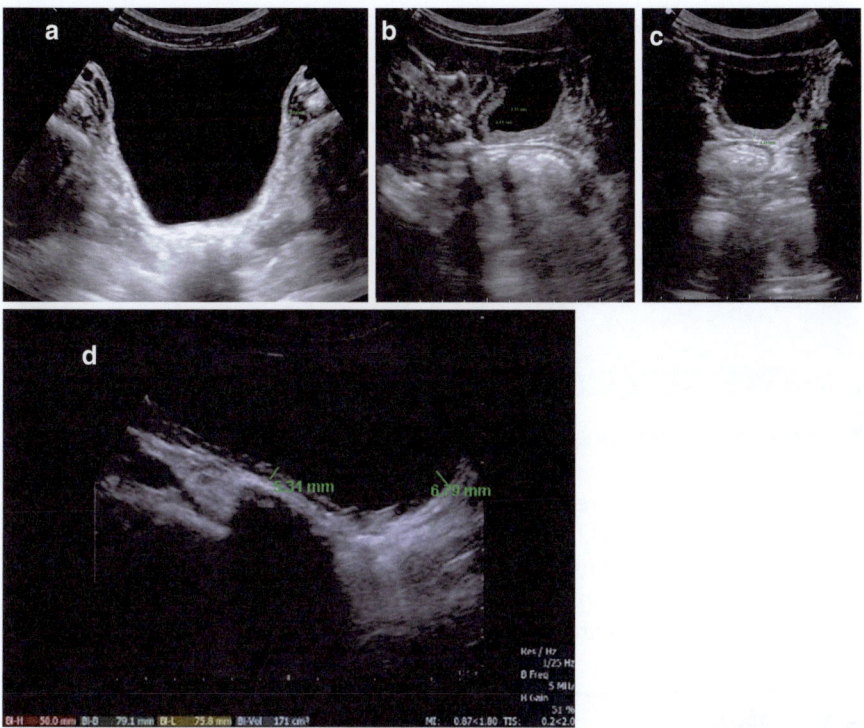

Fig. 5.2 (**a–d**) Ultrasound measure of bladder wall thickness (green measurements): much depends on the location of placing the markers and whether the bladder is full or nearly empty

The voiding diary is important to determine the amount of urine that needs to be in the bladder at the time of measurement. In normal bladders of young children, the bladder wall is <2 mm. A finding >3.5 mm is considered to be abnormal.

When the bladder is filled, it is also worthwhile to look at the bladder neck region (it may be "open" in children with a neurogenic bladder or with sphincteric insufficiency). It may also be helpful to measure urethral length in females with a perineal probe: this requires a lot of experience and is only done in specialized centers [4].

When children are incontinent because of pelvic floor laxity, the US may be used to monitor movement of the bladder and pelvic floor muscles during coughing or straining.

Ultrasound is being used in diagnosing constipation as well: the rectal diameter can be measured behind a filled bladder [5]. Fecal impaction can readily be diagnosed: a diameter > 3.5 cm is considered to be abnormal (Fig. 5.3). One has to remember that this is not the whole story [6]. Some children may only defecate three times a week and not be constipated at all. On the other hand, the diagnostic work-up of children with constipation is rather complex and the pathophysiology multifactorial.

Often there is no agreement between pediatricians and pediatric urologists about the child being constipated or not. When looking at the bowel, it is not only

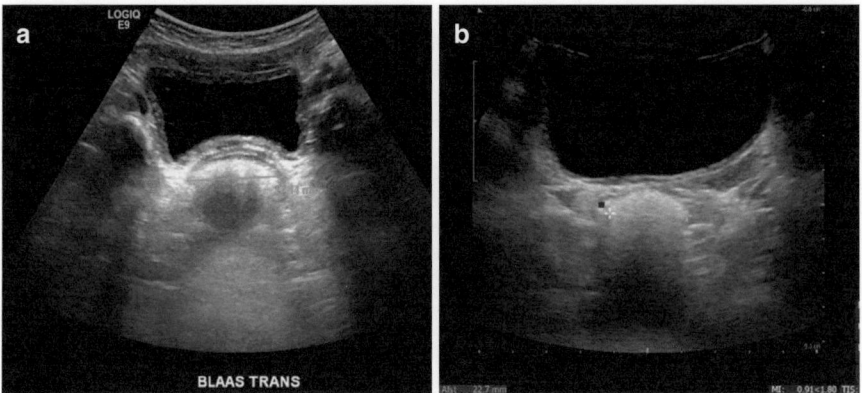

Fig. 5.3 (a–b) Ultrasound measurements of the rectal diameter, to demonstrate constipation

necessary to look at the rectum behind the bladder but also at other parts of the colon: when trying to find the kidneys with the child in supine position, it is sometimes impossible because of an overfilled colon, overlying the kidneys. This in combination with a filled rectum suggests constipation: but it also has to fit in with the history and other signs and symptoms of constipation.

5.3 MRI

MRI studies are most often used in diagnosing an ectopic ureter in a girl with continuous loss of urine while she is otherwise voiding normally. These abnormalities are nowadays diagnosed before birth with an ultrasound study picking up the dilated upper pole of one of the kidneys. After birth the dilatation may disappear, and diagnosing such an (nonfunctioning) upper pole may be difficult.

Even today patient—as well as doctor's delay may be several years. When the diagnosis is made before birth, the problem can be dealt with before the child develops any symptoms. In girls with an ectopic ureter (usually the upper pole of a duplex system) the symptoms may only become evident after the age that normal continence would be present. Only a minority of these children will present with with urinary tract infections, that may prompt an earlier diagnosis. In some children the diagnosis will be made as late as early adulthood.

When the duplex system can be seen with ultrasound studies, it is helpful to see if the child is wet (occasionally some drops of urine may come out of the vagina or be seen in the vestibule). Having the child in supine position for 30 min may show a filled vagina with the ultrasound (this is pathognomonic for an ectopic ureter).

When the kidneys look normal, it is more difficult to show a duplex system and ureteric ectopy. Even cystoscopy may not render the answer; hence, MRI is indicated [7–9].

Figure 5.4 shows several images of an MRI done in a 14-year-old girl with a history of persistent incontinence without infections and negative findings on cystoscopy and normal kidneys on ultrasound.

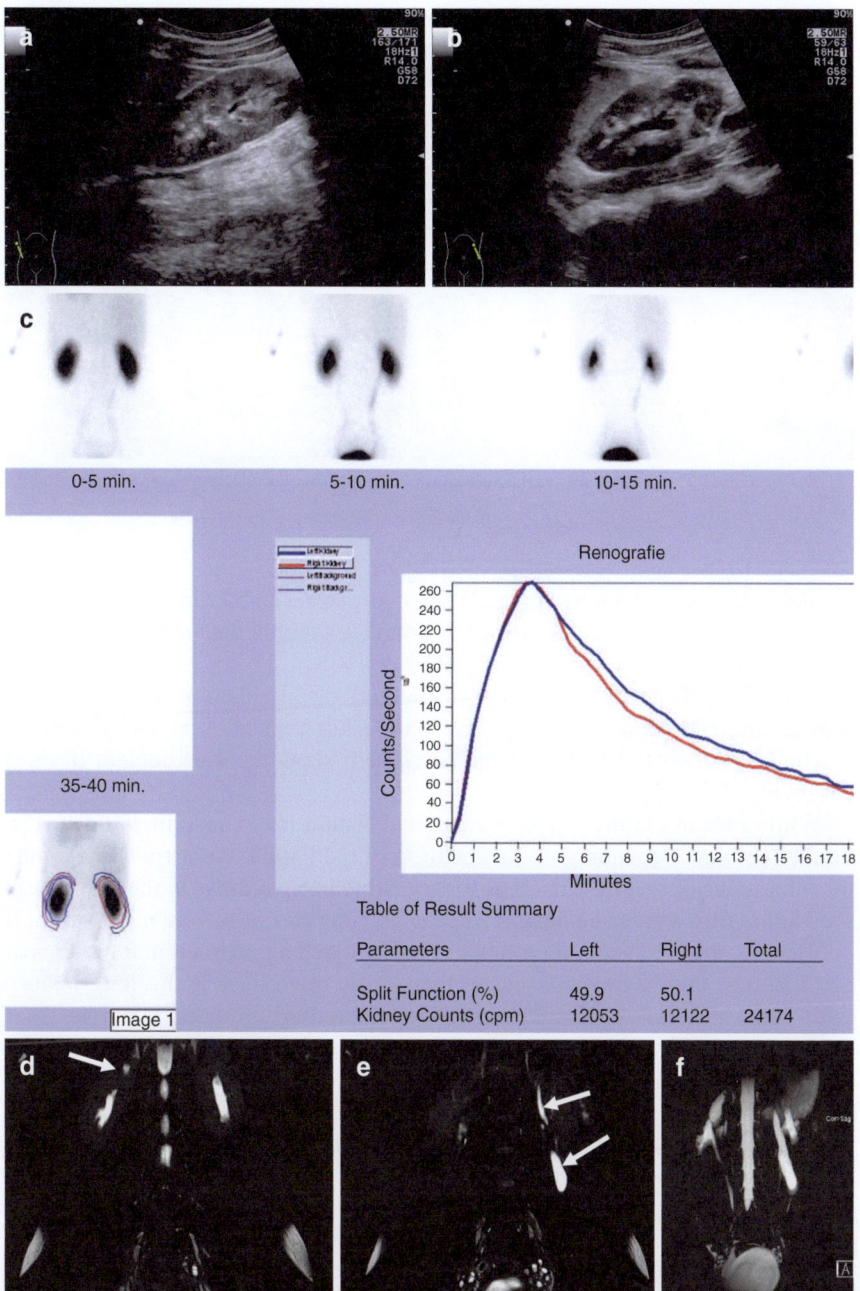

Fig. 5.4 (a–e) US did not show any abnormalities and renography no apparent poor- or nonfunctioning upper poles. The MRI images revealed a bilateral duplex system (indicated by white arrows)

Fig. 5.5 MRI showing urethral diverticulum (white arrow)

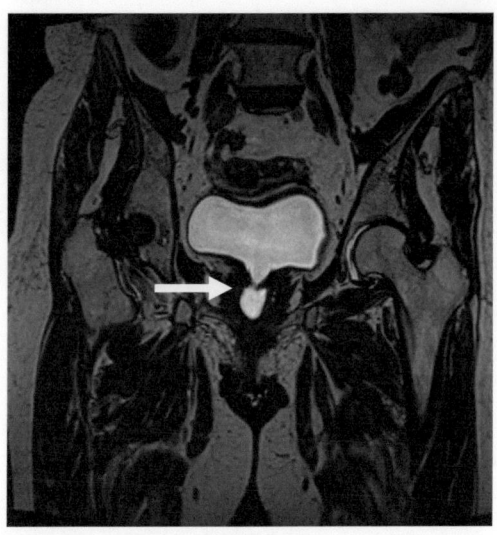

She had a nonfunctioning upper pole on both sides with bilateral ectopic ureters. On physical examination some drops of urine appeared in the vulva after 15 minutes. Following surgery she was completely dry.

Another bothersome problem is a urethral diverticulum in the adolescent female: although more frequently seen in the adult population, it may also occur in younger patients. An MRI of the pelvis will show the diverticulum in most cases (Fig. 5.5) [10].

While rare in children, a urethrovaginal fistula may cause incontinence in young females. Depending on the location of the fistula, the incontinence may be continuous or manifest itself as loss of urine post voiding. In the latter case, the vagina fills with urine during voiding and empties following micturition. It is often regarded as vaginal entrapment and treated as such without much success. Before the diagnosis is made, these girls often have had a long history with many different treatment modalities, including urotherapy, pelvic floor reeducation, and several forms of medical treatment without solving the problem.

In children with complex anomalies or following previous surgery, the MRI may be helpful to plan further surgical interventions (Fig. 5.6).

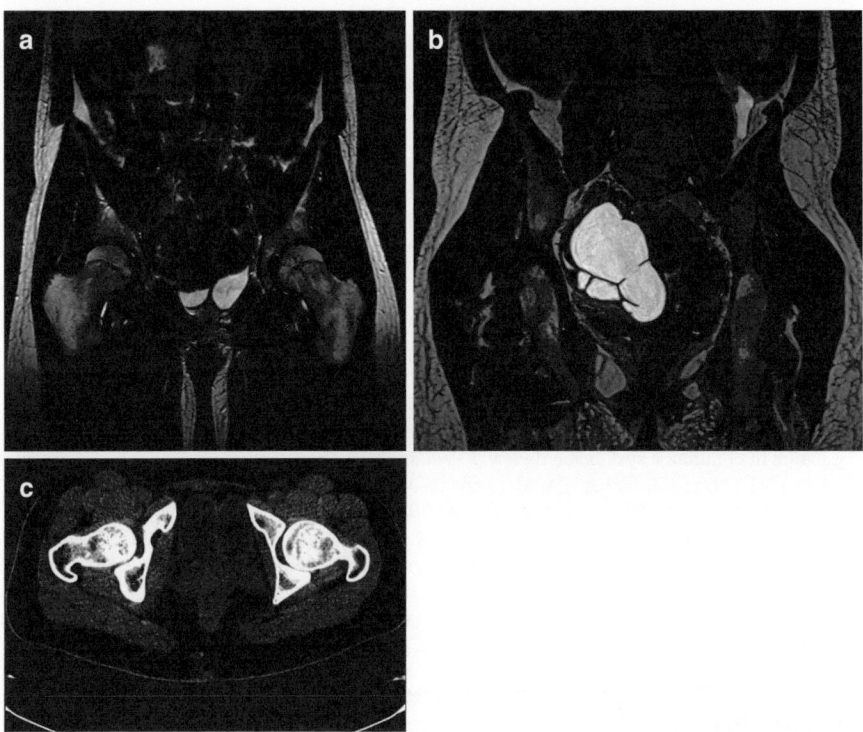

Fig. 5.6 (a–c) MRI in a girl with complete duplication of the bladder and hydrosalpinx on the right side

Conclusion

Both ultrasound and MRI studies can be extremely helpful in the diagnostic process in children with urinary incontinence. The ultrasound is widely available in most hospitals: results may be operator dependent, and one has to be aware that the interpretation of US images may be difficult. The same is true for MRI images of the pelvic region: more and more radiologists are becoming more experienced, thanks to the feedback they receive from the clinicians like pediatric urologists who are more familiar with this anatomic area. Discussing the radiographic findings in relation to the specific complaints really helps both the radiologist and the pediatric urologist to develop a better understanding of an area that is by nature very complex (both anatomically and physiologically).

References

1. Ghani KR, Pilcher J, Rowland D, Patel U, Nassiri D, Anson K. Portable ultrasonography and bladder volume accuracy--a comparative study using three-dimensional ultrasonography. Urology. 2008;72:24–8.
2. Rageth JC, Langer K. Ultrasonic assessment of residual urine volume. Urol Res. 1982;10:57–60.
3. Hwang JY, Byun SS, Oh SJ, Kim HC. Novel algorithm for improving accuracy of ultrasound measurement of residual urine volume according to bladder shape. Urology. 2004;64:887–91.
4. Hirdes MM, de Jong TP, Dik P, Vijverberg MA, Chrzan R, Klijn AJ. Urethral length in girls with lower urinary tract symptoms and forme fruste of female epispadias. J Pediatr Urol. 2010;6:372–5.
5. Klijn AJ, Asselman M, Vijverberg MA, Dik P, de Jong TP. The diameter of the rectum on ultrasonography as a diagnostic tool for constipation in children with dysfunctional voiding. J Urol. 2004;172:1986–8.
6. Berger MY, Tabbers MM, Kurver MJ, Boluyt N, Benninga MA. Value of abdominal radiography, colonic transit time, and rectal ultrasound scanning in the diagnosis of idiopathic constipation in children: a systematic review. J Pediatr. 2012;161:44–50.
7. Chua ME, Ming JM, Farhat WA. Magnetic resonance urography in the pediatric population: a clinical perspective. Pediatr Radiol. 2016;46:791–5.
8. Lipson JA, Coakley FV, Baskin LS, Yeh BM. Subtle renal duplication as an unrecognized cause of childhood incontinence: diagnosis by magnetic resonance urography. J Pediatr Urol. 2008;4:398–400.
9. Figueroa VH, Chavhan GB, Oudjhane K, Farhat W. Utility of MR urography in children suspected of having ectopic ureter. Pediatr Radiol. 2014;44:956–62.
10. Portnoy O, Kitrey N, Eshed I, Apter S, Amitai MM, Golomb J. Correlation between MRI and double-balloon urethrography findings in the diagnosis of female periurethral lesions. Eur J Radiol. 2013;82:2183–8.

Endoscopy

Murat Ucar, Selcuk Keskin, and Selcuk Yucel

6.1 Introduction

Pediatric urologic endoscopy is a minimally invasive urological surgery which is used for diagnosis and treatment with very low complication rates.

Pediatric endoscopy is commonly used in the diagnosis and treatment of diseases of the lower and the upper urinary tract diseases in children who presented with abnormal voiding and storing functions in children. The endoscopy of the lower urinary tract can be identified as the diagnostic examination with the urologic endoscopes of the anterior and posterior urethra, bladder neck, and urinary bladder. Simultaneous endoscopic therapeutic interventions are also possible in majority of cases. The developments in the pediatric endoscopic instruments in recent years have made possible successful diagnostic and therapeutic interventions even in neonates. Pediatric endourological procedures require a complete surgery suit setup and endoscopic instrument collection as well as the surgeon's expertise.

In this section, we will review how to perform endourological procedures for the pathological conditions of pediatric and adolescent age groups, along with their endoscopic examination findings.

6.2 Preparation

Pediatric lower urinary tract endoscopy should be performed in the operation room conditions and general anesthesia.

M. Ucar, M.D.
Department of Urology, Section of Pediatric Urology, Saglik Bilimleri University Tepecik Training and Research Hospital, İzmir, Turkey

S. Keskin, M.D. • S. Yucel, M.D. (✉)
Department of Urology, Acıbadem University School of Medicine, İstanbul, Turkey

© Springer International Publishing AG, part of Springer Nature 2018
G. Mosiello et al. (eds.), *Clinical Urodynamics in Childhood and Adolescence*, Urodynamics, Neurourology and Pelvic Floor Dysfunctions, https://doi.org/10.1007/978-3-319-42193-3_6

The family should be informed about the procedure, and their consent for endoscopic and possible simultaneous therapeutic procedures should be obtained.

Urinalysis should be performed, and active urinary infection should be excluded or properly treated before any urological endoscopic procedure. Preoperative fasting time should be enough, and any antiaggregant or anticoagulant medications should have been stopped preoperatively. Diagnostic procedures generally take about 10–15 min, and the patient is discharged 3–4 h later. However, necessary time should always be spent for proper diagnosis and simultaneous treatment as required.

There are low and medium level recommendations supporting antibiotic prophylaxis for diagnostic urethrocystoscopy. The incidence of symptomatic bacteriuria and urinary tract infection is low after cystoscopy. If the risk factors for urinary tract infection are absent, pre-procedural antibiotic prophylaxis for diagnostic cystoscopy is not recommended [1, 2]. However, if simultaneous treatment is expected following diagnostic endoscopy, prophylaxis is strongly desired.

It is important to have the room temperature close to body heat of the child. Body heat loss decreases the metabolism of the anesthetic medications and increases oxygen consumption. Hypothermia may cause respiratory depression and increase in postoperative complications.

Neonates and toddlers should be brought in heaters, and extremities should be covered properly in order to decrease heat loss (Fig. 6.1).

A heated blanket on the operation table is the most preferable option. Operating room temperature should be around 28–30 degrees Celsius [3].

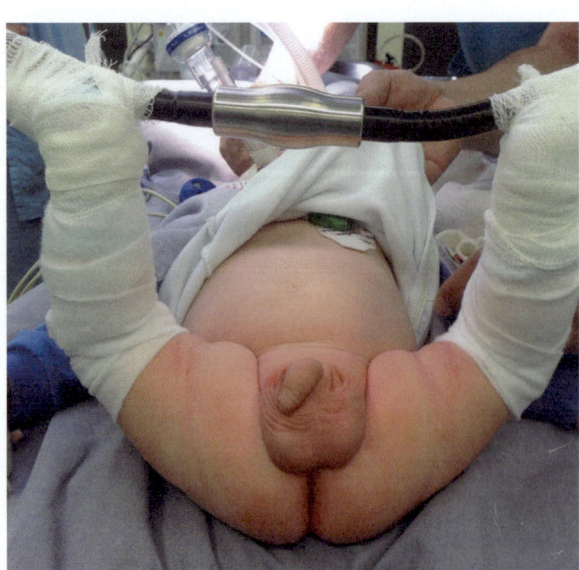

Fig. 6.1 Covering of the extremities

6.3 Endoscopic Tools

Endoscopy can be performed with rigid and flexible endoscopes (Fig. 6.2). The main components of endoscopes are:

- Lens
- Bridge and sheath
- Light source
- Camera

The advantages of using rigid endoscopes are:

- Better vision
- Wider working and irrigation channels

The advantages of flexible endoscopes:

- Can be performed in supine position
- Bladder neck can be negotiated easily
- Examining bladder mucosa from various angles

Different lenses are available for urethrocystoscopy. 0° lens is used for urethra examination and invasive procedures, whereas 30° and 70° are used for the examination of the bladder neck, trigon, and bladder walls as well as treatment of pathologies in the bladder.

The diameters of endoscopic sheaths harboring the lenses vary between 6 and 14.5 Fr. Between the lens and the endoscopic sheath, there is the connecting part called bridge having a room for tools like guidewires, biopsy forceps, ureteral stents,

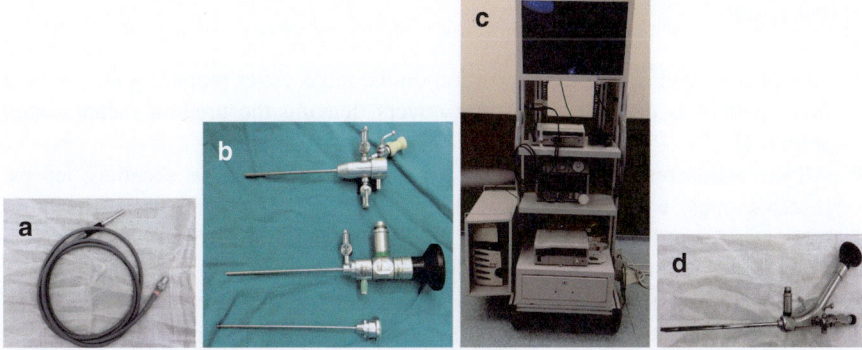

Fig. 6.2 (**a**) Light cable, (**b**) cystoscope, (**c**) camera and recording system, (**d**) compact cystoscope

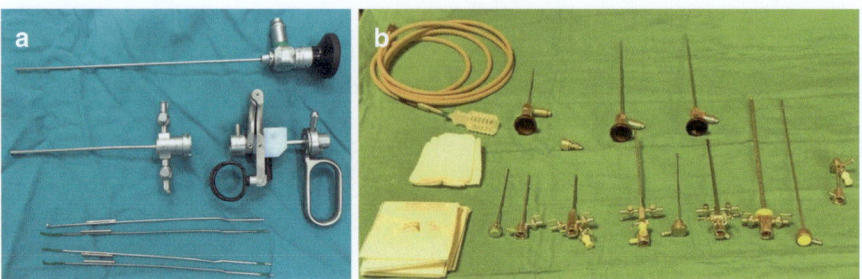

Fig. 6.3 (**a**) Resectoscope set, (**b**) different-sized cystoscope sets

etc. Small compact cystoscopes which are used for neonates and older children do not require placement of a lens, and hence, they are more convenient and durable.

The urethrotome and resectoscopes used for incision or resection during endoscopy are assembled from sheath, lens, working element, and cutting loops. Resectoscope sheaths vary between 8 and 13 Fr. There are cold and hot knife alternatives available used with resectoscopes and urethrotomes (Fig. 6.3).

Irrigation fluid is connected to working sheath. Light wire is placed between the lens and the light source.

Sterile saline or distilled water is used if electrosurgery is not performed. When there is the need for electrosurgery, non-ionized solutions (5% dextrose, glycin, or mannitol) are used. Proper preheated or pump heated solutions will decrease the risk of hypothermia in children who are very prone to hypothermia.

6.4 Technique

Some precautions must be taken in order to achieve a flawless procedure without any mistakes in these procedures which are generally short and have a low risk of complication.

- Patient is placed in lithotomy position on the table. After preparing the surgical field, patient is draped with sterile covers, leaving the urethral meatus open (Fig. 6.4).
- All the endoscopic tools necessary for the operation such as sheaths, lenses, resectoscopes, working elements, loops, light cable, camera head, irrigation tubes, guidewires, injection needles, forceps, and ureteral catheters are placed on the table and connected properly (Fig. 6.5).
- A water-soluble lubricant solution is applied on the endoscope.
- In boys, as the penis is grasped with a sterile gauze pad, endoscope is inserted through the external meatus. The urethra is examined beginning from the outermost part with the endoscope.

6 Endoscopy

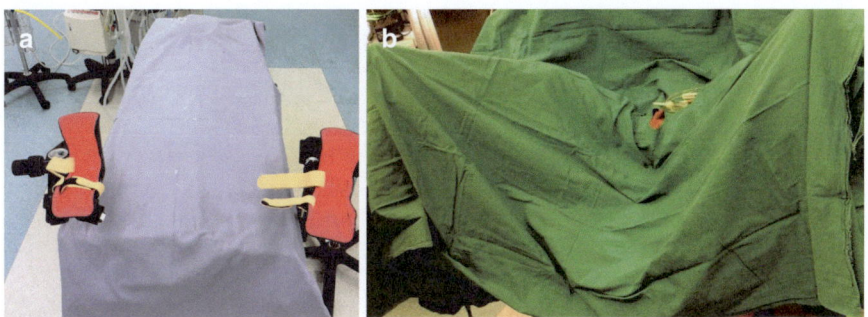

Fig. 6.4 (a) Operation table with pediatric stirrups, (b) lithotomy position for cystoscopy and draping

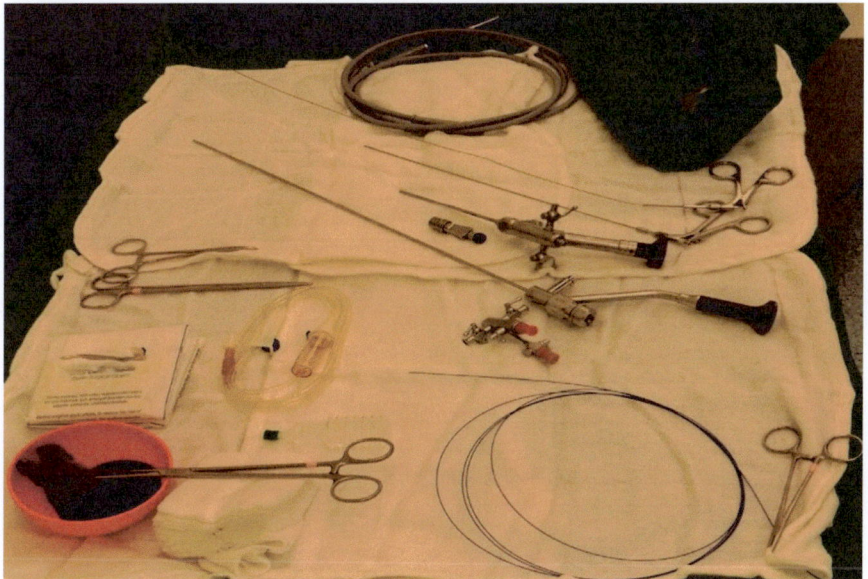

Fig. 6.5 Endoscopic table prepared for operation

- When the cystoscope has reached the membranous urethra, the penis is bent downward to reach the prostatic urethra. After examining the verumontanum, the camera end of the cystoscope is pushed downward, the bladder neck is passed, and then the cystoscope is pushed inside the bladder.
- The bladder mucosa is inspected systematically. Trigon and the localization of the ureteral orifices are examined.
- Since the urethra is short in females, accessing the bladder without any manipulation is possible.

6.5 Indications

The urethrocystoscopy indications for child and adolescent patients are as follows:

- Diagnosis and treatment of urethral stricture
- Diagnosis and treatment of posterior urethral valve
- Anterior urethral valve and urethral diverticulum
- Urethral duplication
- Utricular cyst
- Urethral polyps
- Bladder neck stricture or stenosis
- Diagnosis and treatment of ureterocele
- Evaluation of complete duplicated collecting system
- Endoscopic treatment of vesicoureteral reflux
- Neurogenic bladder
- Bladder diverticula
- Botulinum toxin injection to the bladder
- Evaluation of hematuria

6.6 Contraindications

Endoscopy should be delayed in the presence of active urinary infection until the treatment of the infection and until the antiaggregant or anticoagulant therapy is stopped or condition is properly treated.

6.7 Clinical Conditions

6.7.1 Urethral Stricture

The most common cause of urethral stricture in the pediatric population is the complication of proximal hypospadias surgery. Other causes are transurethral surgery and perineal trauma [4]. 40–68% of urethral strictures in children are after hypospadias surgery, whereas overall urethral stricture after hypospadias surgery is around 6–12% [5–7]. It usually occurs in 6 months after surgery. The symptoms may include weak urine stream, difficulty in voiding, hematuria, and urinary tract infection [5, 8]. In many cases, history, uroflowmetry, retrograde urethrography, or voiding cystourethrography is sufficient for diagnosis, but urethrocystoscopy can also be used for the diagnosis and concomitant treatment. Urethral stricture is observed as narrowing of the urethral lumen during urethrocystoscopy. The most common method for treatment is direct visual urethrotomy (Fig. 6.6). The stricture is cut at 12 o' clock position with a cold knife until fresh and vascular tissue is observed. Holmium:YAG laser has been reported to be an effective energy model for endoscopic stricture incision [7].

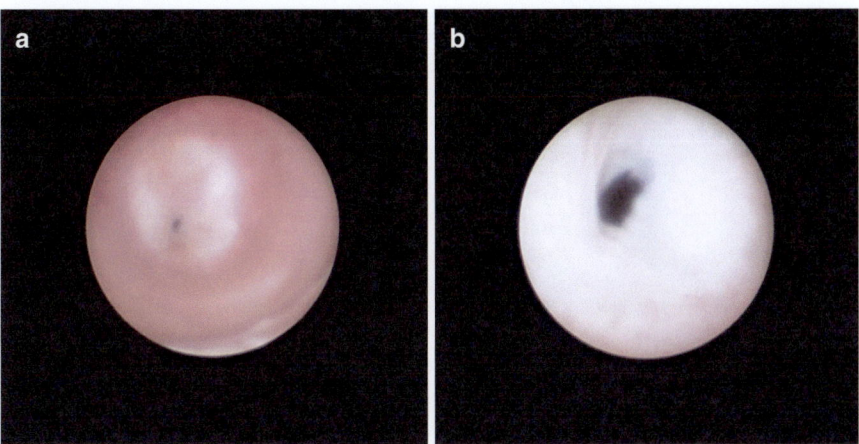

Fig. 6.6 (a, b) Urethral stricture after hypospadias surgery

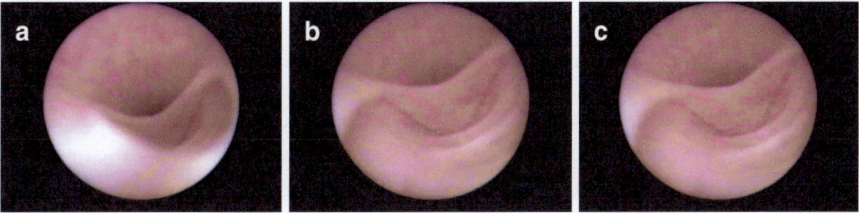

Fig. 6.7 (a–c) Endoscopic view of syringocele [9]

6.7.2 Syringocele (Anterior Urethral Diverticula)

Anterior urethral diverticulum is a rare anomaly of the childhood population. It can be congenital or acquired. It may cause weak stream, straining, hematuria, dysuria, and urinary tract infection. The urethral diverticulum inflates during voiding and compresses the urethra ending with difficulty in voiding and irritative symptoms. Retrograde urethrography, voiding cystourethrography, and urethrocystoscopy can be used for diagnosis.

Open or endoscopic techniques can be used in the treatment (Figs. 6.7 and 6.8). Endoscopic treatment is incision of the syringocele with a cold knife or Holmium:YAG laser.

6.7.3 Anterior Urethral Valve

Congenital anterior urethral valve (AUV) is a rare clinical situation which may cause lower urinary tract obstruction, and it can be seen alone or accompanying a diverticulum [10].

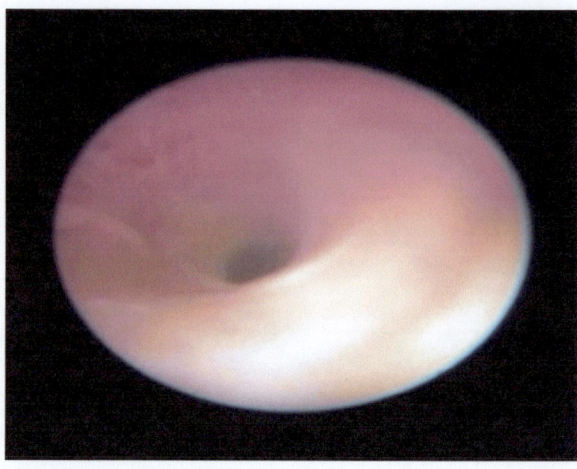

Fig. 6.8 View of the urethra after 2 months of endoscopic treatment of syringocele [9]

The AUV is a generally overlooked pathology mostly and diagnosed in adulthood. Patients may present with difficulty in voiding, urinary incontinence, recurrent urinary tract infections, and hematuria [11]. The patients with AUV may have urethral dilatation, VUR, urinary tract infection, trabeculated bladder, and hydroureteronephrosis [12]. Diagnosis is done with retrograde urethrography, VCUG, and urethrocystoscopy. A cusp-like, semilunar, or iris-shaped valve can be seen in any location of the anterior urethra during urethrocystoscopy [13]. Treatment can be done endoscopically by resection or incision with pediatric resectoscope, or in serious cases open surgery may be applied.

6.7.4 Utricular Cyst

Prostatic utricular cyst is considered as a remnant of the Mullerian duct due to Mullerian-inhibiting substance (MIS) deficiency. It is observed in 4% of newborns and 1% of adults [14]. Although most of the cysts are asymptomatic, some may cause voiding symptoms, epididymitis, and obstructive azoospermia and even may present as palpable masses behind the bladder. Symptoms are related to the size, localization, and degree of obstruction [14]. Prostatic utricular cyst can be seen in 11–14% of distal hypospadias and boys with sexual differentiation disorders, whereas it can be noted up to 50% in the proximal hypospadias patients [15].

Retrograde urethrography, voiding cystourethrography, and MRI can be used for diagnosis. The urethra, cyst, and anatomy of surrounding structures can be examined by contrast material injection from the opening of the utricle.

Small utricles can be treated endoscopically by dilatation of the cyst orifice, incision, or unroofing [16].

6.7.5 Urethral Polyp

Congenital urethral polyp is rare and can cause various symptoms. It is generally localized to the prostatic urethra in males (Fig. 6.9).

Diagnosis can be done with VCUG, but endoscopic evaluation is the gold standard. Generally transurethral resection is sufficient for treatment [17].

6.7.6 Posterior Urethral Valve

Posterior urethral valve (PUV) is a congenital obstructive anomaly which is placed in the posterior urethra of the male children (Fig. 6.10).

PUV may cause upper urinary system dysfunction according to the severity of the obstruction [14]. It is seen in 1 in 5000 to 8000 of male birth [18].

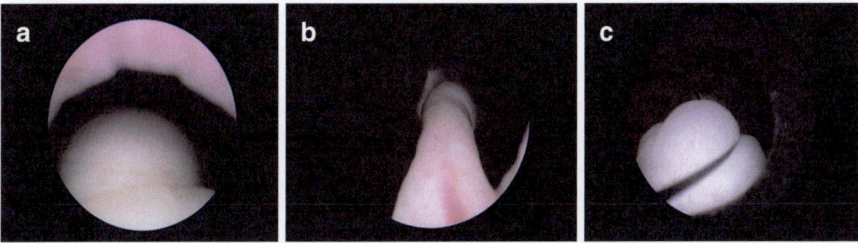

Fig. 6.9 (**a, b**) Endoscopic view of posterior urethral polyp, (**c**) endoscopic treatment of posterior urethral polyp

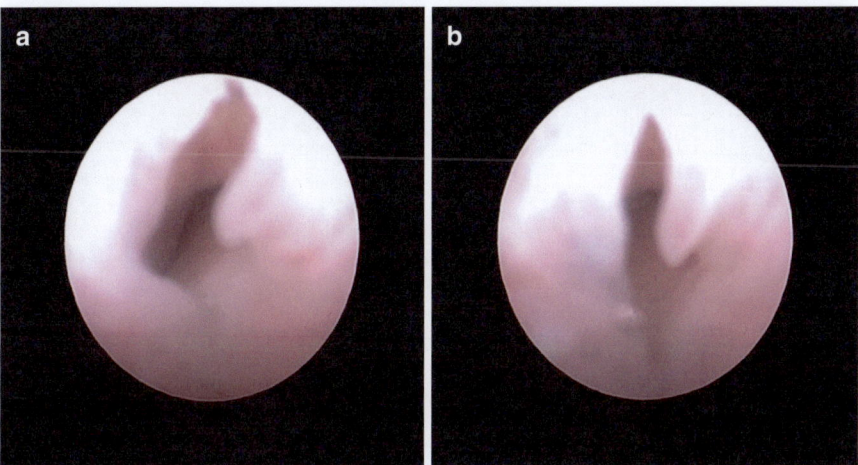

Fig. 6.10 (**a, b**) Endoscopic view of PUV

Young has classified valves according to their relation with the verumontanum. Type 1 is the most common type, and it comprises 95% of posterior urethral valves. Type 3 is less common. Type 2 is believed to be hypertrophy of plica collicula and does not cause obstruction [18, 19]

- Type I: two membranous structures in the posterior urethra originating from the caudal end of the verumontanum rising along the lateral margin of the urethra on each side meeting at 12 o'clock
- Type II: membranes arising from the verumontanum and attached cranially to the bladder neck
- Type III: circular diaphragm in the region of the caudal end of the verumontanum with a central defect

PUV is most commonly diagnosed in prenatal USG with bilateral hydroureteronephrosis, bladder wall thickening, and keyhole sign [20]. Children who are not diagnosed prenatally may present later according to the degree of obstruction. Weak urinary stream and dribbling may be seen in newborns, whereas incontinence, urinary tract infections, renal failure, sepsis, and growth retardation can be seen in older children. PUV is responsible for 17% of end-stage renal disease [18, 20].

Although upper urinary system can be evaluated with USG, VCUG and endoscopy are required for diagnosis.

The patient should be catheterized and stabilized before commencing the treatment of PUV. The treatment of PUV can be done with:

- 6–8 Fr cystoscope with cold knife, bug bee electrode, or laser fiber (Fig. 6.11)
- The Whitaker-Sherwood hook

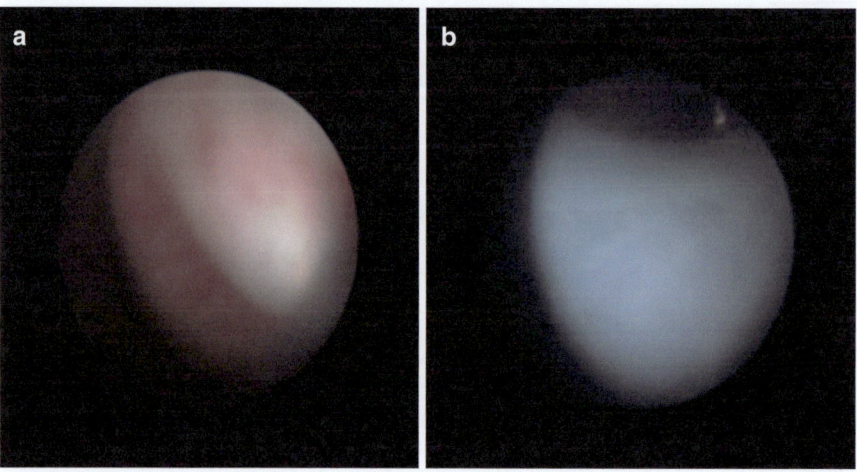

Fig. 6.11 (a, b) Endoscopic view during incision of PUV

- Mohan's valvotomy
- Fogarty balloon catheter or Foley catheter [18]

6.7.7 Endoscopic Evaluation of the Bladder, Trigon, and Orifices

The bladder is accessed by passing the bladder neck which is placed at the end of the prostatic urethra. Bladder mucosa is inspected. The area between the ureteral orifices and urethra is called the trigon.

During the inspection of the bladder mucosa, edema, hyperemia, atrophy, hypertrophy, inflammation, ulcers, necrosis, tumor, stone, and foreign bodies are noted.

The localization of ureteral orifices, ectopic ureter, presence of double collecting system, ureterocele, and diverticula can be examined (Fig. 6.12).

6.7.8 VUR/STI

VUR is the abnormal reflux of the urine from the bladder to the ureter and renal pelvis. Its incidence is 0.4–1.8% in the pediatric population, whereas in the presence of urinary tract infection, it is 10–40% [21]. It can be a benign asymptomatic disease, but on the other hand, it is still one of the leading causes of end-stage renal disease. Its etiology can be primary and secondary. Primary VUR is defined as the anatomical or functional insufficiency of ureterovesical junction. The reflux with accompanying congenital anomalies or conditions affecting the bladder storage and emptying dynamics is called secondary [22, 23].

Ultrasound, VCUG, and DMSA are commonly used in the diagnosis and follow-up of VUR.

The endoscopy is used in the treatment of VUR rather than a diagnostic tool. The anomalies accompanied with VUR such as paraurethral diverticula, ureterocele, and double collecting system can be diagnosed and treated simultaneously as well.

The endoscopic treatment of VUR has boosted after the FDA approval of hyaluronic acid and dextranomere particles in 2001.

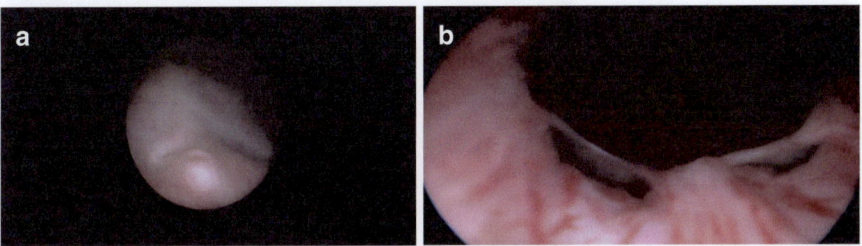

Fig. 6.12 (a) Ureteral orifices of complete duplicated collecting system. (b) Ectopic ureteral orifices of complete duplicated collecting system

Endoscopic injection treatment for VUR is performed with a 8–9.5 Fr cystoscope under direct vision with metal or plastic needles (Puri needle) (Fig. 6.13). STING, HIT, or double HIT techniques can be used [21].

6.7.9 Bladder Diverticula

Congenital or primary diverticulum is defined as the herniation of the bladder mucosa between muscle fibers of the bladder and mostly close to the ureteral hiatus [24]. Moreover, the bladder diverticula can be seen as acquired secondary to neurogenic bladder or bladder outlet obstruction.

Bladder diverticulum is observed in 1.7% of children who have undergone radiological studies because of urological complaints [25]. They are generally unilateral and located paraurethral [26]. They can be either asymptomatic or a reason for recurrent urinary tract infections [26].

Generally USG and VCUG are sufficient for diagnosis.

In endoscopy, they are recognized as blunt sacs with narrow neck opening into the bladder lumen (Fig. 6.14).

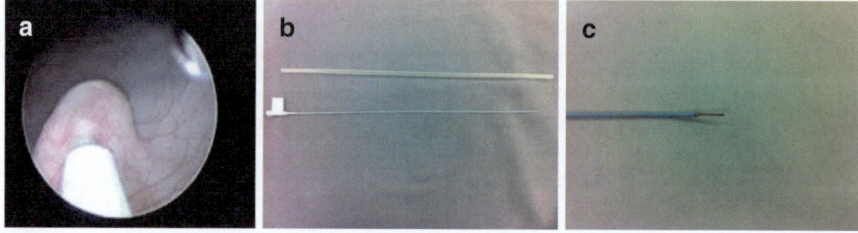

Fig. 6.13 (**a**) STING procedure, (**b**) Puri needle, (**c**) needle tip

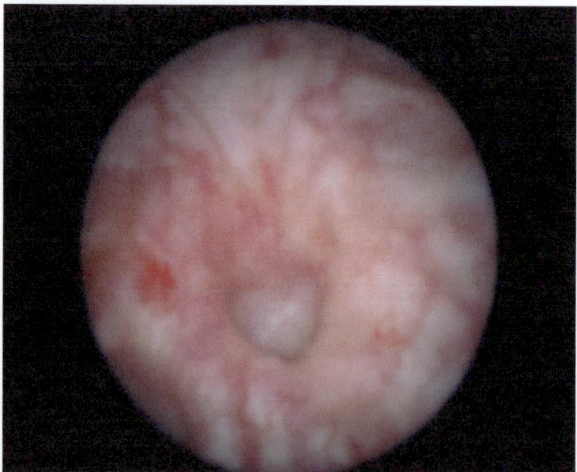

Fig. 6.14 Bladder diverticula

6.7.10 Ureterocele

Ureterocele is a congenital cystic dilatation of the intravesical ureter. It can be seen alone or may accompany as a component of the upper ureter of a complete duplicated collecting system [27].

The real incidence is not known, but it is four times more common in females.

Ureteroceles may be classified as intravesical, extravesical, cecoureterocele, sphincteric, stenotic, and ectopic according to their position and appearance (Fig. 6.15) [27].

The rate of dysplasia and obstructing nephropathy in the upper moiety related to ureterocele is 43–73%. Ipsilateral lower pole reflux is 50% and contralateral VUR is 25% [28].

Most of the patients who are not diagnosed prenatally generally present with recurrent urinary infection.

USG, CT, MRI urography, and VCUG can be used for diagnosis.

Endoscopy can be used both for diagnosis and treatment [29].

During endoscopy, intravesical ureterocele can be observed like a balloon near the ureteral orifice. The fullness of the bladder is important during endoscopic examination. A full bladder may cause compression of the ureterocele, or sometimes ureterocele may disguise to a wide diverticula (everting ureterocele) if the bladder is overdistended.

Endoscopic incision of the ureterocele is an easy and fast outpatient procedure. The success rate of the endoscopic treatment is around 90%, and it is the gold standard treatment option in many cases [30].

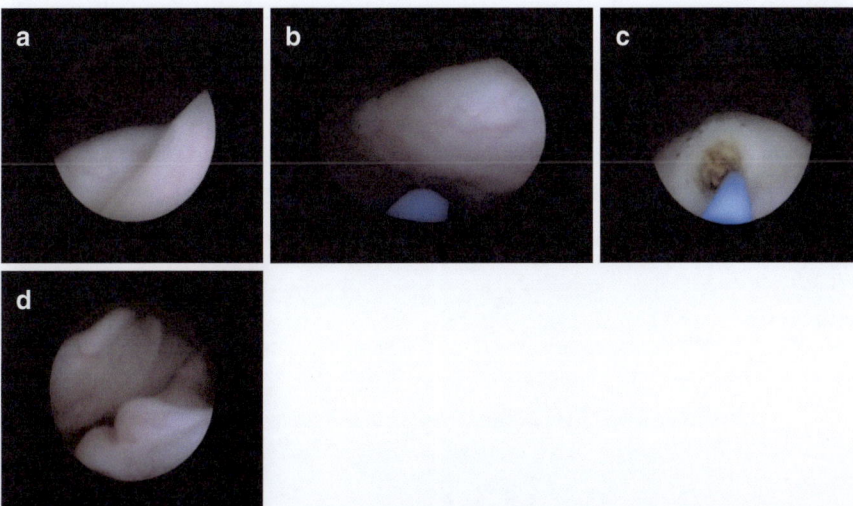

Fig. 6.15 (**a**) Ureterocele, (**b**, **c**) incision of ureterocele with bug bee electrode, (**d**) the view of the lumen after the incision of ureterocele

6.7.11 Neurogenic Bladder

Neurogenic bladder is the abnormality of urinary bladder storage and emptying function due to any congenital or acquired lesion in the peripheral and central nervous system.

The most common cause of neurogenic bladder dysfunction in children is the abnormal development of the spinal canal and inborn damage of the spinal cord.

Incidence is 1/1000 births but has decreased in the last 20 years with the prenatal intake of folic acid and prenatal diagnosis.

There is dysfunction in the lower urinary tract in 40–90% of patients with inborn spinal dysraphism. The child may experience urinary and fecal incontinence and recurrent urinary tract infection leading to end-stage renal disease.

Children with a neurogenic bladder may be complicated with vesicoureteral reflux, recurrent urinary infection, and bladder trabeculation and diverticula. Those trabeculation, cellules, and diverticula can be observed during cystoscopy.

6.7.12 Bladder Tumor

Bladder tumors in children are rare and most of the cases are sarcomas [31]. Epithelial tumors of the urinary bladder are very rare in children, and most of the reported cases are noninvasive, low-grade tumors with a low probability of recurrences and invasion [32].

Although painless hematuria is the presenting symptom in most patients, they can be discovered incidentally during radiological examinations performed for other indications [33].

Bladder tumors can be observed as a small hyperemic lesion or papillary, polipoid well-vascularized exophytic lesions. During endoscopy, the remaining bladder mucosa should be carefully examined, and transurethral resection must be completed simultaneously (Fig. 6.16).

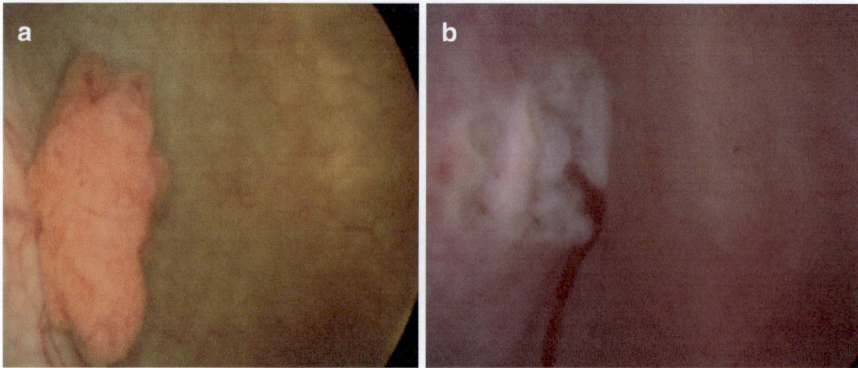

Fig. 6.16 (a) Bladder tumor, (b) after endoscopic resection

6.7.13 Bladder Stone and Foreign Objects

The less commonly observed urethra and bladder stones and foreign objects like retained suture, stent, or catheters can be treated with endoscopic techniques.

According to the size of stone, transurethral or percutaneous cystolithotripsy or open surgery can be performed. If possible, the urethral stones should be pushed back into bladder before fragmentation. Foreign bodies such as indwelling stents may also be removed endoscopically with the help of endoscopic forceps (Fig. 6.17).

6.7.14 Injections into the Bladder, Bladder Neck, and Urethral Sphincter

In the treatment of storage and voiding problems of children, endoscopic injection of bulking agents into the bladder neck and urethra or botulinum toxin injections into the bladder wall and urethral sphincter can be used. Bulking agent injections into the bladder neck are used to increase the bladder neck resistance to increase the bladder volume and void with increasing the intra-abdominal pressure. Lack of bladder outlet resistance can be due to spina bifida, anorectal surgery, or bladder outlet surgery. Injection into the bladder neck is generally done in 2–4 areas until a satisfactory obstructive mound is visible at the bladder outlet.

Moreover, low compliant bladder, high detrusor pressure due to spina bifida, idiopathic detrusor overactivity, and detrusor sphincter dyssynergia can be treated by endoscopic injection of botulinum toxin into the bladder mucosa and/or wall and urethral sphincter (Fig. 6.18) [34].

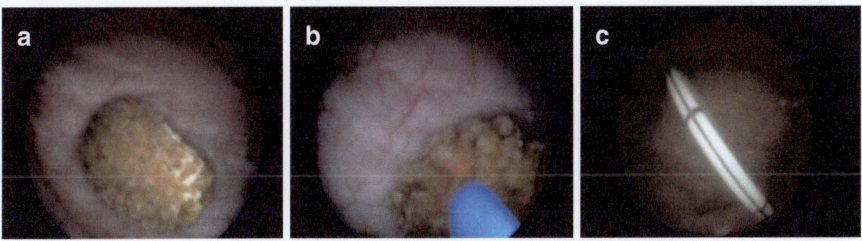

Fig. 6.17 (**a**) Bladder stone, (**b**) laser fragmentation of the bladder stone, (**c**) JJ stent

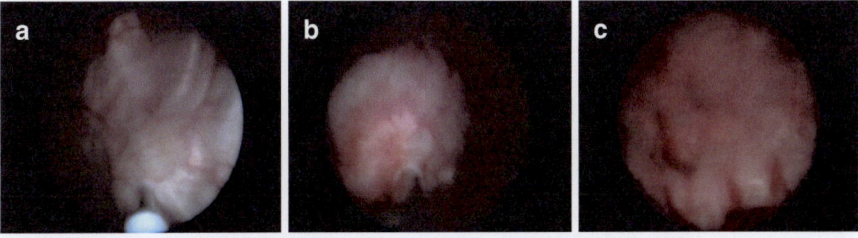

Fig. 6.18 (**a, b**) Bladder Botox injection, (**c**) the view after injection

Onabotulinum toxin A is applied 10 IU/kg with a maximum dose of 300–360 IU. 10 IU of botulinum toxin is diluted in 1 cc saline. It is applied in different locations sparing the trigon to prevent detrusor contractions and increase the bladder volume. Patients and parents must be warned about the urinary retention risk if the patient is not already in clean intermittent catheterization program. Onabotulinum toxin A injection can also be performed into the urethral sphincter at a dose of 100–200 IU to prevent dyssynergic sphincter contraction during voiding either due to neurogenic or idiopathic causes [35–37].

References

1. Mirone V, Franco M. Clinical aspects of antimicrobial prophylaxis for invasive urological procedures. J Chemother. 2014;26(Suppl 1):1–13. https://doi.org/10.1179/1120009X14Z.000000000232.
2. Bootsma AM, Laguna Pes MP, Geerlings SE, Goossens A. Antibiotic prophylaxis in urologic procedures: a systematic review. Eur Urol. 2008;54(6):1270–86. https://doi.org/10.1016/j.eururo.2008.03.033.
3. Walsh PC, Retik AB, Vaughan ED, Wein AJ. Campbell-Walsh Urology. In: Docimo SG, Peters CA, editors. Pediatric Endourology and laparoscopy. 9th ed. Philadelphia: Saunders; 2007. p. 131.
4. Hsiao KC, Baez-Trinidad L, Lendvay T, Smith EA, Broecker B, Scherz H, Kirsch AJ. Direct vision internal urethrotomy for the treatment of pediatric urethral strictures: analysis of 50 patients. J Urol. 2003;170(3):952–5.
5. Snodgrass W, Villanueva C, Bush NC. Duration of follow-up to diagnose hypospadias urethroplasty complications. J Ped Urol. 2014;10:208–11.
6. Gargollo PC, Cai AW, Borer JG, Retik AB. Management of recurrent urethral strictures after hypospadias repair: is there a role for repeat dilation or endoscopic incision? J Ped Urol. 2011;7:34–8.
7. Husmann DA, Rathbun SR. Long-term Followup of visual internal Urethrotomy for Management of Short (less than 1 cm) penile urethral strictures following hypospadias repair. J Urol. 2006;176:1738–41.
8. Launonen E, Sairanen J, Ruutu M, Taskinen S. Role of visual internal urethrotomy in pediatric urethral strictures. J Ped Urol. 2014;10:545–9.
9. Issı Y, Bıçakçı Ü, Yağız B, Germiyanoğlu C, Arıtürk E and Bernay F. Transurethral incision of anterior urethral diverticulum (syringocele) 26th ESPU Congress, Joint Meeting with ICCS + SPU + AAP/SOU + AAPU + SFU. https://www.espu.org/images/documents/mc_Abstract_book_ESPU_2015.pdf
10. Prakash J, Dalela D, Goel A, Singh V, Kumar M, Garg M, Mandal S, Sankhwar SN, Paul S, Singh BP. Congenital anterior urethral valve with or without diverticulum: a single-centre experience. J Ped Urol. 2013;9:1183–7.
11. Kibar Y, Coban H, Irkılata HC, Erdemir F, Seckin B, Dayanc M. Anterior urethral valves: an uncommon cause of obstructive uropathy in children. J Ped Urol. 2007;3:350–3.
12. Routh JC, McGee SM, Ashley RA, Reinberg Y, Vandersteen DR. Predicting renal outcomes in children with anterior urethral valves: a systematic review. J Urol. 2010;184:1615–9.
13. Zia-ul-Miraj M. Anterior urethral valves: a rare cause of Infravesical obstruction in children. J Ped Surg. 2000;35(4):556–8.
14. Desautel MG, Stock J, Hanna MK. Mullerian duct remnants: surgical management and fertility issues. J Urol. 1999;162:1008–14.
15. Coppens L, Bonnet P, Andrianne R, Leval J. Adult mullerian duct or utricle cyst: clinical significance and therapeutic management of 65 cases. J Urol. 2002;167:1740–4.

16. Priyadarshi V, Singh JP, Mishra S, Vijay MK, Pal DK, Kundu AK. Prostatic utricle cyst: a clinical dilemma. APSP J Case Rep. 2013;4(2):16.
17. Akbarzadeh A, Khorramirouz R, Kajbafzadeh AM. Congenital urethral polyps in children: report of 18 patients and review of literature. J Pediatr Surg. 2014;49(5):835–9. https://doi.org/10.1016/j.jpedsurg.2014.02.080.
18. Hodges SJ, Patel B, McLorie G, Atala A. Posterior urethral valves. The Scientific world J. 2009;9:1119–26.
19. Orumuah AJ, Oduagbon OE. Presentation, management, and outcome of posterior urethral valves in a Nigerian tertiary hospital. Afr J Paed Surg. 2015;12:18–22.
20. Hodges SJ, Patel B, McLorie G, Atala A. Posterior urethral valves. The Scientific World J. 2009;9:1119–26.
21. Lopez PJ, Celis S, Reed F, Zubieta R. Vesicoureteral reflux: current management in children. Curr Urol Rep. 2014;15(10):447. https://doi.org/10.1007/s11934-014-0447-9.
22. Fanos V, Cataldi L. Antibiotics or surgery for vesicoureteric reflux in children. Lancet. 2004;364:1720–2.
23. Tekgül S, Riedmiller H, Hoebeke P, Kočvara R, Nijman RJ, Radmayr C, Stein R, Dogan HS, European Association of Urology. EAU guidelines on vesicoureteral reflux in children. Eur Urol. 2012;62(3):534–42. https://doi.org/10.1016/j.eururo.2012.05.059.
24. Rawat J, Rashid KA, Kanojia RP, Kureel SN, Tandon RK. Diagnosis and management of congenital bladder diverticulum in infancy and childhood: experience with nine cases at a tertiary health center in a developing country. Int Urol Nephrol. 2009;41(2):237–42. https://doi.org/10.1007/s11255-008-9443-7.
25. Psutka SP, Cendron M. Bladder diverticula in children. J Pediatr Urol. 2013;9(2):129–38. https://doi.org/10.1016/j.jpurol.2012.02.013.
26. Garat JM, Angerri O, Caffaratti J, Moscatiello P, Villavicencio H. Primary congenital bladder diverticula in children. Urology. 2007;70(5):984–8.
27. Timberlake MD, Corbett ST. Minimally invasive techniques for management of the ureterocele and ectopic ureter: upper tract versus lower tract approach. Urol Clin North Am. 2015;42(1):61–76. https://doi.org/10.1016/j.ucl.2014.09.006.
28. Merlini E, Lelli CP. Obstructive ureterocele-an ongoing challenge. World J Urol. 2004;22(2):107–14.
29. Sander JC, Bilgutay AN, Stanasel I, Koh CJ, Janzen N, Gonzales ET, Roth DR, Seth A. Outcomes of endoscopic incision for the treatment of ureterocele in children at a single institution. J Urol. 2015;193(2):662–6. https://doi.org/10.1016/j.juro.2014.08.095.
30. Shokeir AA, Nijman RJ. Ureterocele: an ongoing challenge in infancy and childhood. BJU Int. 2002;90(8):777–83.
31. Patel R, Tery T, Ninan GK. Transitional cell carcinoma of the bladder in first decade of life. Pediatr Surg Int. 2008;24(11):1265–8. https://doi.org/10.1007/s00383-008-2251-4.
32. Korrect GS, Minevich EA, Sivan B. High-grade transitional cell carcinoma of the pediatric bladder. J Pediatr Urol. 2012;8(3):36–8. https://doi.org/10.1016/j.jpurol.2011.10.024.
33. Aguiar L, Danialan R, Kim C. A case of high-grade transitional cell carcinoma of the bladder in a pediatric patient with turner syndrome. Urology. 2015;85(6):1477–9. https://doi.org/10.1016/j.urology.2014.12.038.
34. Chancellor MB, Elovic E, Esquenazi A, Naumann M, Segal KR, Schiavo G, Smith CP, Ward AB. Evidence-based review and assessment of botulinum neurotoxin for the treatment of urologic conditions. Toxicon. 2013;67:129–40. https://doi.org/10.1016/j.toxicon.2013.01.020.
35. Hassouna T, Gleason JM, Lorenzo AJ. Botulinum toxin A's expanding role in the management of pediatric lower urinary tract dysfunction. Curr Urol Rep. 2014;15(8):426. https://doi.org/10.1007/s11934-014-0426-1.
36. Figueroa V, Romao R, Pippi Salle JL, Koyle MA, Braga LH, Bagli DJ, Lorenzo AJ. Single-center experience with botulinum toxin endoscopic detrusor injection for the treatment of congenital neuropathic bladder in children: effect of dose adjustment, multiple injections, and avoidance of reconstructive procedures. J Pediatr Urol. 2014;10(2):368–73. https://doi.org/10.1016/j.jpurol.2013.10.011.

37. Game X, Mouracade P, Chartier-Kastler E, Viehweger E, Moog R, Amarenco G, Denys P, De Seze M, Haab F, Karsenty G, Kerdraon J, Perrouin-Verbe B, Ruffion A, Soler JM, Saussine C. Botulinum toxin-a (Botox) intradetrusor injections in children with neurogenic detrusor overactivity/neurogenic overactive bladder: a systematic literature review. J Pediatr Urol. 2009;5(3):156–64. https://doi.org/10.1016/j.jpurol.2009.01.005.

Noninvasive Urodynamics and Flowmetry in Children, Adolescents, and Young Adults

7

Mario Patricolo

Urodynamics is frequently confused with what we know as *urodynamic instrumented investigations*. Urodynamic instrumented investigations are a group of physiological tests utilized to investigate lower urinary tract symptoms (LUTS). These investigations are used to analyze lower urinary tract function and dysfunction in order to identify the most appropriate plan for the management of specific clinical conditions. Standards of urodynamic practice and for urodynamic equipment have been published already by the ICS and ICCS [1–3]. It is understood by the majority of professionals dedicated to this area of expertise that the tests must be performed to the highest professional and scientific standard.

The urinary tract is a dynamic system, from the calyces to the urethra. Gravity, diameter of the urinary tract, peristalsis, and urine features are all involved in the dynamic process of urine progress within the urinary tract and voiding/continence. Voiding habits and physical, social, psychological, and environmental factors all influence the urodynamic profile of each individual, in all ages. The urodynamic evaluation becomes more complex, in particular in children, adolescents, and young adults, who display peculiar characteristics and behavior, due to their developmental stages [4]. Urodynamic tests represent only one part of the urodynamics assessment pathway, which should also include history and examination, simple investigations, questionnaires, diaries, charts, etc. The tests should not be performed in isolation but in the context of a full understanding of the clinical problem. When dealing with pediatric patients, one has to deal with different needs and sensitivity, being adaptable to patients' needs while inspiring trust and confidence, at the same time, as well as reassuring their families; the investigator needs to possess detailed knowledge of the lower urinary tract physiology, anatomy, and voiding dysfunction

M. Patricolo
Al Noor Hospital, Abu Dhabi, UAE

© Springer International Publishing AG, part of Springer Nature 2018
G. Mosiello et al. (eds.), *Clinical Urodynamics in Childhood and Adolescence*, Urodynamics, Neurourology and Pelvic Floor Dysfunctions,
https://doi.org/10.1007/978-3-319-42193-3_7

in children and of the most frequent congenital anomalies. All the above is necessary as well as maintaining adherence to the current International Children's Continence Society (ICCS) terminology of lower urinary tract symptoms [5].

The most important step is formulating the "urodynamic question." This will allow the examiner to make a tailored indication and to select the most appropriate investigation to perform. The measurement has to be precise and must undergo control of their value and reliability, and also the report format has to follow standardized criteria.

In children, adolescents, and young adults, the preferred method of investigation, if not the "method of choice," is noninvasive or minimally invasive urodynamics. This approach excludes, by definition, all procedures involving the use of urinary catheters, rectal probes, and needles. Moreover, if we consider also the emotional sphere, then the term "noninvasive" may extend also to procedure that must not involve invasion of patients' privacy and exposure of the genitals to the clinical team, unless this phase of the preparation to the investigation is accepted comfortably by the patient.

As a matter of fact, some patients, especially female children and adolescents as well as adolescents and young adults of both gender, find it very difficult to be investigated by a physician or nurse of the opposite sex. This becomes also a stronger issue, depending on culture and religion, in different areas of the world and leads to sometimes the patient not reporting a LUTS or LUTD, as well as losing patients at follow-up or discontinuation of care, by patient or family choice [6, 7].

The urodynamic assessment starts with accurate history taking and physical examination, a general examination, including phenotype, macroscopically visible congenital anomalies, and neurologic examination, observation of the anal sphincter tone, anal position, bulbous-cavernous reflex, sacral skin anomalies (hair tafts, sacral dimple, discoloration, moles, etc, asymmetry of the buttocks, palpable sigmoid, palpable bladder and/or kidneys, etc. A neurologic examination will always be of advantage and is mandatory in those with ambulation problems and dysfunctional voiding profile. A history of recurring urinary tract infections (UTIs), daytime frequency of urine and/or urgency or urge incontinence, constipation, and fecal soiling has to be investigated and *dug out* thoroughly. Accurate history taking alone is not sufficient. A validated questionnaire will help collect data and record unbiased information from the patient. Three types of questionnaires are already available for the pediatric age, at present: a dysfunctional voiding symptom score (DVSS) [8], a pediatric urinary incontinence quality of life score (PIN-Q) (Bower W.F. et al.) [9], and a short screening instrument for psychological problems in enuresis (SSIPPE) [10].

A 1-week voiding diary is a complex tool, as it requires collecting data for seven nights, regarding wetting episodes and volume of urine voided at night to evaluate nocturnal enuresis. It is recommended, especially in adolescents, who tend to comply less with their self-care, to use a 48-hour voiding chart, not necessarily sampled in to consecutive days.

The weekly bowel diary is crucial for our noninvasive urodynamics approach. As a matter of fact, bowel dysfunction, such as obstinate constipation (*obstipation*) and fecal load and soiling, is associated with LUTS in a large number of cases and can also favor the establishment and recurrence of UTIs due to intestinal flora, therefore contributing to the establishment, persistence, resistance, and recurrence of LUTS. In 1997 Loening-Baucke (London, UK) published a report, advocating that those patients who present LUTS and constipation resolve their symptoms after successfully being treated for constipation, in more than 60% of cases, and those with UTIs resolve the LUTS in approximately 90% of cases, after the eradication of the UTIs [11]. The same center reviewed the previous study after 10 years and in 2007 wrote another article supporting the initial findings from 1997 [12]. The bowel diary needs to contain the dates, the number of bowel motion per day, their consistency (Bristol Stool Scale), the medication taken, the episodes of soiling, the presence of abdominal pain, and any other relevant comment, on a daily basis. All the charts and clinically applicable tools are downloadable from the ICS and ICCS website, for all members of the societies.

7.1 Urinary Flowmetry

A urinary flowmetry is a noninvasive method to obtain data on the rate of urinary flow (mL/s), voided volume, time to maximum flow, voiding time, urinary flow curve profile (voiding pattern), and when a patient is instructed to pass urine into a flowmeter system. Although relatively simple and relatively inexpensive, urinary flowmetry is, in many cases, the only urodynamic test that we can perform in a reproducible noninvasive way, to assess LUTS and LUTD in children, adolescents, and young adults, who dislike any invasive procedure and may not comply with it. Differently from what applies to adult patients, urinary flowmetry, bladder scan or bladder ultrasound (US), and electromyography of the perineal muscles (pelvic floor muscles, PFMs) have high significance in the diagnosis of urinary issues in pediatric age, in non-neuropathic patients, once they are toilet trained, and can undergo the investigation. EMG gives us the opportunity of observing if there is synergy between detrusor contraction and urethral sphincter relaxation and vice versa (Fig. 7.1).

The patient needs to have met the team and the clinician who is performing the test, before. It is rather embarrassing being screened, scanned, and applied surface LED on the perineum by somebody we know, let alone a stranger! Patients and their relatives, especially of underage individuals, need to be informed regarding the details of the procedure, so that no surprise will occur at the time of the investigation. A leaflet with information on noninvasive urodynamics and how to prepare for it including how and when to void and drink before the test has to be given to patients and relatives. The room has to be at average temperature, not too cold and not too hot. If we must choose between hot and warm, warm is better. A clear explanation has to be given again to the patient, regarding the test. The urine must be evaluated in the outpatient setup, just before the test, for the urine concentration may influence the flow rate by up to 5%. A bladder scan or bladder ultrasound (highly preferable) is performed prior to applying the perineal EMG surface (adhesive) LEDs to be sure that the filling of the bladder is not too small and not too much larger than 50% of EBC for age. Once adequate volume has been achieved, the EMG LEDS are applied and tested, and then the patient will be given privacy and asked to pass urine on the commode or stand in front of the uroflowmeter if a male,

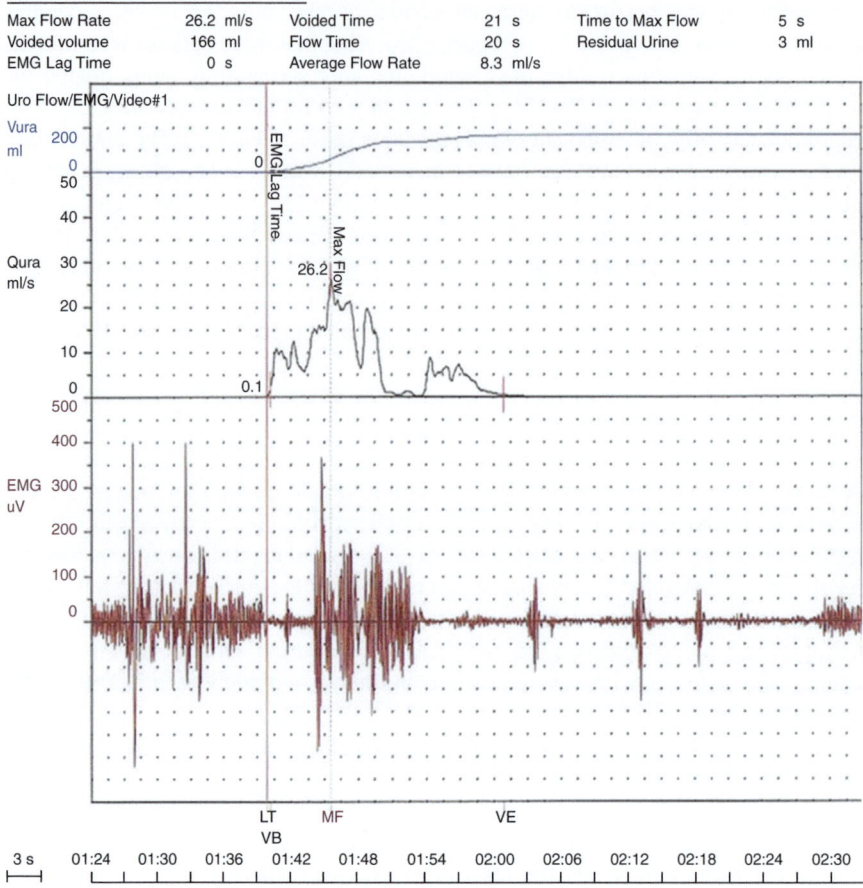

Fig. 7.1 Uroflowmetry-associated surface electromyography of pelvic floor muscles

when he/she feels a normal desire to void. After micturition, the patient resumes a supine or semi-sitted position on the examination bed, to be *scanned* again and to check the post-void residual (PVR). Qmax is the one of the most important data obtained with urinary flowmetry but only second in order of importance to the urinary flowmetry curve profile and to the flowmetry index (FI) (presented by I. Franco at the Annual ICCS Meeting, Kyoto, Japan; June 30–July 2, 2016). Qmax should not include any peak of flow which is shorter than 2 s. Hence, if our machine will not automatically do it, we will need to correct the Qmax result, based on the above concept. Any flow peak, shorter than 2 s, will be excluded from the calculation of Qmax (Schafer W. et al.). A suggested *rule of thumb* is that if the square of the Qmax [(mL/s)^2] is equal to or bigger than the voided volume, then the recorded Qmax is very likely to be normal. Also a standard series of values of Qmax for age and gender has been proposed (Table 7.1).

Apart from Qmax, average flow rate (Qave) and their relation (Qmax/Qave), which are useful to determine indirect signs of bladder outlet obstruction (BOO), in case the value of Qave is higher than 50% of Qmax, the flow curve shape is the most

Table 7.1 Normal value Qmax according to age and gender

Years	Male (mL/s)	Female (mL/s)
4–7	10	10
8–13	12	15
14–18	21	18

important data to observe and analyze. The shape of the urinary flowmetry curve is the result of a series of contributing factors, detrusor contractility, abdominal straining, sphincter relaxation, and anatomical obstruction, from the posterior urethra and bladder neck to the urethral meatus. The normal urinary flowmetry curve is "bell shaped." It is important to mention that a normal urinary flowmetry does not mean that the patient does not have a voiding disturbance. Conversely, an abnormal uroflow curve does not mean necessarily that the patient has a bladder or voiding dysfunction (Bartkowsky DP et al. 2004; Bower W.F. et al. 2004).

A "tower-shaped" curve is the result of explosive voiding and usually a sign of overactive bladder (OAB). "Staccato" voiding curve means that there is a variable, fluctuating flow with peaks and lows but never reaching a flow rate of zero, throughout the void. This pattern is typical of dysfunctional voiding (DV), when detrusor and sphincter are not coordinated in their activity [13]. The same pathophysiological mechanism is defined as detrusor sphincter dyssynergia (DSD) when it occurs in neuropathic patients. Nowadays many professionals commonly call this voiding pattern *DSD*, also in non-neurogenic bladder. In DV and DSD, the relaxation of the sphincter during voiding is intermittent, not continuously relaxed (not continuously contracted). It is important to identify this pattern in a very detailed fashion and explain clearly the dynamic of this phenomenon to the patient and his/her relatives, because the mechanism will be at the basis of future biofeedback sessions, if they will be planned to treat the patient symptoms [14]. An "interrupted" voiding pattern is similar to "staccato" but presents several moments when the flow rate is zero. Usually it is a sign of abdominal strain or underactive bladder or else. This profile can only appear in severe, decompensated, dysfunctional voiding (Fig. 7.2).

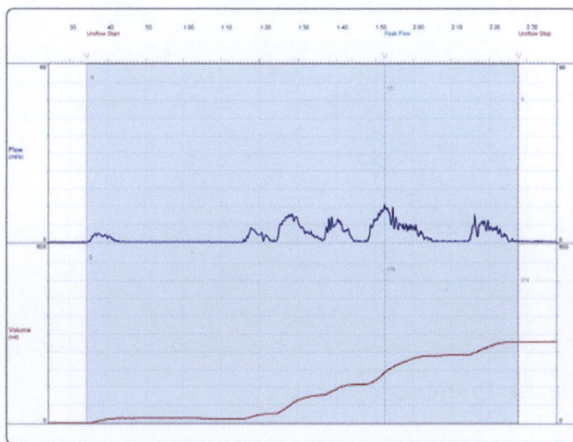

Fig. 7.2 Noninvasive urodynamic evaluation in a dysfunctional voiding

Finally a "plateau" curve is simply a sign of anatomical issues and is a sign of BOO (Fig. 7.3). EMG will help in discriminating dysfunctional voiding from underactive bladder or from anatomical stricture.

Ultrasound and bladder scan are a great component of the noninvasive urodynamic investigation (Fig. 7.4). In fact, bladder filling, pre-void volume at a particular stage of desire to void, bladder wall, surface, lumen aspect, and post-void residual are all relevant data for complex urodynamics in children. Pre- and post-void residual are the only two data that can be obtained with a traditional bladder scanner, as well as the volume at the moment of first desire to void. The

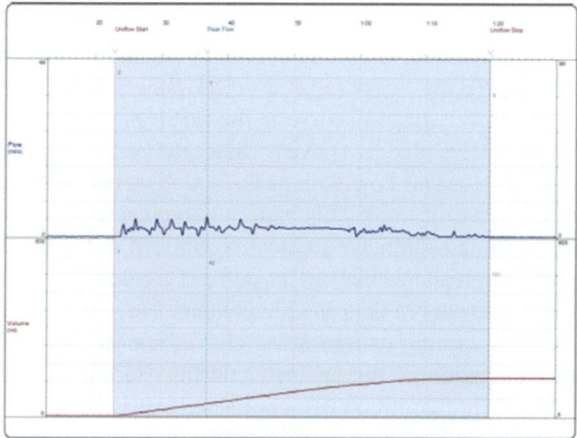

Fig. 7.3 Noninvasive urodynamic investigation results in a urethral meatus stenosis

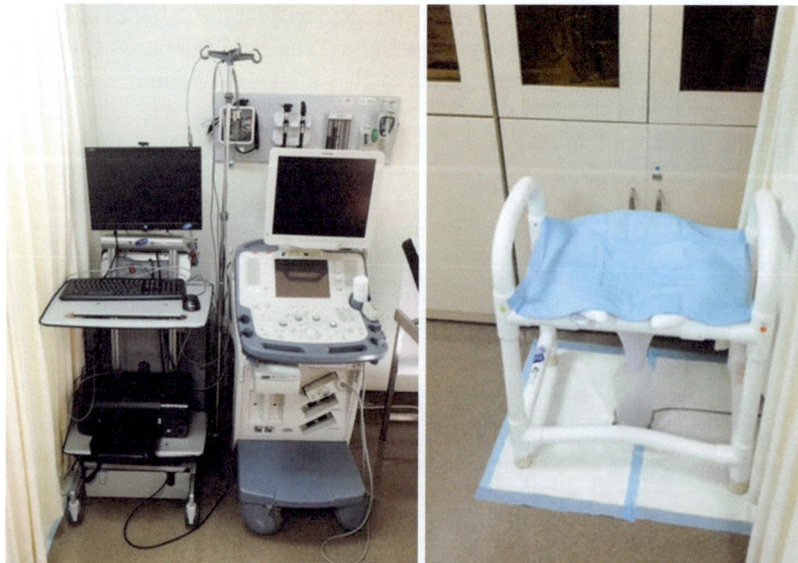

Fig. 7.4 Urodynamic equipment

use of the traditional bladder scanner with no imaging is now considered obsolete by the majority of operators. Numerous studies have been published in the last two decades to highlight the imprecision of bladder scanning and the variables to measurement of pre- and post-void residual volumes, with B-mode ultrasound. This is due to the irregular and unique shape of the urinary bladder. In recent years interest has been directed toward modern portable scanners which measure the bladder volume by a calculation of the automatically detected perimeter and area of the bladder. This new current of thoughts generated from the fact that the traditional calculation of bladder volume via B-mode ultrasound is usually impaired by the variability of bladder shape and by uncertain calculation formulas. Not all formulas are correct, but the one commonly used to calculate bladder volume is longitudinal x horizontal x anteroposterior measure of bladder lumen ×0.72.

The pre-void volume should guarantee that the bladder is not too distended and not under-distended (less than 50% of EBC for age). As a matter of fact, the maximum flow rate, Qmax, is physiologically influenced by bladder volume. A post-void residual at US which is more than 20 mL or more than 10% of EBC for age in a 4–6-year-old patient or more than 20 mL or 15% of EBC for age in a child between 7 and 12 years. is considered pathologic (ICCS Standardization Document of Pediatric Urodynamics). It is crucial that PVR is scanned immediately after micturition, to avoid refilling (as soon as possible, in the first 5 min after the urinary flowmetry).

The accuracy of flow rate signals varies with the uroflowmeter used. There are differences from one system to another, due to the internal signal processing and on the proper periodical calibration of the uroflowmeter (a calibration is recommended every 6 months, in most urodynamics system manuals). Most urodynamics systems nowadays are almost completely automated and even can generate sub-complete reports and corrected curves. For the specific methods needed to operate a non-automated urodynamics system, we suggest the reading of the ICS document on Good Urodynamic Practices, available online on the Society website. Nevertheless we wish to give some advice for everyday practice, extrapolated from the same document and from other available literature [15]:

- Qmax should be rounded to the next whole number (e.g., if the recording is 12.7 mL/s, it should be rounded to 13 mL/s).
- Voided volume and PVR should be rounded to the next 10 mL, above or below.
- The so-called VOID report should be listed as follows: max flow rate (Qmax)/volume voided (VV)/post-void residual (PVR).
- If the numeric data are reported without rounding them or corrected based on the above mentioned approximations, then the term ("raw") has to follow the index (e.g., Qmax.raw).
- The exam should be repeated at least two times and, if possible, three times.
- Urodynamics should be performed only by specialized urodynamics departments. At least 200 studies per annum should be performed within the department.

- A number smaller than 30 patients per age group (children, adolescents, young adults) per annum is inadequate to maintain expertise, and the cases should be referred to a specialized center.
- Some highly specialized Departments, working in relative isolation from other services, or in areas with smaller population then others, it may be impossible to each the suggested numbers. However, these departments will be able to demonstrate their expertise in other ways.
- The team has to be multidisciplinary, and if possible interclinical and collegial meeting and case discussions are strongly encouraged (grand rounds).
- The department should operate under the clear direction of a senior urodynamicist. This will usually be either a urologist with a special interest in LUTS, a urogynecologist, or a nephrologist or a pediatrician specialized in LUTS and certified in urodynamics [15].

A word of caution must be mentioned at the end of this overview on noninvasive urodynamics in children, adolescents, and young adults. Today we "all" perform urodynamics, as opposed to the latter recommendations above from the steering committee on urodynamic training and accreditation. Doctors (urologists, pediatric urologists, nephrologists, pediatricians, physiatrists, etc.), nurses, physiotherapists, and occupational therapists all perform urodynamics and not always after adequate or even more accredited training on the investigation techniques and machinery used. We base our clinical diagnosis and hence care plan, including rehabilitation techniques, invasive procedures like the initiation of clean intermittent catheterization, invasive urodynamics or voiding cystourethrograms, and prescription of medications not always free of side effects or risks (imipramine, alpha-blockers, anticholinergics, botulinum-A-toxin), on a test that so far has only partial accuracy allowing only arbitrary interpretation of data and curves (cit. M. De Gennaro, ICCS Annual Meeting, Kyoto, Japan; 30 June–2 July; 2016). We need to keep this in mind and, unless supported by strong evidences gathered from the history, charts, multidisciplinary team meetings, and accurate review of the documentation of each patient, make a reasoned and ethical decision to maintain safety for our young patients.

References

1. Schaffer W, Abrams P, Liao L, et al. Good urodynamic practices: uroflowmetry, filling Cystometry and pressure-flow studies. Neurourol Urodyn. 2002;21:261–74.
2. Bauer SB, Nijman RJ, Drzewiecki BA, Sillen U, Hoebeke P, International Children's Continence Society Standardization Subcommittee. International Children's continence society standardization report on urodynamic studies of the lower urinary tract in children. Neurourol Urodyn. 2015;34(7):640–7. https://doi.org/10.1002/nau.22783. Epub 2015 May 21.
3. Gammie A, Clarkson B, Constantinou C, et al. International continence society guidelines on urodynamic equipment performance. Neurourol Urodyn. 2014;33(4):370–9. https://doi.org/10.1002/nau.22546. Epub 2014 Jan 4.

4. Bower WF, Christie D, De Gennaro M, et al. The transition of young adults with lifelong urological needs from pediatric to adult services: an international children's continence society position statement. Neurourol Urodyn. 2017;36(3):811–9. https://doi.org/10.1002/nau.23039.
5. Austin PF, Bauer SB, Bower W, et al. The standardization of terminology of lower urinary tract function in children and adolescents: update report from the standardization Committee of the International Children's continence society. Neurourol Urodyn. 2015;9999:1–11.
6. Rizik DEE. Measuring barriers to urinary incontinence care seeking in women: the knowledge barrier. Letter to the editor. Neurourol Urodyn. 2009;28(1):101.
7. Rizk DE, Shaheen H, Thomas L, Dunn E, Hassan MY. The prevalence and determinants of health-care seeking behavior for urinary incontinence in the United Arab Emirates women. Int Urogynecl J Pelvic Floor Dysfunct. 1999;10:160–5.
8. Farhat W, Bägli DJ, Capolicchio G, O'Reilly S, Merguerian PA, Khoury A, McLorie GA. The dysfunctional voiding scoring system: quantitative standardization of dysfunctional voiding symptoms in children. J Urol. 2000;164(3 Pt 2):1011–5.
9. Bower WF, Sit FK, Bluyssen N, Wong EM, Yeung CK. PinQ: a valid, reliable and reproducible quality-of-life measure in children. J Pediatr Urol. 2006;2(3):185–9. https://doi.org/10.1016/j.jpurol.2005.07.004. Epub 2005 Aug 19.
10. Van Hoecke E, Baeyens D, Vanden Bossche H, Hoebeke P, Vande Walle J. Early detection of psychological problems in a population of children with enuresis: construction and validation of the short screening instrument for psychological problems in enuresis. J Urol. 2007;178(6):2611–5. Epub 2007 Oct 22.
11. Loening-Baucke V. Urinary incontinence and urinary tract infection and their resolution with the treatment of chronic constipation in childhood. Pediatrics. 1997;100:228–32.
12. Clayden G, Wright A. Constipation and incontinence in childhood: two sides of the same coin. Archiv Dis Child. 2007;92:372–474.
13. Chase J, Austin P, Hoebeke P, Mc Kenna P, International Children's Continence Society. The Management of Dysfunctional Voiding in children: a report from the standardization Committee of the International Children's continence society. J Urol Vol. 2010;183:1296–302.
14. De Paepe H, Renson C, Van Laecke E, Raes A, Vande Walle J, Hoebeke P. Pelvic-floor therapy and toilet training in young children with dysfunctional voiding and obstipation. BJU Int. 2000;85:889–93.
15. Joint Statement of Minimum Urodynamic Practice in the UK. (Report of the urodynamic training and accreditation steering group: April 2009).

Cystometry, Pressure Flow Study and Urethral Pressure Measurement

Jian Guo Wen

8.1 Introduction

Cystometry, pressure flow study (PFS) and urethral pressure profile (UPP) are core contents of paediatric urodynamic studies (PUDS) which are becoming an increasingly popular tool to evaluate the lower urinary tract dysfunction (LUTD)/lower urinary tract symptoms (LUTS) in clinical practice [1–3]. The aims of these tests are to reproduce symptoms, to identify the underlying causes for symptoms and to quantify related pathophysiological processes.

The International Continence Society (ICS) and International Children's Continence Society (ICCS) describe cystometry as a urodynamic investigation during the filling phase of the micturition cycle and define the PFS (cystometry with flow recording or voiding cystometry) as the procedures to measure the pressure-volume relationship of the bladder, providing information on the voiding function (outflow obstruction, flow pattern, detrusor contractility and sustainability). Obviously, part of their procedure and function is overlapped. Cystometry in combination with perineal EMG skin electrodes provides information regarding pelvic floor activity: both during filling and voiding. Cystometry in combination with fluoroscopy is referred to as a video-urodynamic study (it will not be covered in this chapter).

Urethral pressure profile (UPP) measurement is a procedure used for assessment of the urethral sphincter function (Lose 1997) [4]. It is often done as part of cystometry, uses a special probe or a side hole tube to measure the pressures along the urethra, the canal through which urine flows from the bladder out of the body, and to locate any obstruction. However, the techniques available for recording the UPP

J. G. Wen
Pediatric Urodynamic Center, First Affiliated Hospital of Zhengzhou University, Zhengzhou, China

Pediatric Surgery and Urology, First Affiliated Hospital of Xinxiang Medical University, Xinxiang, China

© Springer International Publishing AG, part of Springer Nature 2018
G. Mosiello et al. (eds.), *Clinical Urodynamics in Childhood and Adolescence*, Urodynamics, Neurourology and Pelvic Floor Dysfunctions,
https://doi.org/10.1007/978-3-319-42193-3_8

are subject to significant pitfalls, interpretation problems and test-retest variation. Therefore, UPP parameters are of limited value in the assessment of the urethral sphincter function [4].

Although these studies developed so quickly during the past decades, there are still some urologists, paediatricians and nurse specialists who do not fully understand how to perform cystometry, PFS and UPP as well as how to interpret the results and don't know how to respond to questions related to these PUDS from children or their parents. In addition, specific characteristics in children, such as normal values for PUDS parameters, are different compared to adults, which then make it difficult to diagnose LUTD. Therefore, it is necessary to prepare this chapter explaining when and how to do these procedures according to ICS and ICCS guidelines and how to interpret results.

Video-urodynamic studies combine the use of real-time X-rays, or fluoroscopy, with cystometry and pressure flow studies. Instead of a fluid such as saline, the bladder is filled with a liquid contrast dye that appears opaque on X-rays and delineates the bladder and urethra on the images [5]. This procedure is reserved for complex cases or when the more standard tests have not yielded satisfactory results. The contents of this chapter will focus on cystometry, PFS and urethral pressure measurement. Video-urodynamic studies will be introduced in other chapters.

8.2 Indication and Preparation

Cystometry, PFS and UPP are used to evaluate LUTD in children who are experiencing problems with urination, such as incontinence, and to pinpoint the cause of the problem. Contemporary guidelines recommend standard multichannel urodynamics as an option for children with a complicated or recurrent LUTD. However, considering the invasive, cystometry and PFS will be only undertaken after history taking, voiding diaries, uroflow and pelvic floor EMG recordings do not answer the questions related to causes nor provide supportive evidence for LUTD.

8.2.1 Indication for Cystometry and PFS

1. Significant post-void residual (PVR) urine with no clear explanation.
2. When non-invasive investigation raises the suspicion of neuropathic detrusor-sphincter dysfunction, such as occult spinal dysraphism; obstruction, such as posterior urethral valves; and genitourinary abnormalities, such as exstrophy and epispadias (Bauer 2015) [6].
3. Profound non-neuropathic detrusor-sphincter dysfunction (i.e. dilating ureter(s), high-grade vesicoureteral reflux, valve bladder syndrome), straining or manual expression during voiding, a weak urinary stream, urge incontinence unresponsive to normal elimination habits or pharmacotherapy, pronounced apparent stress incontinence or new or worsening dilating vesicoureteral reflux (VUR > grade 3 reflux, international classification) and recurrent febrile UTI.

4. In neurogenic bladders, investigation is warranted when recurrent febrile UTI occurs where previously identified or newly diagnosed VUR may indicate a deteriorating bladder.
5. Congenital malformations of the lower urinary tract (i.e. exstrophy, epispadias, ureteroceles, multiple bladder diverticula).
6. The procedure is assumed to affect treatment strategies and for evaluating the treatment response or follow-up.

In summary, the invasive UDS are indicated when non-invasive investigation raises suspicion of neuropathic detrusor-sphincter dysfunction, obstruction, genitourinary abnormalities, profound non-neuropathic detrusor-sphincter dysfunction, or significant PVR of unknown cause.

8.2.2 Indication for UPP

Urethral pressure profile (UPP) is valuable diagnostic tool for children with urinary incontinence (UI), suspected primary sphincter mechanism incontinence, suspected increased urethral tone, reflex dyssynergia, suspected ureteral ectopia, mechanical or functional urethral obstruction and other congenital urethral abnormalities (Goldstein and Westropp 2005) [7]. UPP combined with cystometry and PFS is playing an increasingly significant role in diagnosing various and complex LUTD in children. Considering the clinical relevance static UPP is limited, the simultaneous bladder/urethral pressure measurement is recommended.

8.2.3 Preparation

For monitoring the effect of abdominal pressure on the bladder pressure, it is necessary to record abdominal pressure during PUDS. The abdominal pressure is usually measured via a small rectal balloon catheter. Therefore, to empty the stool in the rectum and colon prior to the study is necessary for accurately assessing the abdominal pressure.

As constipation is a very frequent source of LUTD in children, any defecation problem should be disclosed using a 3-day defecation diary and dealt with before the urodynamic examination. Enema Glycerini is recommended for use when emptying the rectum just before the study. Children who show difficulty emptying the rectum should be given a suppository or oral cathartic the day before the study. Cleaning enema is needed often for severe constipation or fecal incontinence; if a free voiding flowmetry + ultrasound residual measurement is to be carried out before the pressure/flow study, it is recommended that the child drink sufficient quantities of water in order to have a full bladder when they arrive at the urodynamic lab so the uroflow can be accomplished readily.

For the child who is too afraid, an administration of sedative adequately (not anaesthetics) is allowable, but it will be documented. However, any medicine that may affect the LUT function should be avoided at 2 days before the cystometry.

8.3 Cystometry

Cystometry is used to determine the bladder capacity, contractility, compliance, emptying ability and degree of continence. It is used to establish as clearly as possible a baseline, so that changes resulting from treatment and/or growth can be assessed, and to provide some guidance in the choice of treatment (although results of urodynamic test may not necessarily be the deciding factor), and these PUDS should be performed if the outcome is likely to affect treatment or when treatment does not lead to its intended outcome [8]. Filling cystometry is the only method for quantifying the filling function. However, this technique has limited use as a solitary procedure. It is much more effective combined with bladder pressure measurement during micturition (PFS) (Fig. 8.1).

Contemporary guidelines recommend standard multichannel urodynamics as an option for children with voiding dysfunction although nuclear and ambulatory

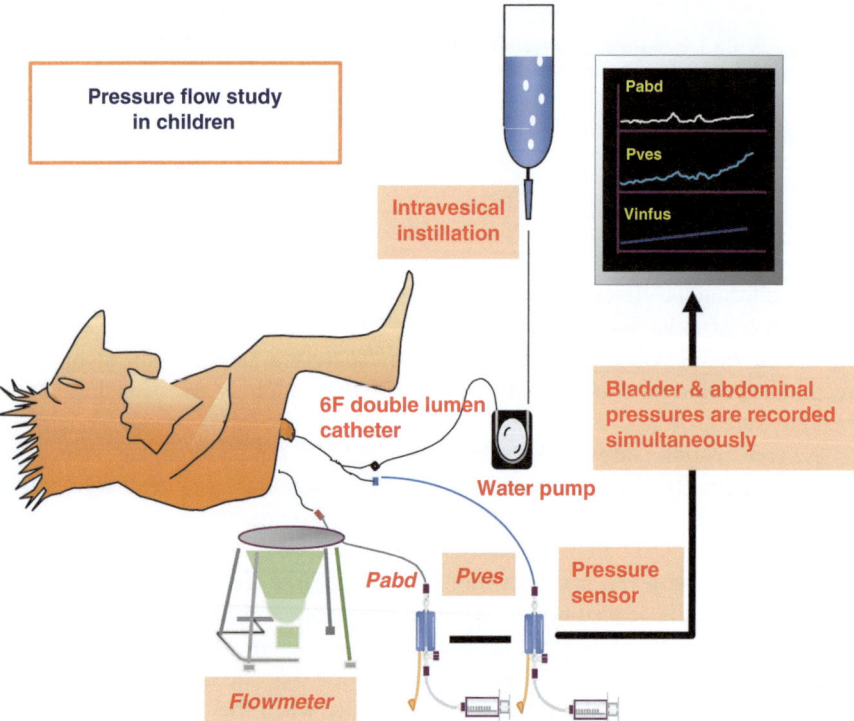

Fig. 8.1 Setting of cystometry and pressure flow study in children

cystometry is reported in the literature. It has been reported that cystometry combined with nuclear cystography precisely identifies when reflux occurs during cystometrography (volume and pressure) as the camera continuously records gamma radiation location of the nucleotide without increased radiation exposure, but it does not provide absolute anatomic detail [9, 10]. Furthermore, the reported advantages must be weighed against costs, radiation exposure and the usually occurring, less comfortable or representative position of the patient that is especially relevant during pressure/flow evaluations.

8.3.1 Procedures

The basic procedures for cystometry and PFS begin from placement of catheter into bladder via either transurethrally or suprapubically immediately after necessary preparation including evacuation of rectum as far as possible. The bladder should be empty at the start of filling. Thereafter, the bladder is filled artificially, and detrusor pressure and flow rate are recorded continually by using the dedicated commuter program.

Prior to inserting the catheter, a free voiding uroflowmetry and PVR to be measured by flowmeter and ultrasound are recommended (Fig. 8.2). This could be the

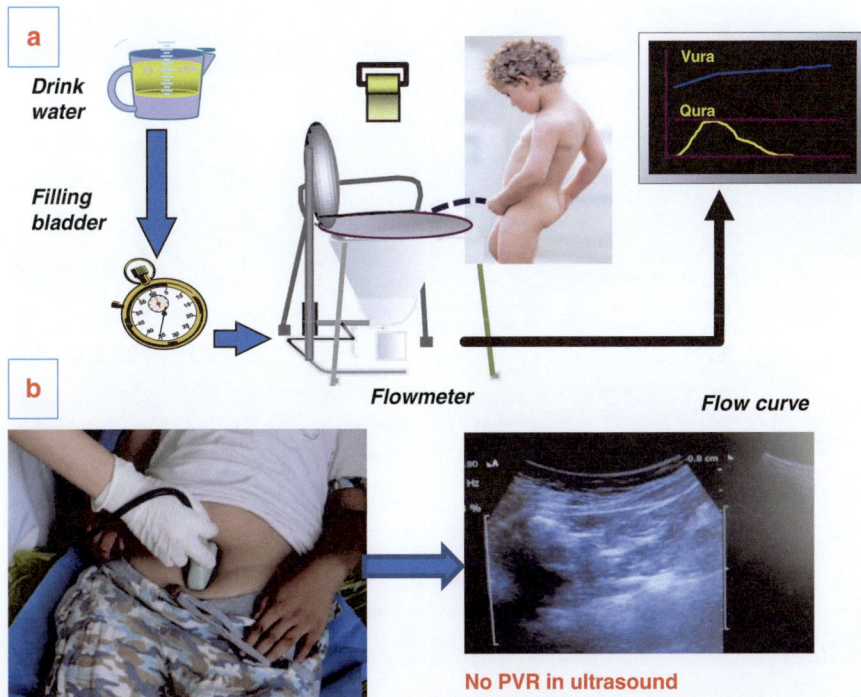

Fig. 8.2 Flowmetry and ultrasound PVR measurement

baseline for follow-up as well as the adjustment criteria for flowmetry during the pressure/flow study. However, a reliable flow rate needs at least two times of uroflow measurements. To identify a staccato voiding curve, three flow measurements are needed. Uroflowmetry with simultaneous EMG is frequently performed in children and may help differentiate DSD from abdominal straining during voiding. The EMG electrodes can be placed on the pelvic floor or on the abdominal muscles. Increased EMG activity secondary to straining is common in children and must be differentiated from true DSD, which is diagnosis of neurogenic bladder dysfunction. EMG is also usually performed concurrently with cystometry.

The steps in performing cystometry and PFS are shown as follows:

1. Setting
    (a) Catheter for recording bladder pressure (detrusor pressure). A transurethral catheter is most often used to measure the pressure within the bladder. When the free uroflowmetry has been completed, a thin double-lumen catheter (used to fill and record bladder pressure; 6Fr is recommended) is inserted transurethrally (Fig. 8.3a, b). Using a lubricant, PVR is measured again by using this catheter. Sometimes, when the bladder is underactive, aspirating it via the catheter is needed to insure the bladder is completely empty. An anaesthetic

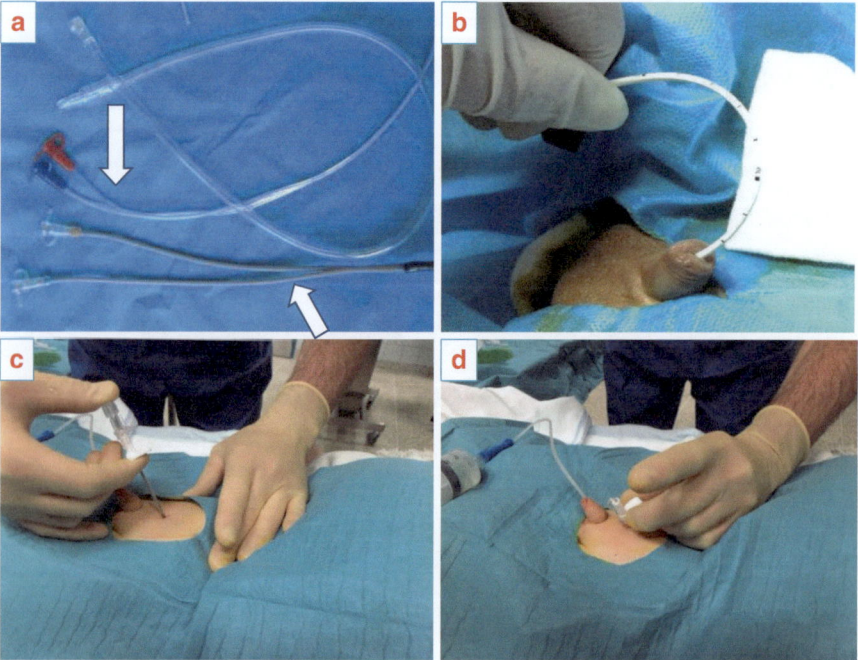

Fig. 8.3 A 6 Fr double-lumen catheter (**a**, arrow) is inserted transurethrally (**b**) using lubricant or anaesthetic gel or suprapubically (**c** and **d**) from Aarhus University Hospital

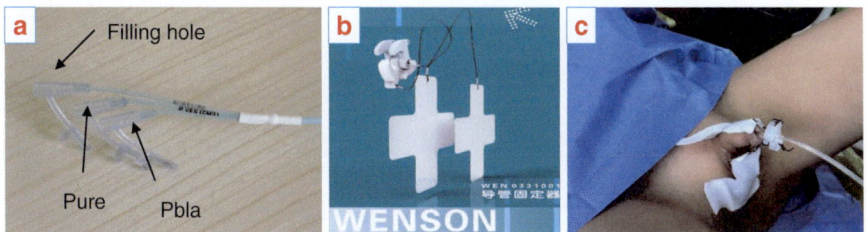

Fig. 8.4 A triple-lumen catheter (**a**) and a 'WENSON Fixation device' (Chinese Patent No: 2010101021670) for fixation of catheter (**b**) were used to record bladder and urethral pressure simultaneously (**c**)

gel may be used to reduce urethral pain induced by catheter placement. However, it may change the voiding pattern due to intact sensation in the proximal part of urethra that is essential for the voiding function. Alternatively, a catheter can be inserted suprapubically to avoid these issues (Fig. 8.3c, d).

(b) Catheter for recording abdominal pressure. An 8 Fr. feeding tube or a small rectal balloon catheter is inserted initially as well to monitor abdominal pressure that can be subtracted from bladder pressure channel recordings in order to get true detrusor pressure and to reduce artefacts of movement. Good Urodynamic Practice recommends, and ICS-2013 confirms, that as thin as possible a transurethral dual lumen catheter should be used for filling and vesical pressure measurement as well as a rectal catheter to monitor intra-abdominal pressure (Fig. 8.4a–c).

(c) Electrodes: surface electrodes are positioned symmetrically left and right from the external anal sphincter to record the reactivity of pelvic floor muscles. Surface patch electrodes are used in most cases, but fine needle electrodes placed directly into the peri-urethral striated sphincter are recombined to diagnose neuropathy; however, this is not normally feasible in children. Recently, a three-lumen catheter was used to record the bladder and urethral pressure simultaneously with diagnosing bladder and urethral function and their coordination, and it may replace EMG recording in the future.

(d) Position and zeroing the pressure: seated in upright position, supination or babies held in mother's arm is acceptable. Placing the child in a sitting position (Fig. 8.5a) and letting him/her watch a video or DVD together with one or both parents is recommended during standard cystometry to minimize anxiety. Young infants may be held in his/her mother's (or caregiver's) arms (Fig. 8.5b) to achieve successful evaluation. It has not been proven that patient position during the procedure has a significant and clinically relevant effect on cystometry. Before filling the bladder, the bladder pressure channel must be zeroed to outside (atmospheric) pressure with the transducer at the level of the pubis whatever the position of the child.

(e) Testing the catheter and sensor: to test the catheter and sensor function, the lower abdomen is pressed (Credéd), whereas older children are encouraged to cough.

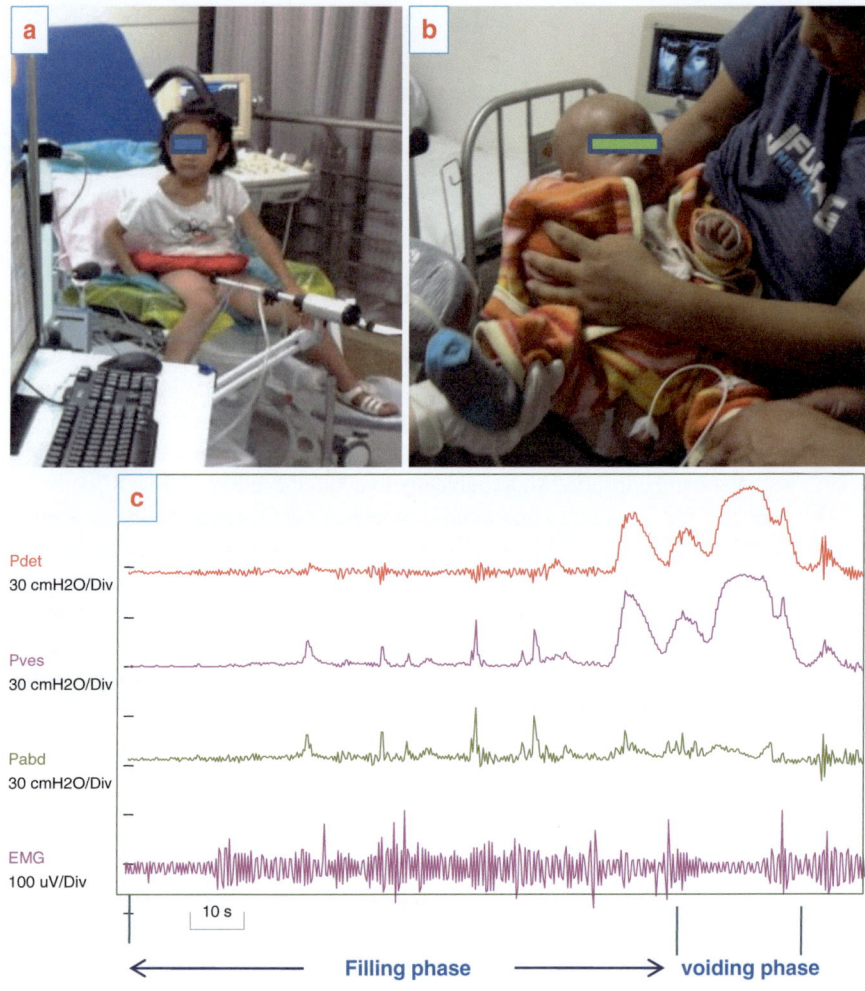

Fig. 8.5 Child in sitting position (**a**) during cystometry. A 2.5-month-old baby held in mother's arms (**b**) with cystometry showing normal voiding curve (**c**)

2. Recording
    (a) A slow filling rate (approximately 5–10% of estimated bladder capacity/min) is recommended, especially in infants and newborn, as compliance (predominantly) and overactivity may be significantly altered by faster rates of filling.
    (b) For retrograde filling, 0.9% saline at body temperature is recommended. However, in practice, most labs used the room temperature saline (25 °C ± 5 °C) to infuse the bladder. In infants, temperature of the filling solution as well as the medium itself may influence bladder capacity and detrusor activity. During the recording, the flowmeter is kept in position so any leakage or incontinence will be shown in the uroflow tracing curve.

(c) When voiding or leakage occurs or there is a very strong desire to void (movement in newborn or infants or curling of toes in older children is observed due to the full bladder), the filling is stopped. Then, as the child is encouraged to urinate, the voiding pressures and uroflow measurements are recorded simultaneously. In practice, it is easier for newborns and younger infants to generate voiding compared to older children during the pressure/flow study. In older children, one frequently encounters resistance to voiding due to irritation in the urethra (pain induced by the catheter). Voiding volume in infants is typically small and thus might not allow for an adequate uroflow curve and satisfactory maximum flow rate as seen in older children.

(d) For children who used the suprapubic catheter, voiding might be easier to generate compared to those who used catheter transurethrally. A suprapubic catheter (5F) is usually inserted at least 24 h before the study.

8.3.2 Quality Control

In newborns, PFS (voiding cystometry) is easy to obtain although it is difficult to define the border of two phases. However, considering a reliable PFS is difficult to record in newborn and infant, it is better to maintain a continuous recording of the filling and voiding phase. This will avoid missing the important transition.

Despite all efforts to achieve normalcy, the test environment is not natural; most children are apprehensive to a degree that can influence findings; a transurethral catheter may affect voiding; and catheter 'irritation' may induce detrusor overactivity. Suprapubic catheterization may eliminate voiding abnormalities associated with a urethral catheter, but detrusor overactivity may result [11].

A two-lumen transurethral catheter can be used to fill the bladder and record bladder pressure in the majority of children. Transurethral catheters (5, 6, 7, and 8 Fr.) do not seem to produce a significant obstructive element in the urethra. Suprapubic catheters may be of value in selected cases. A suprapubic catheter may be inserted beforehand to conduct the study, but this often requires general anaesthesia or conscious sedation, so risks need to be juxtaposed against benefits of this approach.

If infection is strongly suspected from some samples (cloudy, odorous and/or positive nitrites on analysis), the test should be delayed until sterile urine is obtained. For children on clear intermittent catheterization (CIC), colonization is common, so a urine culture and appropriate antibiotics for 3 days prior to the study are preferable. It is also important not to correct P_{abd} during the study, which will result in incorrect P_{det} and P_{abd} measurements. Finally, these mistakes will result in studies that cannot be compared between hospitals or between patients, as normal values will not be attainable.

For EMG recording, surface electrodes are widely used in children to study pelvic floor activity. However, considering the resistances in electrical current across skin electrode interface, the skin should be degreased (alcohol) and desquamated skin removed (abrasive paper) before applying a conductive gel and the electrodes.

It has been established that filling rate and filling medium have an impact on bladder function. Paradoxically, the faster the bladder is filled, the larger its volume; this may be due to the fact that saline may impact on detrusor contractility [12]. It is unnecessary to use warm infusion solution on a routine basis for urodynamic studies in children. However, for children younger than 2 years, warm solution is recommended [13]. Considering the temperature of the infusate may influence bladder capacity and detrusor activity; however, its clinical relevance remains unknown. Finally, two cycles of cystometry is necessary for making sure the result is repeatable.

Cooperation is important for successful cystometry and PFS. The following steps might be valuable for achieving this success. Firstly, the lab should be built like a kindergarten; animation wall with a TV is helpful. Dedicated and knowledgeable staff should be employed to give patients an explanation about procedure and aim of urodynamic studies and if possible engage the infants to cooperate. The child should have a well-cleansed rectum. To reduce anxiety, the study is best performed with the child seated, watching a video or DVD, accompanied by one or both parents. Only essential equipment should remain in the room. The urodynamic evaluation approach should start minimally involved tests as possible ending up with invasive investigations, if needed. Avoid general anaesthesia, as this affects the natural state and eliminates the chance for voiding. Intranasal midazolam may be administered in certain situations where high anxiety levels cannot be mollified, as this drug does not appear to have a significant effect on outcome of the study. Administration of sedative should be performed adequately (not anaesthetics), and documenting follows when child was too afraid. Prior application of 1% lidocaine jelly or a liquid solution instilled into the urethra as a topical anaesthetic may aid in catheter passage. After putting the catheter in the bladder, if agitated, keep him/her away from the examination room until calm. Toys, eating or drinking during the examination as needed.

8.3.3 Interpretation of the Storage Phase

Cystometry (or a cystometrogram) involves instilling fluid through a catheter into the bladder and evaluating the bladder's muscle and nerve function. Various parameters are measured during the storage phase: the pressure within the bladder or intravesical pressure (P_{ves}), the filling detrusor pressure ($P_{det.fill}$), abdominal pressure (P_{abd}) and detrusor pressure ((P_{det}) or ($P_{abd}-P_{ves}$)), the sensation of urgency that you feel when your bladder is full, muscle contractions by the bladder wall or detrusor activity, maximum bladder capacity ($V_{blad.max.cap}$) and the detrusor compliance ($\Delta C = \Delta V/\Delta P$).

The filling detrusor pressure ($P_{det.fill}$) is the detrusor during filling. The detrusor pressure increases very little (<5 cmH$_2$O) immediately at the start of filling and incrementally with further filling of the bladder; it reaches a maximum just before the urge to void (normally, <15 cmH$_2$O). It has been noted that the risk of renal damage increases significantly if $P_{detr.fill.max} > 40$ cmH$_2$O.

Maximum bladder capacity ($V_{blad.max.cap}$) indicates maximum bladder volume just at the time voiding begins. It is calculated using voiding volume and PVR measured immediately after urination. In most instances, the maximum filling volume or maximum voided volume is very similar to the maximum bladder capacity. In cases of sphincter incompetence or lack of bladder sensation, maximum cystometric capacity is difficult to determine. A Foley balloon catheter can occlude the bladder outlet to determine capacity. Presence of a sensory lesion warrants stopping filling when resting detrusor pressure reaches (exceeds) 30 cmH$_2$O. The predicated maximum bladder volume can be calculated by $V_{blad.max.cap}$(mL) = 30 + 30 × age (y) in a child >1 year of age and $V_{blad.max.cap}$ (mL) = 38 + 2.5 × age(months) or $V_{blad.max.cap}$ (mL) = 25 + 3 × age (month) in males and $V_{blad.max.cap}$ (mL) = 19 + 2.6 × age (month) in females, for infants <1 year old.

Bladder sensation is very difficult to evaluate in young children. It is a relevant parameter in toilet-trained children. Terminologies like 'first desire to void' and 'strong desire to void' although useful in adults have little value in children. Normal desire to void is not relevant in infants but can be a guide in toilet-trained children >4 years. Normal desire to void should be considered as the volume at which some unrest is noted, i.e. wiggling of toes usually indicates voiding is imminent. In the older child when fear of discomfort may result in smaller than expected volumes during initial cystometrography. or when detrusor overactivity is anticipated but not seen. Two cycles of filling are recommended (personal observation). Bladder sensation can be classified as normal, increased (hypersensitive), reduced (hyposensitive) or absent.

The detrusor compliance ($\Delta C = \Delta V/\Delta P$) is one of the most important parameters that measure the elasticity of the bladder. With a filling rate in 10% of predicted or known bladder volume, per minute, $\Delta C < 10$ mL/cmH$_2$O indicates decreased bladder compliance. Pressure curves during filling may determine when it is best to measure ΔC (Fig. 8.6). The end-filling pressure (just before voiding) should be less than 15 cmH$_2$O. It seems to be an accurate parameter to predicate the ΔC, but a full characterization of compliance may be helpful, as some children have varying compliance factors throughout filling. This variability depends on several factors: rate of

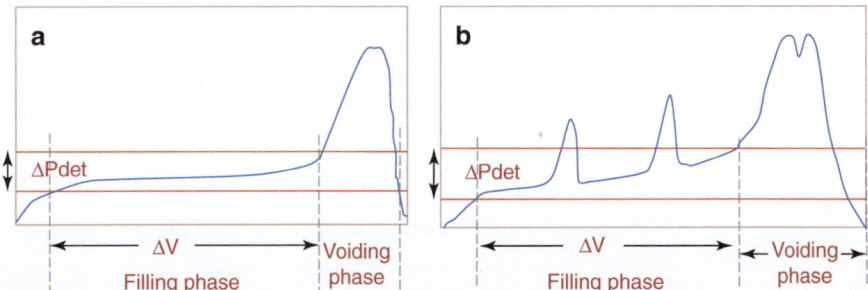

Fig. 8.6 Detrusor compliance (ΔC) = $\Delta V/\Delta P_{det}$. (**a**) The non-linear portions—the beginning and end of the V/P_{det} diagram do not contribute to compliance. (**b**) $\Delta V/\Delta P_{det}$ essentially captures the angle of the line describing the incremental increase in resting pressure

filling, which part of the curve is used for compliance calculation, shape (configuration) of the bladder, thickness and mechanical properties of the bladder wall, contractility, relax ability of the detrusor and degree of bladder outlet resistance. When reporting compliance the rate of bladder filling, the volumes between which compliance is calculated, and which part of the curve used to derive this number should be noted. When severe detrusor overactivity is present, it may be difficult to determine compliance.

Detrusor activity is interpreted from measuring P_{det}. During the storage phase, it may be normal, overactive or underactive. In normal children, a minimal rise in detrusor pressure occurs throughout filling. This process is called accommodation. Even after provocation, there should be no involuntary contractions. The normal detrusor is described as stable. Involuntary detrusor contractions during filling (spontaneous or provoked) are characteristic of 'detrusor overactivity (DO)'. The child may not completely suppress these contractions; usually, an increase in pelvic floor EMG activity is noted as a counteractive guarding reflex. Involuntary detrusor contractions may also be provoked by alterations in posture, coughing, laughing, walking, jumping, suprapubic tapping or compression and other triggering stimulants.

Detrusor sphincter dyssynergia (DSD) during filling phase happens when increased sphincter activity occurs with an increased detrusor pressure as it may be a conscious attempt to prevent voiding (Fig. 8.7); it is considered a 'guarding reflex' and is normal. When it occurs unconsciously, it is considered DSD and is abnormal.

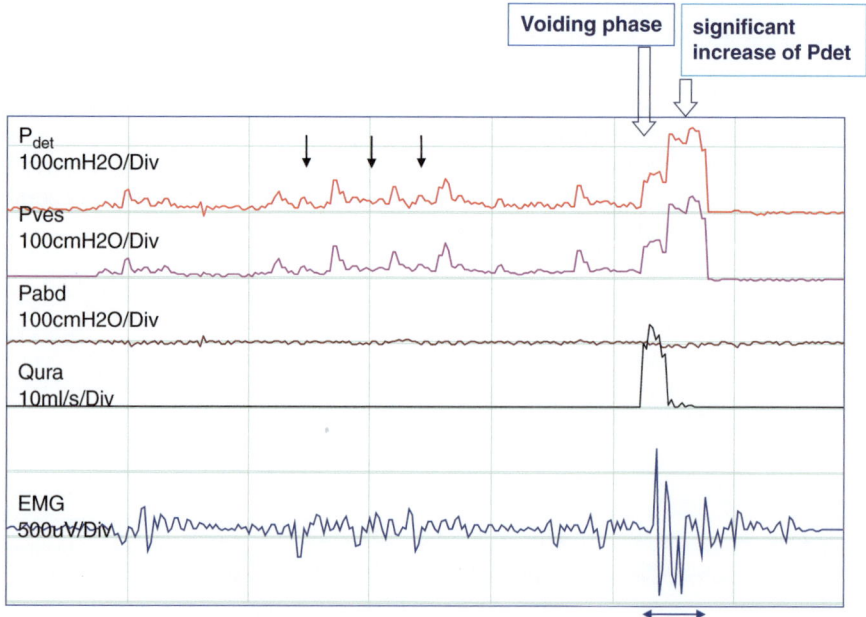

Fig. 8.7 DSD occurs during the voiding phase induced significant increase of P_{det} and increase PVR in a 6-year-old girl with OAB and increase PVR

When sphincter activity decreases in response to an increase in detrusor pressure, it may be a normal response signalling the true cystometric capacity; leakage occurs until the child makes an effort to stop the urination. Uroflowmetry with simultaneous EMG is frequently used to differentiate DSD from abdominal straining during voiding. Increased EMG activity secondary to straining is common in children and must be differentiated from true DSD, which is diagnostic of neurogenic bladder dysfunction.

Incontinence indicates the unconscious loss of urine during the filling phase when it occurs before the expected bladder capacity is reached, and it is called leakage.

Bladder leak point pressure (BLPP) indicates the bladder pressure at which leakage occurs. Similarly, *detrusor leak point pressure (DLPP)* indicates the detrusor pressure at which leakage occurs. DLPP is measured by subtracting P_{abd} from P_{ves} at the moment of leakage when the first drops of urine pass through the meatus in the absence of raised abdominal pressure or an involuntary detrusor contraction. A pressure < 40 cmH$_2$O is considered acceptable for those with a fixed resistance who cannot generate a detrusor contraction. DLPP >40 cmH$_2$O implies a high likelihood of subsequent renal damage.

Electromyographic studies are used to evaluate the function of the external urinary sphincter and pelvic floor muscles, which help to control the outflow of urine from the bladder. Several sensors, or electrodes, are used to measure the electrical activity of these muscles at rest, during contraction and during urination. These tests are usually done simultaneously with cystometry and pressure flow studies.

Possible pathological findings at cystometry include DO, low bladder compliance, abnormal bladder sensations, incontinence, an incompetent or relaxing urethra and DLPP. The presence of these contractions does not necessarily imply a neuropathic disorder. In infants, detrusor contractions may occur in 10% of normal children during filling. Occasionally, overactive contractions may be seen very near the maximum capacity, which should be interpreted as normal. In children with VUR, detrusor overactivity is seen in more than half the infants. Overactivity due to a disturbance of the nervous system is called neuropathic detrusor overactivity. In the absence of any neuropathology, it is called idiopathic detrusor overactivity. Any leakage occurring during an involuntary detrusor contraction is labelled detrusor overactive incontinence. If overactivity occurs regularly, it is called detrusor phasic contractions. This usually occurs in the latter part of the filling phase in those with NBD.

8.4 Pressure Flow Study

PFS is defined as measuring the detrusor pressure and uroflow during the micturition or voiding phase. It reflects the coordination between detrusor and urethra or pelvic floor during the voiding phase. It is even more powerful if combined with filling cystometry and with video-urodynamics. LUT function must be recorded during the voiding phase.

8.4.1 Procedures

It begins when the child and the urodynamist decide that 'permission to void' has been given or when uncontrollable voiding begins [14]. This occurs when the maximum cystometric capacity (MCC) has been reached in children with no voiding dysfunction [15]. During this phase the detrusor contracts, producing voiding detrusor pressure. At the completion of voiding, the detrusor relaxes, and the urethra/bladder outlet 'closes'. At this phase, the detrusor pressure increases with the urethral pressure decrease (EMG of the sphincter activity decrease), and voiding occurs. The pressures are recorded through the same catheter used at cystometry. During the recording, a flowmeter connected to the urodynamic equipment allows flow rate parameters to be juxtaposed against pressure data and correlated with one another.

During voiding the detrusor may be classified as *normal*, *underactive* or *acontractile*. Normal voiding is achieved by a voluntarily initiated detrusor contraction; it is sustained and cannot be suppressed easily once it has begun. In the absence of bladder outlet obstruction, a normal contraction will lead to complete emptying. A high pressure with a low urine flow indicates obstruction; low pressure with a low flow indicates a problem with the bladder itself, such as nerve or muscle dysfunction.

8.4.2 Interpretation of Voiding Phase

During PFS, Q_{max} and voided volume (bladder functional capacity) are recorded. Pressures that can be obtained during the voiding phase are pre-micturition pressure, opening pressure, the intravesical opening pressure, opening time, maximum pressure, pressure at maximum flow, closing pressure and minimum voiding pressure (Fig. 8.8).

Normal voiding (*normal detrusor function*) is achieved by a voluntary, continuous detrusor contraction which leads to complete emptying of the bladder within an acceptable time span. *Detrusor underactivity* is defined as a contraction of reduced strength and/or duration, resulting in prolonged bladder emptying and/or a failure to achieve complete bladder emptying within a normal time span. This often results in an increase of PVR at the completion of voiding. *An acontractile detrusor* does not demonstrate any contractile activity during urodynamic assessment. Some children cannot or will not generate a detrusor contraction in the laboratory setting. This could be mistaken for a wrong diagnosis. Spending extra time encouraging the child to void, dripping water on the pubic area or lower extremity and/or having the mother or caregiver helps in the process may induce the child to void and obviate this phenomenon. The acontractile detrusor demonstrates no activity during voiding. If acontractility is neurologically induced, it is called detrusor areflexia. It denotes the complete absence of a centrally coordinated contraction. Terms such as hypotonic, autonomic or flaccid are to be avoided.

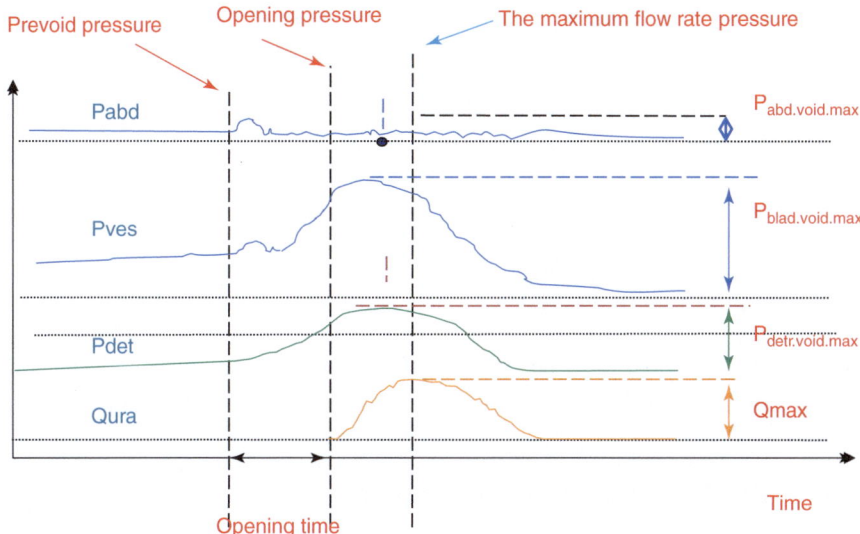

Fig. 8.8 The parameters recorded during voiding phase

Maximum voiding detrusor pressure ($P_{detr\cdot void.max}$) is defined as the maximum detrusor pressure during the voiding (voiding phase). The $P_{detr\cdot void.max}$ is clinically relevant in determining the presence of bladder outlet obstruction (BOO) or a poorly contractile detrusor. *High voiding detrusor pressures* may be induced by significant resistance as is seen in BOO where the detrusor overcompensates for BOO. Conversely if urethral resistance is low, this may be reflected by a low pressure contraction. In addition, $P_{detr.void.max}$ is significantly higher in the presence of pelvic floor overactivity than in its absence (105 ± 44 (45–214) cmH$_2$O vs. 69 ± 22 (40–100) cmH$_2$O, $P < 0.001$). It is not difficult to understand that a $P_{detr.void.max}$ in children (DSD is quite common during voiding in children) is higher than that of adults (118–127 cmH$_2$O for boys and 72–75 cmH$_2$O for girls [16]. High $P_{detr.void.max}$ in infants or a staccato detrusor pressure curve during voiding indicates the existence of DSD (Fig. 8.7).

DSD is noted when there is either a sustained or increased response or intermittent changes in urethral sphincter activity at capacity or during the voiding phase. DSD is usually evaluated by a pressure/flow/EMG study or with simultaneous bladder/urethral pressure measurements.

The most important parameters to note for flowmetry are maximum flow rate (Q_{max}) and PVR. Normal PVR values have been established in children of varying ages when two consecutive uroflows have been performed (<20 mL for children 4–6 years of age and <10 mL for children aged >6–<12 years). In another study, the PVR of <10 mL for all children aged <12 years has been reported when two consecutive measurements were obtained immediately after voiding. The uroflow and PVR are considered normal if bladder empties at least once during at least two cycles of PFS. These two parameters should be verified by free flowmetry and PVR measurement performed just before PFS. If a PVR is not demonstrated during free-flow uroflowmetry, then any raised PVR during the urodynamic assessment can be considered as an artefact due to the artificial circumstances of the test and the presence of an in situ urethral catheter. Voiding efficiency is calculated by functional bladder capacity ($V_{\text{fun.max.cap}}$)/maximum bladder capacity ($V_{\text{max.cap}}$).

A post-voiding contraction indicates a detrusor contraction which occurs immediately after micturition has ended. Its clinical relevance is still unclear, but it may be related to detrusor overactivity.

Possible pathological findings at PFS include detrusor underactivity, DSD, a high urethral resistance and residual urine. Most types of obstruction caused by neuro-urological disorders are due to DSD, non-relaxing urethra or non-relaxing bladder neck. Pressure flow analysis mostly assesses the amount of mechanical obstruction caused by the urethra's inherent mechanical and anatomical properties.

8.5 Urethral Pressure Measurement

The status of urethral sphincter (activity) may be recorded by electromyography (EMG) of the pelvic floor or urethral pressure profile (UPP). UPP is defined as the continual recording of pressure through a hole in the side of a small catheter as it is pulled (at a constant rate, although either water or a gas is infused through the hole) from a point within the bladder, through the vesical neck, down to the entire urethra and a form of resistance measurement that gives a tracing indicative of the functional length of the urethra and the points of maximal urethral resistance.

Obviously, UPP is a record of the pressure exerted by the urethral wall on a recording catheter as it is withdrawn from the bladder to the external meatus. It must be stressed that the UPP is a 'static' measurement: it records urethral closure pressures with the bladder at rest and does not measure, and may bear no relationship to, the resistance offered by the urethra during voiding (Harrison 1976) [17]. It has been found that UPP parameters do not (1) discriminate stress incontinence from other disorders, (2) provide a measure of the severity of the condition and (3) return to normal after successful incontinence surgery (Lose, 1997) [4].

Recently, simultaneous bladder pressure and urethral pressure is encouraging, which is able to assess the synergy between the bladder and urethral sphincter mechanisms during filling and voiding phase.

8.5.1 Procedures

Similar to detrusor pressure that indicates the bladder function, urethral pressure shows bladder outlet function. Two methods are used to direct recording the urethral pressure, one is a 'static' measurement, recording urethral closure pressures with the bladder at rest by the urethral wall on a recording catheter as it is withdrawn from the bladder, and another is simultaneous bladder and urethral pressure measurement, recording at one point of urethral (the point of external sphincter) over a period of time (filling phase and/or voiding phase).

8.5.1.1 UPP

The UPP may be performed independently by inserting a catheter with a side hole transurethrally, and then, withdraw the catheter at constant rate with simultaneous recording of the pressure. Practically, it is usually performed after PFS by recording the UPP continuously through the bladder catheter (with a hole in the side) as it is pulled out at a constant rate. The details of procedures are shown as follows:

1. Insert the pressure-recording catheter into the bladder transurethrally (the procedures are same as cystometry and PFS). Two side holes at the same level placed 5 cm to the end of catheter are recommended. Clinically, two lumen catheters (one lumen for filling bladder, another with two side holes for bladder pressure recording, also used for later UPP recording) are often used.
2. After cystometry and PFS, the bladder is filled to one third of expected capacity and then the catheter withdrawn at constant rate of 1 mm/sec with simultaneous recording of the pressure. Meanwhile, the water is infused through the hole (1 mL/min) for preventing side holes is blocked during the pressure recording. It is a form of resistance measurement that gives a tracing indicative of the functional length of the urethra and the points of maximal urethral resistance.

8.5.1.2 Simultaneous Bladder and Urethral Pressure Measurement

1. Insert the pressure-recording catheter into the bladder transurethrally (the procedures are the same as UPP). Three lumen catheters (one lumen for filling bladder, one for bladder pressure recording, one for urethral pressure recording) are often used. The side hole for urethral pressure recording is placed around 5–10 cm to the end of the catheter according to its used in male or female cases.
2. After zeroing the pressure and testing the catheter as well as sensor, the catheter is pulled out slowly until the maximum urethral pressure appears (the urethral pressure side hole is just located in the place of the external sphincter or the place need to record pressure), and then the catheter is fixed. A fixer has been used to fix the catheter firmly during the measurement (Fig. 8.4c).
3. The cystometry with simultaneous urethral pressure recording is then performed. Similar to UPP the water is infused through the urethral pressure tube (1 mL/min) for preventing the pressure recording hole is blocked during recording.

8.5.2   Interpretation

8.5.2.1 Terminology and Clinical Significance

By measurement of UPP, the relevant parameters are showed in Fig. 8.9.

The normal urethral closing mechanism maintains a positive urethral closure pressure (guarding reflex) (Park 1997) [18]. Shortly before micturition, the normal closure pressure decreases to allow flow out. An *incompetent closure mechanism* is defined as one that allows leakage of urine in the absence of a detrusor contraction. In genuine stress incontinence, leakage occurs when P_{ves} exceeds P_{ure} (intraurethral resistance) as a result of an increase in intra-abdominal pressure, often in

Fig. 8.9 Diagram of a female urethral pressure profile (static) in children

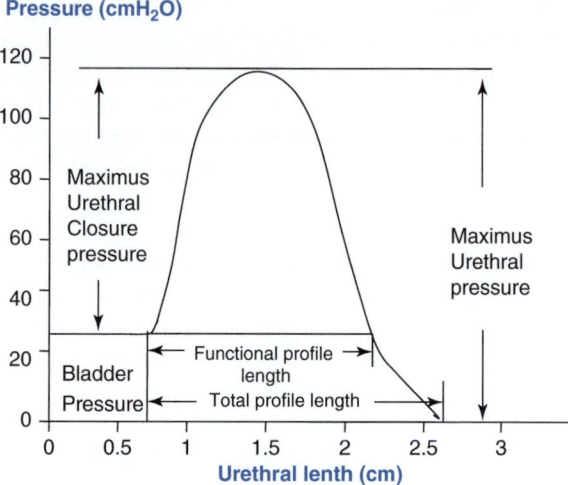

Fig. 8.10 Simultaneous bladder urethral pressure measurement indicates urethral instability during filling phase (arrow in black) and at the time of detrusor overactivity (arrow in white). (Pura. clos: urethral closure pressure)

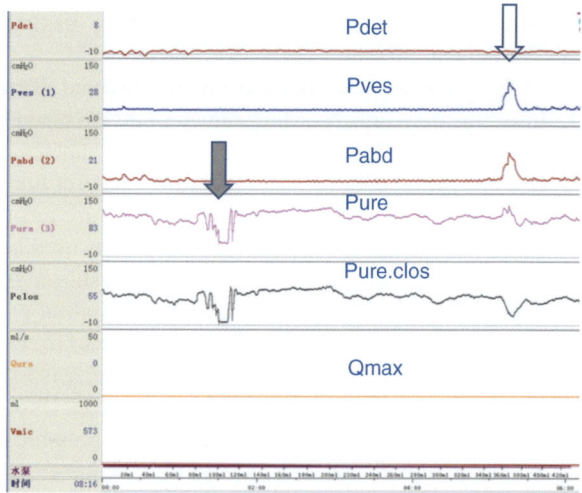

conjunction with low P_{ure} (Fig. 8.10). Although common in multiparous females, it is exceedingly rare in paediatrics but may be noted in athletically active teenage girls.

If detrusor contractility is inadequate in magnitude and duration to effectively empty the bladder, it is referred to as *detrusor underactivity during voiding*. The urethra during voiding may be *normal* or *obstructive*. The urethra opens during voiding to allow the bladder to empty at normal pressures without any loss of kinetic energy. Obstructive urethral function may be due to overactivity of the sphincteric mechanism or anatomical obstruction (posterior urethral valves, urethral stricture, ectopic ureterocele). DSD is noted when there is either a sustained or increased response or intermittent changes in urethral sphincter activity at capacity or during the voiding phase.

An anatomic obstruction is a fixed narrow diameter in a urethral segment that does not expand during voiding, resulting in a plateau-shaped flow pattern, with a low and constant maximum flow, despite high detrusor pressure and complete relaxation of the external urethral sphincter (EUS). Functional obstruction is the active contraction of the EUS during voiding that creates a narrowed urethral segment, either constantly or intermittently. Functional and anatomic obstructions can be differentiated by measuring EUS activity during voiding with simultaneous recordings of pressure and flow (urethral resistance at the EUS), or EMG activity of the striated EUS, using needle or patch electrodes. Video UDS is helpful as pelvic floor muscle activity can be observed during voiding and anatomic obstruction can be differentiated from functional obstruction.

In some children fearful of voiding, 'urethral overactivity' may be a natural reaction resulting in elevated voiding pressures, intermittent emptying and/or substantial PVR. Increased activity occurs as the child senses the need to urinate. In neurogenic DSD, the detrusor contraction and involuntary contraction of the urethral and/or periurethral striated muscles occur simultaneously during micturition. When overactivity of the external urethral sphincter occurs during voiding in neurologically normal children, it is termed dysfunctional or discoordinated voiding.

Conclusion

Cystometry and PFS are useful tools for evaluating LUTD in children. UPP may be useful in disclosing local pathology, in assessment of changes with intervention in the individual patient and in selecting patients with 'low pressure urethra' which may have therapeutic implications. However, the techniques may subject to significant pitfalls, interpretation problems and test-retest variation. Simultaneous bladder and urethral pressure measurement may replace the UPP to evaluate the urethral function in the future due to reliable recording of the dynamic function of the urethra and its coordination with the bladder.

These tools should be considered as one procedure, but not the only one, to clarify the diagnosis and to make therapeutic decisions as well as to follow up treatment responses to the voiding dysfunction when less invasive studies are inconclusive. To understand the characteristics in PUDS, normal voiding parameters and following good urodynamic practice (GUP) recommendations [19] are the basis of successful testing. In addition, the urodynamics should be performed by very experienced personnel; usually it is best performed by very well-educated urotherapists with a very good sense for the child's symptoms and reactions. To establish cooperation with the child is fundamental, and sometimes it is better to postpone an investigation than to force one. And it has to be taken into consideration that the child may have to undergo a new urodynamic examination at a later time.

It must be emphasized that less invasive tests should be undertaken first, before these more sophisticated studies are ordered. The majority of children with lower urinary tract problems can be dealt with non-invasive investigations as supplement to the physical examination. Multiple spontaneous flow plus ultrasound estimation of post-void residual is fundamental and so is a voiding diary for at least 3 days together with a registration of fluid intake. Also, urine cultures and estimation of bladder wall thickness should be performed before urodynamics are contemplated.

References

1. Wen JG, Lu YT, Cui LG, Bower WF, Rittig S, Djurhuus JC. Bladder function development and its urodynamic evaluation in neonates and infants less than 2 years old. Neurourol Urodyn. 2015;34(6):554–60.
2. Austin PF, Bauer SB, Bower W, Chase J, Franco I, Hoebeke P, Rittig S, Walle JV, von Gontard A, Wright A, Yang SS, Nevéus T. The standardization of terminology of lower urinary tract function in children and adolescents: update report from the standardization committee of the international Children's continence society. Neurourol Urodyn. 2016;35(4):471–81. https://doi.org/10.1002/nau.22751. [Epubahead of print] PubMed PMID: 25772695.
3. Austin PF, Bauer SB, Bower W, Chase J, Franco I, Hoebeke P, Rittig S, VandeWalle J, von Gontard A, Wright A, Yang SS, Nevéus T. The standardization of terminology of lower urinary tract function in children and adolescents: update report from the standardization Committee of the International Children's continence society. J Urol. 2014;191:1863–5.
4. Lose G. Urethral pressure measurement. Acta Obstet Gynecol Scand Suppl. 1997;166:39–42.
5. Wen JG, Yeung CK, Djurhuus JC. Cystometry techniques in female infants and children. Int Urogynecol J Pelvic Floor Dysfunct. 2000;11:103–12.
6. Bauer SB, Nijman RJ, Drzewiecki BA, Sillen U, Hoebeke P. International Children's continence society standardization report on urodynamic studies of the lower urinary tract in children. Neurourol Urodyn. 2015;34:640–7.
7. Goldstein RE, Westropp JL. Urodynamic testing in the diagnosis of small animal micturition disorders. Clin Tech Small Anim Pract. 2005;20:65–72.
8. Groen J, Pannek J, Castro Diaz D, Del Popolo G, Gross T, Hamid R, Karsenty G, Kessler TM, Schneider M, 't Hoen L, Blok B. Summary of European Association of Urology (EAU) guidelines on Neuro-urology. Eur Urol. 2016;69(2):324–333. pii: S0302-2838(15)00740-X. https://doi.org/10.1016/j.eururo.2015.07.071.
9. Maizels M, Weiss S, Conway JJ, Firlit CF. The cystometric nuclear cystogram. J Urol. 1979;121:203–5.
10. Sfakianakis GN, Smuclovisky C, Strauss J, Hourani M, Lockhart G, Zilleruelo G, Freundlich M, Gorman H, Politano V, Serafini A. Improving the technique of nuclear cystography: the manometric approach. J Urol. 1984;131:1061–4.
11. Andersson S, Bjerle P, Hentschel J, Kronström A, Niklasson U. Continuous and stepwise cystometry through suprapubic catheters--effect of infusion pattern and infusion rate on the cystometrogram of the normal human bladder. Clin Physiol. 1989;9:89–96.
12. Sørensen SS, Nielsen JB, Nørgaard JP, Knudsen LM, Djurhuus JC. Changes in bladder volumes with repetition of water Cystometry. Urol Res. 1984;12:205–8.
13. Chin-Peuckert L, Rennick JE, Jednak R, Capolicchio JP, Salle JL. Should warm infusion solution be used for urodynamic studies in children? J Urol. 2004;172:1657–61.

14. Chapple CR, MacDiamid SA, Patel A. Urodynamics made easy. Third ed. London: Elsevier Churchill Livngstone. p. 83–102. ISBN:978-0-443-06886-7.
15. Wen JG, Tong EC. Cystometry in infants and children with no apparent voiding symptoms. Br J Urol. 1998;81:468–73.
16. Wen JG, Yeung CK, Chu WC, Shit FK, Metreweli C. Video cystometry in young infants with renal dilation or a history of urinary tract infection. Urol Res. 2001;29:249–55.
17. Harrison NW. The urethral pressure profile. Urol Res. 1976;10(4):95–100.
18. Park JM, Bloom DA, McGuire EJ. The guarding reflex revisited. Br J Urol. 1997;80:940–5.
19. MacLachlan LS, Rovner ES. Good urodynamic practice: keys to performing a quality UDS study. Urol Clin North Am. 2014;41(3):363–73.

Videourodynamic in Children

Valerio Iacovelli, Giuseppe Farullo, Andrea Turbanti, and Enrico Finazzi Agrò

9.1 Introduction

Urodynamic studies (UDS) have become a major tool in evaluating lower urinary tract dysfunction in children with neurogenic or non-neurogenic bladder. Lower urinary tract dysfunctions (LUTD) in children frequently occur in combination with other disorders of the lower part of the body. By definition of the International Children's Continence Society (ICCS) standardization paper on LUTD in children [1], any item that gives information on the function of the urinary tract and the bowel is part of UDS.

Following the European Association of Urology (EAU), videourodynamic (VUD) can be defined as the combination of filling cystometry and pressure flow study with imaging. It is the gold standard for urodynamic investigation in neuro-urological disorders (grade of recommendation A; GR, A) [2]. Besides this, the American Urological Association (AUA) guideline on urodynamics notes that when available, clinicians may perform fluoroscopy at the time of urodynamics (VUD) in patients with relevant neurologic disease at risk for neurogenic bladder or in patients with other neurologic disease and elevated post-void residual or urinary symptoms [3].

Videourodynamic is useful to evaluate any pathological findings including all those described in the cystometry and the pressure flow study sections and any morphological pathology of the lower urinary tract (LUT) and reflux to upper urinary tract (UUT) [4]. In pediatric neuro-urology, VUD is often considered a second-line treatment in the case of resistance to initial treatment or in the case of former failed treatment. A reevaluation of these cases is warranted and further videourodynamic (VUD) studies may be considered. Sometimes, there are minor, underlying,

V. Iacovelli • G. Farullo • A. Turbanti • E.F. Agrò (✉)
Department of Experimental Medicine and Surgery, Urology Division,
Tor Vergata University of Rome, Rome, Italy
e-mail: e.finazzi@tin.it

urological or neurological problems, which can only be suspected using VUD. In these cases, structured psychological interviews to assess social stress should be added (GR, A) [2, 5].

9.2 Initial Assessment and Technique

As mentioned above, VUD is considered a second-line invasive treatment. Initially it is imperative to formulate an "urodynamic question(s)" following a comprehensive history, careful physical examination, and standard urologic investigations. Validated questionnaires are helpful in structuring history taking and providing checklists for gathering data [6–8].

A proper initial first-line evaluation comprehends a frequency/volume chart (FVC) or bladder diary which is a detailed recording of fluid intake and urine output over specified 24-h periods and a uroflowmetry. Uroflowmetry is an indispensable, first-line noninvasive test for most children with suspected LUT dysfunction. Objective, quantitative information, which helps to understand both storage and voiding symptoms, is obtainable. FVC in combination with repeated (two) uroflowmetries and measurements of post-void residual (PVR) urine volume provides noninvasive, objective information that help formulate the urodynamic question and determine the need for invasive tests, that is, filling cystometry with or without fluoroscopy (VUD) or pressure flow studies [8]. Although ultrasound or magnetic resonance VUD exams have been described in literature [9, 10], the fluoroscopy technique is still the most common.

Following the ICCS guidelines, invasive UDS are second-line noninvasive tests [8]. According to the ICS, in these children, UDS is recommended for characterization of non-neurogenic bladder dysfunction (NNBD) and/or to rule out NBD [11]. Combing UDS with voiding fluoroscopic cystourethrography (VCUG), a VUD study provides useful both functional and anatomical information.

9.2.1 Setting

To reduce anxiety, the study is best performed with the child seated, watching a video or DVD accompanied by one or both parents. Only essential equipment should remain in the room. Both the child and his/her parents need adequate preparation about every aspect of the study before it is undertaken. If the initial investigation is inconclusive and/or inconsistent with the history or prior uroflowmetry, repeating it two to three times may be necessary. Children who are not yet toilet trained or unable to support themselves sitting upright may lay supine for the voiding phase, thus excluding recording accurate flow rate data. In newborns, only storage function can be evaluated. Voiding may be observed, but reliable pressure flow studies are difficult to perform [8, 12].

9.2.2 Procedure

Most children readily accept a 6 or 7 Fr double-lumen transurethral catheter to fill the bladder and record pressure. In selected cases, a suprapubic catheter may be inserted under general anesthesia, the previous day or several hours earlier on the same day, but risks need to be juxtaposed against benefits of this approach [13]. Before inserting a catheter, a uroflow is obtained (the child is instructed to arrive with a full bladder). After voiding is completed, a transurethral catheter is inserted in a timely manner and residual urine measured and cultured. If infection is strongly suspected (this sample is cloudy, odorous, and/or has positive nitrites on analysis), the test should be delayed until a sterile urine is obtained. For children on CIC, colonization is common, so a culture and appropriate antibiotics beginning 3 days prior to the study are preferable [8].

A water-filled 8 Fr catheter connected to a pressure transducer is inserted into the rectum for pressure measurement. All pressures are measured using a transducer and recorded on a computer. The bladder is filled through the transurethral catheter using diluted contrast medium with sterile water. Two filling cycles may be useful in order to allow correct radiographic urethral assessment. Detrusor activity, bladder sensation, capacity, and compliance can be measured during filling cystometry. Voiding phase consists of recording pressures in the bladder sphincter and abdomen with simultaneous urinary flow measurement when possible (pressure/flow study). Cystometry combined with fluoroscopy (VUD) is able to provide simultaneous VCUG. The VCUG also provides information on the behavior of the bladder neck, which is not assessed by conventional cystometry [14].

9.3 Indications

9.3.1 UDS General Considerations

ICCS standardization subcommittee provided a uniform guideline on measurement, quality control, and documentation of urodynamic studies in children [8]. Following the ICCS, invasive UDS are indicated when noninvasive investigation raises suspicion of neuropathic detrusor-sphincter dysfunction (occult spinal dysraphism), obstruction (i.e., posterior urethral valves), genitourinary abnormalities (i.e., exstrophy, epispadias), profound non-neuropathic detrusor-sphincter dysfunction (children with dilating VUR and recurrent febrile UTI), or significant PVR of unknown cause.

Indications for invasive UDS in *non*-neurogenic conditions include:

- Voiding frequency ≤3 per day
- Straining or manual expression during voiding
- A weak urinary stream
- Urge incontinence unresponsive to proper elimination habits or pharmacotherapy
- Pronounced apparent stress incontinence or new or worsening dilating vesicoureteral reflux (VUR, ≥grade 3 reflux, international classification).

In children with *neurogenic* bladders, investigation is warranted when recurrent febrile UTI occurs where previously identified or newly diagnosed VUR may indicate a deteriorating bladder.

Recently, an ICI-RS think tank (International Consultation on Incontinence-Research Society) reviewed the evidence with the aim of identifying the indications for adding video to the UDS [15]. The think tank has firstly recommended that standardized ALARA ("as low as reasonably achievable") principles should be adopted for VUD in children. The risk-benefit balance of X-ray exposure needs to be better evaluated and defined. The think tank also underlined that VUD combines functional and anatomical observations. In order to better describe the role of VUD in children, the authors divided patients in those having:

1. Dysfunction without relevant neurological abnormalities (non-neurogenic dysfunctions, NND)
2. Dysfunction with relevant or suspect neurological abnormalities (neurogenic dysfunctions, ND)

9.3.2 VUD in Patients with Dysfunction Without Relevant Neurological Abnormalities: NND

Hoebeke et al. reported that in children presenting with a thickened bladder wall on ultrasound with depressed flow patterns suggesting obstruction or dysfunction, dilated lower ureters suggesting reflux, suspected bladder neck dysfunction, failure of empirical therapy, or anatomical problems, a full urodynamic evaluation, including video fluoroscopy when available, should be administered [16]. Many reports do specifically consider recurrent UTIs as relevant for further invasive investigations. These may also be considered for children with repeated nonfebrile UTIs who failed standard urotherapy [17, 18].

Agreement exists that no VUD or VCUG is necessary when only one UTI has occurred [19]. The EAU guidelines on pediatric urology [20] on "daytime LUT" conditions recommend "In case of therapy resistance, re-evaluation will be required which may consist of video-urodynamics etc…" Regarding the diagnostic work-up in children with VUR, this guideline mentions "Video-urodynamic studies are only important in patients in whom secondary reflux is suspected, such as those with spina bifida or boys in whom VCUG is suggestive of posterior urethral valves." Neither the recommendation nor the background text is referenced for evidence.

9.3.3 VUD in Patients with Dysfunction with Relevant or Suspect Neurological Abnormalities: ND

VUD enables the diagnosis of bladder neck abnormalities in patients with neurogenic bladder. It also may help identify the etiology of neurogenic bladder with respect to the underlying neurologic disease [3] and treat the patient earlier. Clinical validity of VUD for children with meningomyelocele/spinal dysraphism (MMC/SD) has been established [21]. Early treatment to reduce those elevated pressures in children with neurogenic LUTD (e.g., spina bifida aperta) has been demonstrated to be beneficial [22]. However, there is still little good quality evidence between standard urodynamics versus the addition of fluoroscopic imaging [23].

> **Conclusion**
> Much of the evidence regarding VUD is separated into investigations for obvious congenital abnormalities such as ectopia vesicae or anorectal malformations, MMC/SD, tethered cord, and UDS for children without such abnormalities. VUD combines functional and anatomical observations. Anatomical abnormalities affecting the pelvis or lower part of the body will almost certainly have consequences for LUT function. Although many reports promote VUD in children, with relevant neurological abnormalities or not, the precise indication for the test has not been ascertained because of the predominantly retrospective and heterogeneous single-center studies reported. Further studies are necessary to better clarify the role of VUD in children.

References

1. Austin PF, Bauer SB, Bower W, et al. The standardization of terminology of lower urinary tract function in children and adolescents: update report from the standardization Committee of the International Children's continence society. J Urol. 2014;191(6):1863.
2. Groen J, Pannek J, Castro Diaz D, Del Popolo G, Gross T, Hamid R, Karsenty G, Kessler TM, Schneider M, 't Hoen L, Blok B. Summary of European Association of Urology (EAU) guidelines on Neuro-urology. Eur Urol. 2016;69(2):324–33.
3. Winters JC, Dmochowski RR, Goldman HB, Herndon CD, Kobashi KC, Kraus SR, Lemack GE, Nitti VW, Rovner ES, Wein AJ, American Urological Association, Society of Urodynamics, Female Pelvic Medicine & Urogenital Reconstruction. Urodynamic studies in adults: AUA/SUFU guideline. J Urol. 2012;188(6 Suppl):2464–72.
4. Marks BK, Goldman HB. Videourodynamics: indications and technique. Urol Clin North Am. 2014;41(3):383–91, vii–viii.
5. van Gool JD, de Jong TP, Winkler-Seinstra P, Tamminen-Möbius T, Lax H, Hirche H, Nijman RJ, Hjälmås K, Jodal U, Bachmann H, Hoebeke P, Walle JV, Misselwitz J, John U, Bael A, European Bladder Dysfunction Study (EU BMH1-CT94-1006). Multi-center randomized controlled trial of cognitive treatment, placebo, oxybutynin, bladder training, and pelvic floor training in children with functional urinary incontinence. Neurourol Urodyn. 2014; 33:482.
6. Van Gool JD, Hjalmas K, Tamminen-Mobius T, et al. Historical clues to the complex of dysfunctional voiding, urinary tract infection and vesicoureteral reflux—the international reflux study in children. J Urol. 1992;148:1699–702.
7. Bower WF, Wong EMC, Yeung CK. Developlment of a validated quality of life tool specific to children with bladder dysfunction. Neurourol Urodyn. 2006;25:221–7.
8. Bauer SB, Nijman RJ, Drzewiecki BA, Sillen U. Hoebeke P; international Children's continence society standardization subcommittee. International Children's continence society standardization report on urodynamic studies of the lower urinary tract in children. Neurourol Urodyn. 2015;34(7):640–7.

9. Borghesi G, Simonetti R, Goldman SM, Szejnfeld J, Srougi M, Ortiz V, Bruschini H. Magnetic resonance imaging urodynamics. Technique development and preliminary results. Int Braz J Urol. 2006;32(3):336–41; discussion 341.
10. Ozawa H, Igarashi T, Uematsu K, Watanabe T, Kumon H. The future of urodynamics: non-invasive ultrasound videourodynamics. Int J Urol. 2010;17(3):241–9.
11. Neveus T, von Gontard A, Hoebeke P, Hjalmas K, Bauer S, Bower W, et al. The standardization of terminology of lower urinary tract function in children and adolescents: report from the standardisation Committee of the International Children's continence society. J Urol. 2006;176:314e24.
12. Chin-Peuckert L, Komlos M, Rennick JE, et al. What is the variability between 2 consecutive cystometries in the same child? J Urol. 2003;170:1614–7.
13. Reynard JM, Lim C, Swami S, et al. The obstructive effect of a urethral catheter. J Urol. 1996;155(3):901.
14. Spinoit AF, Decalf V, Ragolle I, Ploumidis A, Claeys T, Groen LA, Van Laecke E, Hoebeke P. Urodynamic studies in children: standardized transurethral video-urodynamic evaluation. J Pediatr Urol. 2016;12(1):67–8.
15. Anding R, Smith P, de Jong T, Constantinou C, Cardozo L, Rosier P. When should video and EMG be added to urodynamics in children with lower urinary tract dysfunction and is this justified by the evidence? ICI-RS 2014. Neurourol Urodyn. 2016;35(2):331–5.
16. Hoebeke P, Bower W, Combs A, et al. Diagnostic evaluation of children with daytime incontinence. J Urol. 2010;183:699–703.
17. Hoebeke P, Van Laecke E, Van Camp C, et al. One thousand video-urodynamic studies in children with non-neurogenic bladder sphincter dysfunction. BJU Int. 2001;87:575–80.
18. Glazier DB, Murphy DP, Fleisher MH, et al. Evaluation of the utility of videourodynamics in children with urinary tract infection and voiding dysfunction. Br J Urol. 1997;80:806–8.
19. Coulthard MG, Lambert HJ, Vernon SJ, et al. Guidelines to identify abnormalities after childhood urinary tract infections: a prospective audit. Arch Dis Child. 2014;99:448–51.
20. Tekgul S, Dogan HS Hoebeke P, et al. EAU guidelines on Pediatric Urology 2016: European Society for Paediatric Urology and European association of urology. uroweb.org/wp-content/uploads/22-Paediatric-Urology_LR.pdf.
21. McGuire EJ, Woodside JR, Borden TA, et al. Prognostic value of urodynamic testing in myelodysplastic patients. J Urol. 1981;126:205–9.
22. Dik P, Klijn AJ, van Gool JD, et al. Early start to therapy preserves kidney function in spina bifida patients. Eur Urol. 2006;49:908–13.
23. Marks BK, Goldman HB. Videourodynamics: indications and technique. Urol Clin North Am. 2014;41:383–91.

The Neurophysiological Testing

Giorgio Selvaggio and Roberto Cordella

The neurophysiological testing plays an important role in evaluation of patients affected by detrusor sphincter dysfunction. Despite this concept the tests are not used routinely. These studies require particular and expensive equipment and clinical experience of neurophysiologist. In addition to this, the neurophysiological tests present in pediatric patient limits related to age, child, and parents compliance.

Electromyography (EMG), nerve conduction latency studies, reflex latencies, and sensory evoked potential are classic tests. In pediatric patients their service is not all indicated. EMG and sensory evoked potential have clinical application.

10.1 Electromyography

The EMG is recording related electrical potentials to the depolarization of striated muscle fibers. The striated urethral sphincter keeps continuous motor unit activity. During bladder storage phase, the activity has an increment as coughing and other maneuvers that increases intra-abdominal pressure. In voiding phase the first step is an inhibition of motor unit activity by detrusor contraction and urine emission.

The EMG should be used during cystometry, pressure/flow study, and noninvasive urodynamic study (Fig. 10.1). The study could be used to detect either detrusor/sphincter dyssynergia in neurological patients or dyscoordination in functional patients. In non-neurological patients, who present a dysfunctional voiding, the

G. Selvaggio, M.D. (✉)
Department of Pediatric Surgery, Children's Hospital "V.Buzzi", Milan, Italy
e-mail: giorgio.selvaggio@asst-fbf-sacco.it

R. Cordella, M.Sc., Ph.D.
Department of Neurosurgery, Fondazione IRCCS Istituto Neurologico "Carlo Besta", Milan, Italy

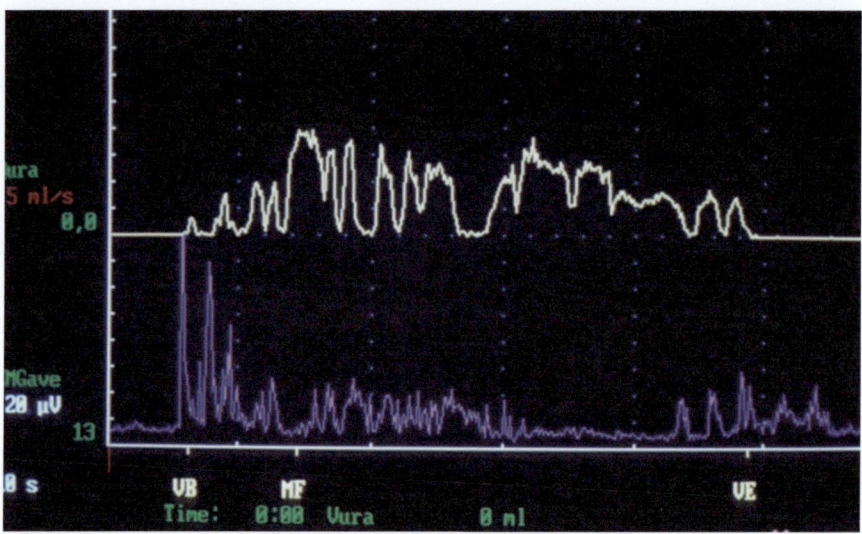

Fig. 10.1 Noninvasive urodynamic study: dyscoordinated micturition in functional patient. External sphincter contraction during the flow

EMG could be used as a part of biofeedback to improve the pelvic floor relaxation during the micturition.

Detrusor sphincter dyssynergia (DSD) is characterized by involuntary contractions of the external urethral sphincter during a hyperreflexic detrusor contraction. It is caused by neurological lesions above the sacral levels to the pontine micturition center. Three main types of DSD are well established. In type 1 there is an increase of sphincter EMG activity during detrusor contraction. At the peak of the detrusor contraction, the sphincter suddenly relaxes and voiding occurs. Type 2 DSD is characterized by clonic contractions of the external urethral sphincter during the detrusor contraction (Fig. 10.2). In type 3 DSD, there is a crescendo-decrescendo pattern of sphincter contraction, which results in urethral obstruction throughout the entire detrusor contraction [1].

The perfect EMG study would be unit action potentials from single muscle fibers of striated sphincter. The standard urodynamic equipment is not created for this application, and it records a quantitative EMG. Vaginal electrode and catheter with ring electrode are not suitable in pediatric age. Two types of electrode can be used during a standard urodynamic study. The surface silver chloride electrodes, which are fixed on left and right perianal skin, or needle electrode inserted transperineally in midline (male) and in lateral parameatal site (female). A neutral electrode placement is necessary. Both recording systems present limits, problems, and artifacts. The urethral sphincter is a part of muscle complex.

Therefore the electromyographic signal is the result of all the activities of pelvic muscles, and we know that there is a significant discrepancy in electric activity between the anal and urethral sphincters though the same innervations from the sacral segments. Despite these argumentations, in pediatric age, the EMG is registered in almost all of the patients through surface electrode. The needle placement

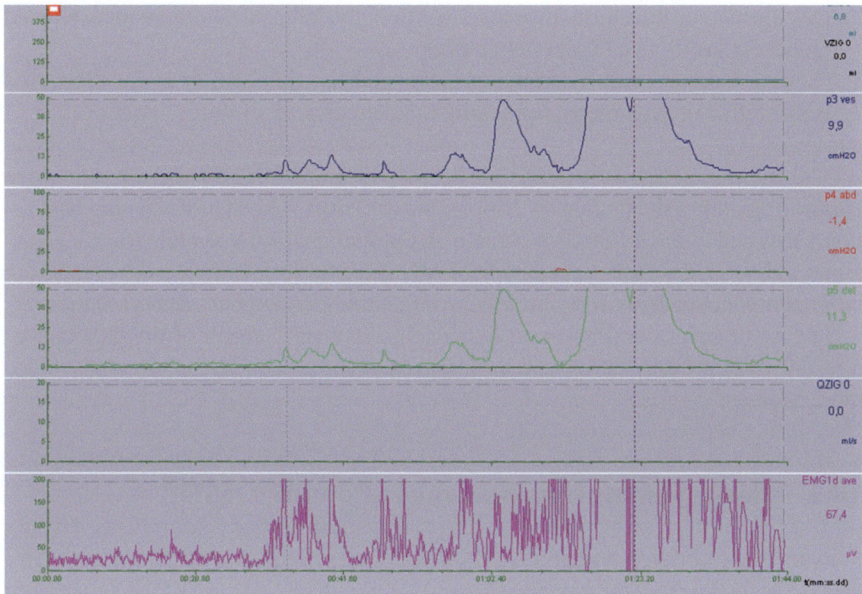

Fig. 10.2 Cystometrogram: detrusor sphincter dyssynergia (DSD) type 2

presents dramatic problem of tolerance. The use of this electrode is dedicated only to neurological nonsensitive patients. In many cases the surface electrode does not permit a correct registration because of detachment during urodynamic test. To elevate the recording quality, it is essential to degrease and dry the perianal skin. Electrode covering with waterproof tape reduces the risk of dislodgement, especially from sitting position to standing position, and short circuit during the urinary flow.

The urodynamic/videourodynamic study is considered a gold standard testing for children affected by lower urinary tract dysfunction. Simple uroflowmetry is inadequate to determine obstruction vs hypocontractility. The EMG/uroflowmetry only adds data about functional urethral sphincter obstruction. Nevertheless, uroflowmetry is commonly used with electromyography for the evaluation of non-neurogenic patients.

In normal children and adolescents with lower urinary tract symptoms, Van Batavia et al. [2] have shown that four lower urinary conditions can be defined using noninvasive study with specific attention to pelvic floor activity during voiding and to EMG lag time. These conditions can be urodynamically defined:

1. Dysfunction voiding—active pelvic floor electromyography during voiding with or without staccato flow
2. (a) Idiopathic detrusor overactivity disorder-A—a quiet pelvic floor during voiding and shortened lag time (>2 s)
    (b) Idiopathic detrusor overactivity disorder-B—a quiet pelvic floor during voiding with normal lag time

3. Detrusor underutilization disorder—volitionally deferred voiding with expanded bladder capacity but a quiet pelvic floor
4. Primary bladder neck dysfunction prolonged lag time (>6 s) and a depressed right shifted uroflowmetry curve with a quiet pelvic floor during voiding.

The authors successively published positive data over the efficacy of noninvasive monitoring during the treatment. Despite the criticism, related to ICCS standardization terms and to the difficulty to obtain an optimal inter-rater agreement using current criteria [3], the uroflowmetry with EMG is useful for noninvasive evaluation in non-neurogenic patients without urinary infection or/and upper urinary dilation.

In case of several artifacts and nonconclusive results, much of the data can be inferred from a cystometrogram, or alternatively a videourodynamic study is far more accurate.

10.2 Nerve Somatosensory Evoked Potential (SSEP)

Somatosensory evoked potential (SSEP) provides information of the afferent conduction pathway from the peripheral nerves to the dorsal portion of the spinal cord and sensory cortex in response to electric stimuli at peripheral site.

The pudendal nerve motor branches innervate the urethral and anal sphincters as well as other muscles of the pelvic floor. On the other hand, its sensory branches innervate the dorsal penis, clitoris, distal urethra, and vulvar labia. Electrical stimulation of sensory receptors generates potentials traveling through the peripheral nerve and spinal cord to the cortex [4, 5]. Recording is taken during a series of stimuli in average method. In women the stimulation is performed with the cathode placed adjacent to the clitoris, and the anode is placed between the labia minora and labia majora. The former is placed 2–3 cm proximal to the latter. In man, the cathode and anode stimulate the dorsal portion of the penis. Clitoral/penis sensory threshold is defined as the intensity necessary for the patient to first realize the stimulus. Stimulus parameters are 0.2 milliseconds (ms) in duration and frequency of 3–4 hertz (Hz) increasing the intensity until two to three times the sensory threshold. Recording is obtained placing either needle or surface electrodes positioned according to the international 10–20 EEG system. Needle electrodes are placed subdermally over the scalp: the active site is usually Cz' placed 2 cm posterior to Cz and Fpz as reference. It is important to keep the impedance below 2Kohms. The sampling window is set at 10 ms per division, 1 mV/div. The amplifier band pass ranged between 1 and 5 Hz and 2/3 KHz. Between 200 and 500, responses are averaged to obtain the evoked potentials from the cortical background noise, and it analyzed the latency of the positive deflection at around P40. Additional recording sites are C3'/C4' at the scalps and L2/L3 at the spinal level (Fig. 10.3). According to the study of Cavalcanti et al. [6] in healthy woman, the mean P40 latency had a latency of about 37 ms. Similar latencies are reported in normal men [7]. These latencies are comparable to the latency recorded during posterior tibial nerve stimulation.

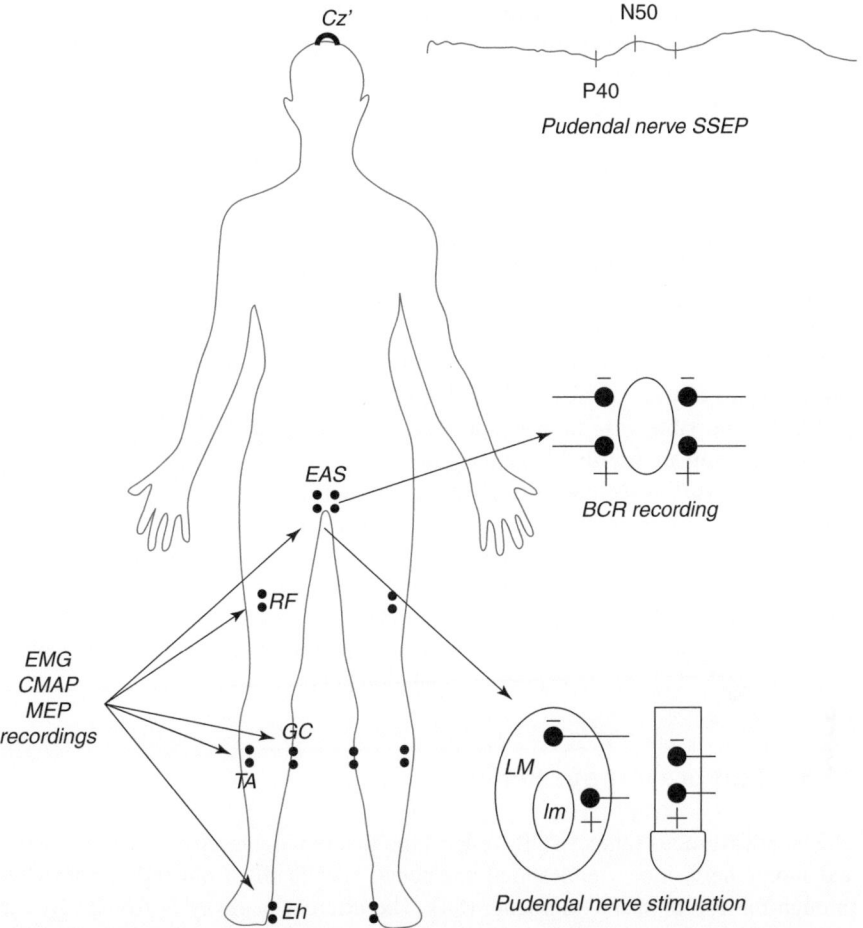

Fig. 10.3 Illustration of stimulating and recording electrode placement employed for intraoperative neurophysiological monitoring in cono-cauda surgical procedures. Abbreviations: *BCR* bulbocavernous reflex, *CMAP* compound muscle action potentials, *LM* labra majora, *lm* labra minora, *MEP* motor evoked potentials, *EAS* external anal sphincter muscle, *RF* rectus femoris, *TA* tibialis anterior, *GC* gastrocnemius, *EH* extensor hallucis

Unfortunately, no relevant information is present in the literature regarding pudendal SSEP in pediatric population, and part of the reason is, as well as for EMG registration by needle electrodes, that pudendal SSEP presents limits related to child compliance.

Occult spina bifida causes progressive neurological deterioration due to the "tethered cord syndrome"; the time of spontaneous deterioration is unknown, and there is much controversy regarding whether to perform surgery before or after the onset of such possible progression. This mechanism leads to motor deficits and spasms, sensory problems, and urodynamic/anorectal changes. Later on, orthopedic deformations may also occur due to the strength disequilibrium on feet and calves.

In diagnosis and monitoring of patients affected by tethered cord, the posterior tibial nerve somatosensory evoked potential is widely used. Posterior tibial SSEP has been shown to be a sensitive indicator of neurophysiological deterioration related to ischemia of the lower conus due to traction of the spinal cord occurring with growth and flexion [8]. In addition SSEP is a more sensitive diagnostic test than the clinical data, and improvement after detethering has been documented [7, 9]. Stimulation should be delivered to the posterior tibial nerve at the ankle, posterior to the medial malleolus, through needle or surface electrode. The pulse should be increased with a sufficient intensity to cause a plantar flexion of the toes. The recording electrode should be placed on the ipsilateral knee, the low back, the cervical region, and on the scalp.

In recent years, due to child compliance and artifacts, the neurophysiological test has lost a part of value in diagnosis and monitoring in tethered and retethered cord. The MR, if possible, also in prone position to check anterior mobility, and urodynamic follow-up are useful for the purpose.

Nevertheless, this technique might be useful during surgical procedures involving the S2–S4 nerve roots. In pediatric population, a possible field of application could be in detethering cord procedures. However, in young children and under general anesthesia, lower limb SSEP monitoring is reported to be challenging and far from being a reliable source of information for the surgeon [10]. Pudendal nerve SSEP has been applied during sacral nerve stimulation (SNS) which lead to positioning in adults but also in pediatric population [11].

10.3 Bulbocavernous Reflex

The bulbocavernous reflex (BCR) reflects the functional integrity of sacral sensory and motor nerve fibers and spinal segments, specifically from the second (S2) through the fourth sacral segments (S4). The afferent pathway is formed by the sensory fibers of the pudendal nerves, and the efferent pathway is made by the motor fibers to the pelvic floor or external anal sphincter muscles.

The integrity of this reflex arc might be clinically investigated by means of gentle squeezes of either the glans penis or clitoris evoking EMG responses from pelvic floor muscles, including the external anal sphincter. The sphincter contraction as response is visually well evident also in young patients. BCR has been also evoked through electrical stimulation of the dorsal portion of the penis or clitoris. Although BCR cannot be lateralized in clinical practice, electro-stimulation has allowed latency measurement and sophisticated electro-clinical comparison studies. For example, in the study by Niu et al. [12], BCR latencies were significantly longer in patients suffering from cauda equina syndrome when compared to those of healthy volunteers. Cauda equina syndrome is a consequence of injuries of the cauda equina, spinal nerve roots, and anterior horn of the sacral spinal cord. Its usual clinical features are lower back and leg pain, lower extremity weakness and sensory loss, perineal anesthesia, sphincter dysfunction, and erectile dysfunction. It is worth to add that the abnormal BCR latencies were also associated with significant longer latencies in pudendal SSEP. Stimulation sites and arrangements, for both male and female, are similar to those of the above-described, pudendal SSEP (Fig. 10.3). Stimulation parameters may range from single pulse at 1/5 Hz [13], double pulse (ISI 3 ms) train [13], to the train of five method [14] with pulse width of 0.1/0.2 ms. Recording site is the external anal sphincter muscle, bilaterally, at the mucocutaneous junction. The sampling window is set at 3–10 ms msec per division, 20–50 µV/div. The amplifier band pass ranged between 10 and 20 and 2\3 kHz. Signals might be averaged (10–20 stimuli) or a single stimulus response is also reported. The latency is the clinical parameter mainly considered. As well as for pudendal SSEP, no relevant literature is presented for the BCR in pediatric population. The necessity of electrical stimulation limits the compliance of very young children for BCR, too. However, intraoperative neurophysiological monitoring, especially in neurosurgical procedures involving the cono-cauda structures, is employing BCR in pediatric population. Intraoperative neurophysiological monitoring is also a basic step of pelvic surgery. In pediatric age sacrococcygeal teratoma, particularly totally intrapelvic retrorectal type IV, and pelvic neuroblastoma, a cause of position of the mass, represent a risk condition for nerve injuries. It is well known that neurological impairment of the bladder and rectum can be the dramatic consequences of pelvic surgery. This complication has been underestimated for a long time. The ideal medical process should require a preoperative urodynamic evaluation and especially a urodynamic monitoring after the surgery to prevent upper urinary tract deterioration. BCR is feasible to be recorded in pediatric population during sacral plexus surgical procedures, and the great advantage of the BCR is its presumed ability to detect conduction block at both the peripheral somatic (afferent or efferent) and central (neuronal) levels. Because parasympathetic fibers are intimately associated with somatic sacral roots of the cauda equina, BCR affords surrogate testing of major bowel, bladder, and sexual vegetative functions.

All the available literature is from a limited number of studies in adult population; thus generalization to pediatric population is questionable; however the increasing role of the intraoperative neurophysiological monitoring might be important in investigating sensory/motor pathways innervating the pelvic floor also in very young patients.

References

1. Blaivas JG, Sinha HP, Zayed AA, Labib KB. Detrusor-external sphincter dyssinergia: a detailed electromyiographic study. JUrol. 1981;125(4):545–8.
2. Van Batavia JP, Combs AJ, Hyun G, Bayer A, Medina-Kreppein D, Schlussel RN, Glassberg KI. Simplifying the diagnosis of 4 common voiding conditions using uroflow/electromyography, electromyography lag time and voiding history. J Urol. 2011;186(4 Suppl):1721–6.
3. Faasse MA, Nosnik IP, Diaz-Saldano D, Hodgkins KS, Liu DB, Schreiber J, Yerkers EB. Uroflowmetry with pelvic floor electromyography: inter-rater agreement on diagnosis of pediatric non neurogenic voiding disorders. J Pediatr Urol. 2015;11(4):198.e1–6.
4. Opsomer RJ, Guerit JM, Wese FX, Van Cangh PJ. Pudendal cortical somatosensory evoked potentials. J Urol. 1986;135:1216–8.

5. Vodusek DB. Evoked potential testing. Urol Clin North Am. 1996;23:427–46.
6. Cavalcanti GA, Bruschini H, Manzano GM, Nunes KF, Giuliano LM, Nobrega JA, Srougi M. Pudendal somatosensory evoked potentials in normal women. Int Braz J Urol. 2007;33(6):815–21.
7. Kale SS, Mahapatra K. The role of somatosensory evoked potentials in spinal dysraphism-do they have a prognostic significance? Childs Nerv Syst. 1998;4(7):325–30.
8. Pang D. Tethered cord syndrome: newer concepts. In: Wilkins RH, Rengachary SS, editors. Neurosurgery update. New York: McGraw-Hill; 1991. p. 336–44.
9. Polo A, Zanette G, Manganotti P, Bertolasi L, De Grandis D, Rizzuto N. Spinal somatosensory evoked potentials in patients with tethered cord syndrome. Can J Neurol Sci. 1994;21(4):325–30.
10. Sala F, Squintani G, Tramontano V, Arcaro C, Faccioli F, Mazza C. Intraoperative neuro physiology in tethered cord surgery: techniques and results. Childs Nerv Syst. 2013;29:1611–24.
11. Valentini LG, Selvaggio G, Erbetta A, Cordella R, Pecoraro MG, Bova S, Boni E, Beretta E, Furlanetto M. Occult spinal dysraphism: lessons learned by retrospective analysis of 149 surgical cases about natural history, surgical indications, urodynamic testing, and intraoperative. Childs Nerv Syst. 2013;29:1657–69.
12. Niu X, Wang X, Ni P, Huang H, Zhang Y, Lin Y, Chen X, Teng H, Shao B. Bulbocavernosus reflex and pudendal nerve somatosensory evoked potential are valuable for the diagnosis of cauda equina syndrome in male patients. Int J Clin Exp Med. 2015;8(1):1162–7.
13. Podnar S. Predictive value of the Penilo-Cavernosus reflex. Neurourol Urodyn. 2009;28:390–4.
14. Pedersen E, Harving H, Klemar B, Torring J. Human Anal Reflexes. J Neurol Neurosurg Psychiatry. 1978;41:813–8.

Diagnostic Tests for Defecation Disorders

11

Peter Christensen

11.1 Introduction

It should be emphasised that diagnostic tests for defecation disorders in childhood and adolescence should be restricted to those rare cases not responding to a structured clinical approach based on careful patient history taking, targeted therapy, systematic evaluation of treatment response and subsequently modified therapy. This has been outlined within the most recent NICE guidelines [1] and in a recent consensus review [2]. However, additional diagnostic tests have to be considered if requested by specialist services to rule out rare secondary causes and/or before more invasive treatment modalities are introduced.

11.1.1 Patient History

As for any medical condition, a careful patient history is essential in the evaluation of disordered defecation. The nature of the disorder should be characterised including onset, frequency, duration, diurnal variation, bowel frequency, stool consistency, faecal incontinence, previous management, coexisting urinary incontinence, relation to food intake and physical activity and the impact on social relations and overall well-being [1, 2].

Special attention should be paid to 'red flag' findings such as onset from birth or the first few weeks, delayed passage of meconium, abdominal distension and vomiting, failure to thrive and familial or social factors raising concerns over possibility of child maltreatment [1, 2].

P. Christensen
Pelvic Floor Unit, Department of Surgery, Aarhus University Hospital, Aarhus, Denmark
e-mail: petchris@rm.dk

© Springer International Publishing AG, part of Springer Nature 2018
G. Mosiello et al. (eds.), *Clinical Urodynamics in Childhood and Adolescence*, Urodynamics, Neurourology and Pelvic Floor Dysfunctions,
https://doi.org/10.1007/978-3-319-42193-3_11

The patient history should be supported by patient-reported outcome measures (PROMs) to quantify patient symptoms and convert individual experiences into data. Thereby grading of the severity of disordered defecation is possible, and treatment can be monitored for quality control and for scientific purpose. A bowel habit diary can be used for daily registration of bowel habits [3, 4]. Traditionally this has been done on paper forms, but current initiatives are undertaken to convert bowel habit diaries into smartphone apps [5].

11.1.2 Physical Examination

Perineal inspection is mandatory to assess abnormal appearance or position of the anus including anal fistula, multiple fissures, anterior placed anus, perianal skin erosions and absent anal wink. The inspection should be extended to the back to look for asymmetry or flattening of the gluteal muscles, evidence of sacral agenesis, discoloured skin, naevi or sinus, hairy patch, lipomas and scoliosis. At the front, the abdomen should be palpated and inspected for gross abdominal distension [1, 2].

11.2 Digital Rectal Examination

The necessity of a digital rectal examination is highly controversial [1, 2]. Some advocate for the examination to confirm the diagnosis of rectal impaction, but the ability of the digital examination to discriminate between radiographically constipated and non-constipated has been poor [6]. Others argue that the examination adds to the unpleasant experiences by the passage of stools keeping the child in the virtuous cycle of retention. If a digital examination should be undertaken in the presence of any 'red flag' findings, this should only be by healthcare professionals competent to interpret features of anatomical abnormalities and competent to initiate treatment [1]. If necessary the examination should be under general anaesthesia.

11.2.1 Anorectal Physiology Tests

Anorectal physiology testing may in rare cases be used in disordered defecation in childhood and adolescence before sophisticated treatment modalities are introduced. However, as for anorectal physiology tests in adults, the prognostic value of each test has been questioned, and it should be emphasised that anal physiology test cannot stand alone in the clinical decision-making [7].

Anorectal manometry can either be done by water-perfused [8], solid state or by fibre optic catheters. High-resolution manometry of the anal canal provides detailed spatial information about anal pressures [9]. The technique is increasingly used, but it remains to be established whether the rather expensive equipment provides better guidance towards therapy than standard manometry [10, 11]. Fibre optic catheter for colonic manometry has also been used in children but not outside a strict research setting [12, 13].

Anorectal manometry determines the anal resting pressure, the anal squeeze pressure, rectal sensation, rectal compliance, defecation dynamics and for special interest in childhood and adolescence of the rectoanal inhibitor reflex to rule out Hirschsprung's disease. The normal physiological response to rectal distension is relaxation of the internal anal sphincter, thereby enable defecation to take place. In Hirschsprung's disease the ganglion cells in the myenteric plexus (Auerbach's plexus) are absent, and the reflex cannot be mediated leading to aperistalsis.

11.3 Rectal Biopsy

Although a beautiful example of applied neurophysiology in clinical practice, the absence of the rectoanal inhibitory reflex often is not imperative to Hirschsprung's disease, since false negative results often are seen. Therefore the definitive diagnose require a full thickness rectal biopsy with the absence of ganglion cells in the myenteric plexus. However, positive rectoanal inhibitor reflex exclude the diagnosis [2].

In general, Hirschsprung' s disease is a rare disease (1:5000 new births) and rectal biopsies are not recommend unless any of the following clinical features are/have been present: delayed passage of meconium, constipation since first few weeks of life, chronic abdominal distension plus vomiting, family history of Hirschsprung's disease or faltering growth in addition to any of the previous features [1].

11.4 Rectal Biomechanics

In adults, rectal capacity and compliance can be tested with a rectal balloon gradually filled with either air or water. Rectal sensibility is also assessed during balloon filling. A barostat may be used in order to measure rectal compliance and is recognised as the golden standard [14, 15]. Increased rectal compliance has been found to correlate with subgroups of constipation in adolescence [16, 17]. Advanced measurement of rectal motility using impedance planimetry failed to find correlation between constipated children and rectal compliance but found that constipated children had more frequent episodes of rectal phasic contractions than did healthy children [18]. The use of rectal motility measures outside a research setting seems to be limited.

11.4.1 Transcutaneous Ultrasonography of the Rectum

As digital rectal examination to determine rectal faecal impaction seems to be of limited value and more advance rectal motility measures requires sophisticated technology, transcutaneous ultrasonography of the rectal diameter seems to be a valuable tool to identify faecal impaction [19, 20]. The method uses a normal surface ultrasonography probe approx. 2 cm above the symphysis and a child with a full bladder. The transverse rectal diameter is then measured. Constipated children have significantly larger rectal diameter than healthy children. When constipation is treated, the rectal diameter is reduced significantly [20]. It is likely that this non-invasive examination can replace digital rectal examination for faecal impaction, when this information is needed.

11.5 Colonic Transit Times

The use of plain abdominal X-ray to access faecal impaction has gained popularity and different scoring systems have been suggested [21–23]. The individual scoring is however investigator dependent [24], and each X-ray exposes the child for radiation.

More detailed and useful information can be achieved by adding per oral ingested radiopaque markers to the investigation allowing for the calculation of both total and segmental colonic transit times. Different protocols for marker intake and calculation exist [25–27], and they show good correlation to either number of defecations or the ability to discriminate between children with or without clinical constipation [24, 26, 28]. Moreover, a normal CTT in a child with suspected constipation either indicate a non-retensive faecal incontinence or an unreliable medical history [2].

Colonic transit time can also be determined by wireless motility capsules measuring intraluminal pH and temperature [10]. More advanced capsules also detect specific motor patterns [29]. Both concepts have not yet found its place within paediatric gastroenterology. Also colonic scintigraphy can be used but it is expensive, implies exposure to radiation and there is limited access to the technology.

References

1. Constipation in children and young people: diagnosis and management. 2010.
2. Tabbers MM, DiLorenzo C, Berger MY, Faure C, Langendam MW, Nurko S, et al. Evaluation and treatment of functional constipation in infants and children: evidence-based recommendations from ESPGHAN and NASPGHAN. J Pediatr Gastroenterol Nutr. 2014;58(2):258–74. https://doi.org/10.1097/MPG.0000000000000266.
3. Pless CE, Pless IB. How well they remember. The accuracy of parent reports. Arch Pediatr Adolesc Med. 1995;149(5):553–8.
4. van der Plas RN, Benninga MA, Redekop WK, Taminiau JA, Buller HA. How accurate is the recall of bowel habits in children with defaecation disorders? Eur J Pediatr. 1997;156(3):178–81.
5. Myint M, Adam A, Herath S, Smith G. Mobile phone applications in management of enuresis: the good, the bad, and the unreliable. J Pediatr Urol. 2015;12(2):112.e1–6.
6. Beckmann KR, Hennes H, Sty JR, Walsh-Kelly CM. Accuracy of clinical variables in the identification of radiographically proven constipation in children. WMJ. 2001;100(1):33–6.
7. Hill K, Fanning S, Fennerty MB, Faigel DO. Endoanal ultrasound compared to anorectal manometry for the evaluation of fecal incontinence: a study of the effect these tests have on clinical outcome. Dig Dis Sci. 2006;51(2):235–40.
8. McHugh SM, Diamant NE. Anal canal pressure profile: a reappraisal as determined by rapid pullthrough technique. Gut. 1987;28(10):1234–41.

9. Banasiuk M, Banaszkiewicz A, Albrecht P. Pp-9 normal values of 3d high-resolution anorectal manometry in children. J Pediatr Gastroenterol Nutr. 2015;61(4):523–4. https://doi.org/10.1097/01.mpg.0000472237.44732.84.
10. Belkind-Gerson J, Tran K, Di Lorenzo C. Novel techniques to study colonic motor function in children. Curr Gastroenterol Rep. 2013;15(8):335. https://doi.org/10.1007/s11894-013-0335-3.
11. Ambartsumyan L, Rodriguez L, Morera C, Nurko S. Longitudinal and radial characteristics of intra-anal pressures in children using 3D high-definition anorectal manometry: new observations. Am J Gastroenterol. 2013;108(12):1918–28. https://doi.org/10.1038/ajg.2013.361. Epub Oct 29
12. Dinning PG, Wiklendt L, Maslen L, Gibbins I, Patton V, Arkwright JW, et al. Quantification of in vivo colonic motor patterns in healthy humans before and after a meal revealed by high-resolution fiber-optic manometry. Neurogastroenterol Motil. 2014;26(10):1443–57. https://doi.org/10.1111/nmo.12408. Epub 2014 Aug 11
13. Sintusek P, Mutalib M, Thapar N, Lindley K. Op-2 the diagnostic value of radiological colonic transit study compared with high-resolution colonic manometry. J Pediatr Gastroenterol Nutr. 2015;61(4):509. https://doi.org/10.1097/01.mpg.0000472206.16023.ae.
14. Vanhoutvin SA, Troost FJ, Kilkens TO, Lindsey PJ, Hamer HM, Jonkers DM, et al. The effects of butyrate enemas on visceral perception in healthy volunteers. Neurogastroenterol Motil. 2009;21(9):952–e76. https://doi.org/10.1111/j.365-2982.009.01324.x. Epub 2009 May 19
15. van den Berg MM, Di Lorenzo C, van Ginkel R, Mousa HM, Benninga MA. Barostat testing in children with functional gastrointestinal disorders. Curr Gastroenterol Rep. 2006;8(3):224–9.
16. van den Berg MM, Voskuijl WP, Boeckxstaens GE, Benninga MA. Rectal compliance and rectal sensation in constipated adolescents, recovered adolescents and healthy volunteers. Gut. 2008;57(5):599–603. Epub 2007 Oct 26
17. van den Berg MM, Bongers ME, Voskuijl WP, Benninga MA. No role for increased rectal compliance in pediatric functional constipation. Gastroenterology. 2009;137(6):1963–9. https://doi.org/10.1053/j.gastro.2009.08.015. Epub Aug 21
18. Moeller Joensson I, Hagstroem S, Fynne L, Krogh K, Siggaard C, Djurhuus JC. Rectal motility in pediatric constipation. J Pediatr Gastroenterol Nutr. 2014;58(3):292–6. https://doi.org/10.1097/MPG.0000000000000203.
19. Bijos A, Czerwionka-Szaflarska M, Mazur A, Romanczuk W. The usefulness of ultrasound examination of the bowel as a method of assessment of functional chronic constipation in children. Pediatr Radiol. 2007;37(12):1247–52. Epub 2007 Oct 19
20. Joensson IM, Siggaard C, Rittig S, Hagstroem S, Djurhuus JC. Transabdominal ultrasound of rectum as a diagnostic tool in childhood constipation. J Urol. 2008;179(5):1997–2002. https://doi.org/10.1016/j.juro.2008.01.055. Epub Mar 20
21. Barr RG, Levine MD, Wilkinson RH, Mulvihill D. Chronic and occult stool retention: a clinical tool for its evaluation in school-aged children. Clin Pediatr. 1979;18(11):674.
22. Moylan S, Armstrong J, Diaz-Saldano D, Saker M, Yerkes EB, Lindgren BW. Are abdominal x-rays a reliable way to assess for constipation? J Urol. 2010;184(4 Suppl):1692–8. https://doi.org/10.1016/j.juro.2010.05.054. Epub Aug 21
23. Cunha TB, Tahan S, Soares MF, Lederman HM, Morais MB. Abdominal radiograph in the assessment of fecal impaction in children with functional constipation: comparing three scoring systems. J Pediatr. 2012;88(4):317–22. https://doi.org/10.2223/JPED.199.
24. Benninga MA, Buller HA, Staalman CR, Gubler FM, Bossuyt PM, van der Plas RN, et al. Defaecation disorders in children, colonic transit time versus the Barr-score. Eur J Pediatr. 1995;154(4):277–84.
25. Arhan P, Devroede G, Jehannin B, Lanza M, Faverdin C, Dornic C, et al. Segmental colonic transit time. Dis Colon Rectum. 1981;24(8):625–9.
26. Gutierrez C, Marco A, Nogales A, Tebar R. Total and segmental colonic transit time and anorectal manometry in children with chronic idiopathic constipation. J Pediatr Gastroenterol Nutr. 2002;35(1):31–8.

27. Abrahamsson H, Antov S, Bosaeus I. Gastrointestinal and colonic segmental transit time evaluated by a single abdominal x-ray in healthy subjects and constipated patients. Scand J Gastroenterol Suppl. 1988;152(72–80):72–80.
28. Zaslavsky C, da Silveira TR, Maguilnik I. Total and segmental colonic transit time with radio-opaque markers in adolescents with functional constipation. J Pediatr Gastroenterol Nutr. 1998;27(2):138–42.
29. Hedsund C, Joensson IM, Gregersen T, Fynne L, Schlageter V, Krogh K. Magnet tracking allows assessment of regional gastrointestinal transit times in children. Clin Exp Gastroenterol. 2013;6:201–8. https://doi.org/10.2147/CEG.S51402. eCollection 2013

Part II
Pathological Conditions

Lower Urinary Tract Dysfunction in Children and Young Adults: An Introduction

12

Tryggve Nevéus

12.1 Introduction, Scope of the Chapter

This chapter will give an overview of the panorama of lower urinary tract (LUT) disturbances in childhood, including their aetiology, epidemiology and clinical presentation, as well as which words to use when describing them. The reader is also provided with the warning signs to look out for in the initial evaluation of children with LUT problems in order not to miss conditions that may impair renal function or need invasive evaluation without delay. Finally, the two areas of comorbidity which cannot be ignored regardless of which kind of LUT disorder is at hand—i.e. bowel function and issues related to psychiatry and behaviour—are briefly dealt with.

12.2 Definitions

Before discussing the paediatric LUT and its disturbances, we need to agree upon which words to use. Much research and clinical practice in this scientific field has been hampered by ambiguous terms and conflicting terminologies. This situation has, however, been ameliorated during the last decade by the introduction of a globally accepted terminology by the International Children's Continence Society (ICCS) [1, 2], which will be strictly adhered to in this chapter.

Incontinence is subdivided into continuous and intermittent variants, the former expression being reserved for urine leakage that is constantly dribbling without any dry intervals. *Continuous incontinence* is pathological in all ages since it is often a

---

T. Nevéus, M.D. Ph.D.
Uppsala University Children's Hospital, Uppsala, Sweden
e-mail: Tryggve.Neveus@kbh.uu.se

sign of an underlying anatomic malformation. *Intermittent incontinence* means that urine leaks in discrete portions. This term is relevant from the age of presumed bladder control or 5 years and is subdivided into daytime incontinence and enuresis. *Enuresis*—i.e. (intermittent) nocturnal incontinence—is further subdivided into monosymptomatic and nonmonosymptomatic varieties depending on whether symptoms of daytime bladder dysfunction are also present. 'Diurnal enuresis' is an obsolete term previously used for children with (intermittent) *daytime incontinence*. *Urgency* is the term used for the sudden, imperative need to go to the toilet. Children who experience this symptom are said to suffer from *overactive bladder*, and the term *urge incontinence* is used if they also have (intermittent) daytime incontinence. Urgency is typically, but not universally, indicative of underlying *detrusor overactivity*, a term that may be used if, during cystometric examination, uninhibited involuntary detrusor contractions have been observed.

Dysfunctional voiding is a term used for the children who habitually contract the sphincter during bladder emptying, usually resulting in a staccato uroflow curve. Please note that the use of this term, or 'voiding dysfunction', as an umbrella term for all kinds of LUT disturbances is strongly discouraged. *Voiding postponement* are the words used for children who, by the use of various *holding manoeuvres*, try to delay micturition as long as possible. Children with dysfunctional voiding or voiding postponement often suffer from daytime incontinence and/or overactive bladder as well. *Underactive bladder* means that raised intraabdominal pressure needs to be used in order to void, and *detrusor underactivity* means that weak or insufficient detrusor contractions have been detected on cystometry.

When assessing the storage function of the bladder, volumes are usually taken from a bladder diary. It is important then to use the term *voided volume*, not bladder volume or bladder capacity—these latter terms are reserved for when the amount of urine actually within the bladder has been measured (using ultrasound, for instance). When comparisons with expected or 'normal' bladder storage ability are needed, we use the term *expected bladder capacity* (EBC) which is expressed in millilitres and calculated according to the following formula: EBC = (age in years +1) * 30 [3].

12.3 Functional Disturbances of Urine Storage

Incontinence—during the day or the night—is extremely common. In a normal school class of 20 7-year-olds, two to three children can be expected to regularly wet their beds and/or clothes [4].

12.3.1 Enuresis

Bedwetting, or enuresis, is not, as was previously thought, primarily a psychiatric disorder. Instead, it has been shown that the enuretic child wets his or her bed because the nocturnal urine production is too high and/or there are uninhibited nocturnal detrusor contractions, combined with the fact that the arousal signals from the distended or overactive detrusor for some reason fail to awaken the child [5]. The condition is often inherited.

The enuretic child may present with just the bedwetting, i.e. monosymptomatic enuresis or concomittant daytime symptoms such as daytime incontinence or urgency, i.e. nonmonosymptomatic enuresis. If a careful history is taken, it will be found that the latter group represents the majority.

For unknown reasons enuresis is more common among males than females [4]. The prevalence among 7-year-olds is approximately 5% [4]. By teenage it has dropped to approximately 1–2% [6], whereas in adulthood the figure is around 0.5–1% [7, 8]—still a common disorder. Thus, there is a clear tendency for spontaneous remission, but it may be incomplete and/or delayed and constitutes no reason to postpone active treatment, since the consequences of delayed dryness are not trivial [9].

Even though enuresis is not a primarily psychiatric disorder, behavioural comorbidity is common, especially in nonmonosymptomatic enuresis [10, 11].

12.3.2 Overactive Bladder and Daytime Incontinence

In the majority of cases, daytime incontinence in childhood is caused by detrusor overactivity. In the typical case, the child has urgency symptoms as well and a bladder diary will often, but by no means always, show that voidings are frequent and voided volumes are small. Some incontinent children also have voiding postponement or dysfunctional voiding, and the combination of daytime incontinence and enuresis is quite common [4]. The overrepresentation of constipated children among those with daytime incontinence of urine is extra important to take into account [12, 13] since in these cases the constipation may have a clear causative role.

Daytime incontinence is also very common—approximately 5–10% of children at school start [4] and 3–5% in teenage [14]—but here the girls are more commonly afflicted than the boys [4, 14]. The wetting may continue into adulthood and individuals who have been incontinent in childhood are at increased risk for almost any kind of LUT problems later in life [15].

12.3.3 Unusual Functional Disorders of Urine Storage

Vaginal reflux is a self-explanatory term; urine is trapped in the vagina during normal voiding and then soon afterwards leaks into the child's underclothes. The prevalence is unknown but the disorder is not rare [16]. The condition is easy to treat and will otherwise spontaneously disappear at puberty.

True *giggle incontinence* is rare, but the condition is probably often both over- and underdiagnosed. The term should only be used for patients, most often girls or young women, who have a completely normal LUT function except for the fact that laughter tends to elicit a complete bladder emptying. The natural history of the condition is poorly known, but it may certainly persist for many years [17]. Pathogenesis is a mystery.

Another condition of unclear pathogenesis is the appropriately named *extraordinarily daytime urinary frequency syndrome*, which usually starts in children 3–5 years of age and causes them to have to go to the toilet extremely often during daytime, whereas nocturnal bladder function is completely normal. Prevalence figures are not available but spontaneous remission appears to be the rule [18, 19].

12.4 Functional Disturbances of Bladder Emptying

12.4.1 Voiding Postponement

There is indirect evidence for voiding postponement being a primarily behavioural disorder. The child has somehow learnt to ignore the urge to go to the toilet [20]. This may or may not be in response to underlying detrusor overactivity and can in severe cases proceed to underactive bladder (see below). The prevalence among the population at large is unknown but voiding postponement may be very common among children with incontinence admitted to specialised clinics [21]. Constipation is very often present as well, and there is an increased risk for psychiatric comorbidity [21].

12.4.2 Dysfunctional Voiding

As mentioned above, dysfunctional voiding means that the child contracts the sphincter during micturition, causing a nonstructural outflow obstruction. The pathogenesis is unclear but the disorder is probably multifactorial, often includes a behavioural component [22] and may coexist with detrusor overactivity and/or incontinence. Prevalence in the general population is unknown, but among children with daytime incontinence, figures between 4 and 32% have been reported [22].

Since voiding is often incomplete in the child with voiding dysfunction, it should come as no surprise that the risk for recurrent UTI is high [23]. This is also one of the LUT disturbances which very often coincides with constipation [24].

12.4.3 Underactive Bladder, Detrusor Underactivity

Dysfunctional voiding may in severe cases proceed to detrusor underactivity, which increases the risk for UTIs even more and may be harmful for kidney function. The condition may also arise de novo, with unclear pathogenesis. It is extremely important to differentiate functional bladder underactivity from neurogenic bladder or anatomic outflow obstruction. Prevalence is unknown.

12.4.4 Severe Bladder and Bowel Dysfunction

At the most severe end of the spectrum of functional disorders of bladder emptying lies the condition that was previously called the *Hinman bladder* [25] or given the confusing name *non-neurogenic neurogenic bladder*. We now use the term severe bladder and bowel dysfunction when we describe the children with dysfunctional voiding, detrusor underactivity and constipation. The upper urinary tracts are often affected as well, recurrent UTIs are the rule and there is a very real risk of renal failure [26]. This condition will not resolve spontaneously, and bladder function will never normalise. Pathogenesis is frustratingly unclear but may possibly in some cases start as vicious circles arising from poor bladder behaviour [26]. It may also be associated with Down's syndrome [27] or the inheritable association of severe LUT dysfunction and an inability to smile known as the Ochoa syndrome [28].

12.5 Lower Urinary Tract Dysfunction Due to Neurogenic or Anatomic Causes

12.5.1 Neurogenic Bladder

Any damage to the parts of the central nervous system involved in LUT function may result in the neurogenic bladder. By far the most common cause in childhood is myelomeningocele [29]. The incidence has been decreasing in the industrialised world due to folic acid supplementation during pregnancy. The neurogenic bladder is characterised cystometrically by dyscoordination of the sphincter and detrusor and various combinations of under- or overactivity of both. Before the discovery of clean intermittent catheterisation (CIC), children with this condition usually had repeated febrile UTIs and progressive renal failure due to these and to high intravesical pressure. When LUT function is impaired for neurological reasons, bowel function is usually also affected. Thus, these children need aggressive treatment of concomittant constipation [30].

12.5.2 LUT Dysfunction Due to Anatomical Obstruction

The most common cause of anatomic obstruction to urine outflow is the posterior urethral valve (PUV), which only occur in boys. The aetiology is unclear but usually not genetic [31]. In the most severe cases, the child may succumb neonatally due to congenital renal failure and pulmonary hypoplasia, whereas milder cases may present later in life with symptoms such as therapy-resistant urinary incontinence, voiding difficulties, recurrent UTIs and/or polyuric renal failure. Even though the valve as such is usually easily surgically corrected, bladder function will never normalise, and the situation may deteriorate especially at puberty due to adherence issues and growth of the prostate [32, 33].

12.5.3 Ureteral Ectopia

When the ureter, usually belonging to the upper moiety of a duplex system, joins the LUT distal to the sphincter, there will be continuous, dribbling incontinence, starting already in the neonatal period. This rare malformation is most common in girls [34].

12.6 Warning Signs

When meeting a child with LUT problems, it is of utmost importance to detect without delay the few underlying disturbances that may lead to deterioration of kidney function and/or need of surgical treatment. These conditions include the neurogenic bladder, detrusor underactivity, severe bladder and bowel dysfunction, anatomic obstruction, ureteral ectopia and polyuric renal failure. If keeping in mind a few warning signs, these children can usually be detected early and the correct radiological and/or urodynamic examinations be performed without delay (Table 12.1). Importantly, this also has the consequence that in the rest of the patients invasive or complicated examinations will *not* have to be performed.

12.7 Relevant Comorbidity

Just as the child cannot be treated in isolation from his or her family, the LUT cannot be viewed as an isolated organ. Comorbidities within certain spheres are common enough to warrant consideration regardless of what kind of LUT dysfunction is at hand.

12.7.1 Constipation

The LUT and the bowel are closely interrelated organs, both functionally and anatomically. Disturbances in the one are often linked to disturbances of the other [24]. There are several potential and/or confirmed causes for this comorbidity:

Table 12.1 Signs indicating underlying serious conditions, or the need for radiological or urodynamic evaluation, in a child with LUT dysfunction

Warning sign	Possible background
Continuous incontinence	Ureteral ectopia, anatomic obstruction, neurogenic bladder
Weak stream, voiding difficulties	Detrusor/bladder underactivity, anatomic or functional obstruction, neurogenic bladder
Recurrent febrile UTIs	Detrusor/bladder underactivity, anatomic or functional obstruction, neurogenic bladder
Excessive thirst with a need to drink at night	Polyuric renal failure (or diabetes)

1. The LUT and the bowel are innervated from the same parts of the CNS. This is relevant at least in children with spinal dysraphism.
2. Constipation means that the rectum—which should normally be a signal space, not a storage organ—is dilated for prolonged periods of time. The distended rectum compresses and dislocates the posterior bladder wall, which may lead to detrusor overactivity and/or voiding difficulties [35]. This is probably the main reason for the strong link between constipation and functional daytime urinary incontinence.
3. If, for psychological reasons, emptying of the bladder is habitually deferred, the same may be true for bowel emptying as well, and vice versa. This mechanism can be assumed to be relevant among children with voiding postponement and constipation [36].

Approximately 50% of children with functional daytime incontinence can be expected to have concomittant constipation [37], whereas the figure is lower in children with monosymptomatic nocturnal enuresis [38].

12.7.2 Psychiatry and Behavioural Issues

Although the old assumption that all children who wet themselves have underlying psychiatric or behavioural issues causing the incontinence has now been abandoned, there are anyway strong links between LUT problems and psychiatry/psychology [39]. The types of comorbidity can be classified as follows:

1. The LUT disturbance causes psychological problems. The most obvious way this can happen is via low self-esteem. This has been clearly shown to be the case for many children with daytime incontinence or enuresis [40]. Another more subtle mechanism in nocturnal enuresis may be by the adverse effects of disturbed sleep on daytime cognitive function [41].
2. Psychiatrical problems or behavioural issues cause LUT dysfunction. This is much more rare than was previously thought. Still, incontinence may sometimes be part of the posttraumatic stress disorder, and, as mentioned above, in some cases of dysfunctional voiding, voiding postponement or severe bladder and bowel dysfunction, this mechanism may be active.
3. The LUT dysfunction and the behavioural problems may share an underlying cause. This is probably the case for the association between neuropsychiatric disorders such as attention deficit hyperactivity disorder (ADHD) and day- or nighttime incontinence [11]. The exact reason for this association is unclear.
4. The two kinds of disorders may appear in the same individual just by coincidence. It should be kept in mind that neuropsychiatrical problems and other behavioural issues are very common in the general population, as is incontinence.

In children with functional incontinence, the psychiatric comorbidity is strongest among those who have secondary daytime incontinence and weakest among children with primary monosymptomatic nocturnal enuresis. Children with non-monosymptomatic or secondary enuresis hold intermediate positions in this regard [39].

It is important to be aware of the risk for psychiatric comorbidity since this may influence the chance for successful treatment of the LUT dysfunction. It may, as an example, be difficult to comply with the enuresis alarm therapy for a child with untreated ADHD [39]. Another reason to take these matters into account is, of course, the risk for long-term psychological consequences.

References

1. Nevéus T, von Gontard A, Hoebeke P, Hjälmås K, Bauer S, Bower W, et al. The standardization of terminology of lower urinary tract function in children and adolescents: report from the standardisation committee of the International Children's Continence Society (ICCS). J Urol. 2006;176(1):314–24.
2. Austin P, Bauer S, Bower W, Chase J, Franco I, Hoebeke P, et al. The standardization of terminology of lower urinary tract function in children and adolescents: update report from the standardization committee of the international Children's continence society. J Urol. 2014;191(6):1863–5.
3. Koff SA. Estimating bladder capacity in children. Urology. 1983;21:248.
4. Hellström A-L, Hansson E, Hansson S, Hjälmås K, Jodal U. Incontinence and micturition habits in 7-year-old Swedish school entrants. Eur J Pediatr. 1990;149:434–7.
5. Nevéus T. Nocturnal enuresis – theoretic background and practical guidelines. Pediatr Nephrol. 2011;26(8):1207–14.
6. Bakker E, van Sprundel M, van der Auwera JC, van Gool JD, Wyndaele JJ. Voiding habits and wetting in a population of 4,332 Belgian schoolchildren aged between 10 and 14 years. Scand J Urol Nephrol. 2002;36(5):354–62.
7. Hirasing RA, van Leerdam FJ, Bolk-Bennink L, Janknegt RA. Enuresis nocturna in adults. Scand J Urol Nephrol. 1997;31(6):533–6.
8. Baek M, Park KH, Lee HE, Kang JH, Suh HJ, Kim JH, et al. A nationwide epidemiological study of nocturnal enuresis in korean adolescents and adults: population based cross sectional study. J Korean Med Sci. 2013;28:1065–70.
9. Coyne KS, Kaplan SA, Chapple CR, Sexton CC, Kopp ZS, Bush EN, et al. Risk factors and comorbid conditions associated with lower urinary tract symptoms: EpiLUTS. BJU Int. 2009;103:24–32.
10. Equit M, Klein AM, Braun-Bither K, Gräber S, von Gontard A. Elimination disorders and anxious-depressed symptoms in preschool children: a population-based study. Eur Child Adolesc Psychiatry. 2014;23(6):417–23.
11. von Gontard A, Equit M. Comorbidity of ADHD and incontinence in children. Eur Child Adolesc Psychiatry. 2015;24(2):127–40.
12. Chung JM, Lee SD, Kang DI, Kwon DD, Kim KS, Kim SY, et al. An epidemiologic study of voiding and bowel habits in Korean children: a nationwide multicenter study. Urology. 2010;76(1):215–9.
13. Veiga ML, Lordêlo P, Farias T, Barroso C, Bonfim J, Barroso UJ. Constipation in children with isolated overactive bladder. J Pediatr Urol. 2013;9:945–9.

14. Hellström A, Hanson E, Hansson S, Hjälmås K, Jodal U. Micturition habits and incontinence at age 17 - reinvestigation of a cohort studied at age 7. Br J Urol. 1995;76:231–4.
15. Kuh D, Cardozo L, Hardy R. Urinary incontinence in middle aged women: childhood enuresis and other lifetime risk factors in a British prospective cohort. J Epidemiol Community Health. 1999;53(8):453–8.
16. Mattsson S, Gladh G. Urethrovaginal reflux--a common cause of daytime incontinence in girls. Pediatrics. 2003;111(1):136–9.
17. Berry AK, Zderic S, Carr M. Methylphenidate for giggle incontinence. J Urol. 2009;182(4 Suppl):2028–32.
18. Bergmann M, Corigliano T, Ataia I, Renella R, Simonetti GD, Bianchetti MG, et al. Childhood extraordinary daytime urinary frequency - a case series and a systematic literature review. Pediatr Nephrol. 2009;24:789–95.
19. Chen WF, Huang SC. Pollakiuria: extraordinary daytime urinary frequency a common problem in pediatric practice. Changgeng Yi Xue Za Zhi. 1995;18(2):115–9.
20. von Gontard A, Lettgen B, Olbing H, Heiken-Lowenau C, Gaebel E, Schmitz I. Behavioural problems in children with urge incontinence and voiding postponement: a comparison of a paediatric and child psychiatric sample. Br J Urol. 1998;81(Suppl 3):100–6.
21. Zink S, Freitag CM, von Gontard A. Behavioral comorbidity differs in subtypes of enuresis and urinary incontinence. J Urol. 2008;179(1):295–8.
22. Chase J, Austin P, Hoebeke P, McKenna P. The management of dysfunctional voiding in children: a report from the standardisation committee of the International Children's Continence Society. J Urol. 2010;183(4):1296–302.
23. Ramamurthy HR, Kanitkar M. Recurrent urinary tract infection and functional voiding disorders. Indian Pediatr. 2008;45(8):689–91.
24. Burgers R, de Jong TP, Visser M, Di Lorenzo C, Dijkgraaf MG, Benninga M. Functional defecation disorders among children with lower urinary tract symptoms. J Urol. 2013;189(5):1886–91.
25. Hinman F, Bauman FW. Vesical and ureteral damage from voiding dysfunction in boys without neurologic or obstructive disease. J Urol. 1973;109:727–32.
26. Varlam DE, Dippell J. Non-neurogenic bladder and chronic renal insufficiency in childhood. Pediatr Nephrol. 1995;9(1):1–5.
27. Handel LN, Barqawi A, Checa G, Furness PD 3rd, Koyle MA. Males with Down's syndrome and nonneurogenic neurogenic bladder. J Urol. 2003;169(2):646–9.
28. Ochoa B. Can a congenital dysfunctional bladder be diagnosed from a smile? The Ochoa syndrome updated. Pediatr Nephrol. 2004;19:6–12.
29. de Jong TP, Chrzan R, Klijn AJ, Dik P. Treatment of the neurogenic bladder in spina bifida. Pediatr Nephrol. 2008;146:113–7.
30. Rawashdeh YF, Austin P, Siggaard C, Bauer SB, Franco I, de Jong TP, et al. International children's continence society's recommendations for therapeutic intervention in congenital neuropathic bladder and bowel dysfunction in children. Neurourol Urodyn. 2012;31(5):615–20.
31. Schreuder MF, van der Horst HJ, Bökenkamp A, Beckers GM, van Wijk JA. Posterior urethral valves in three siblings: a case report and review of the literature. Birth Defects Res A Clin Mol Teratol. 2008;82(4):232–5.
32. Hensle TW, Deibert CM. Adult male health risks associated with congenital abnormalities. Urol Clin North Am. 2012;39(1):109–14.
33. López Pereira P, Martinez Urrutia MJ, Jaureguizar E. Initial and long-term management of posterior urethral valves. World J Urol. 2004;22(6):418–24.
34. Hanson GR, Gatti JM, Gittes GK, Murphy JP. Diagnosis of ectopic ureter as a cause of urinary incontinence. J Pediatr Urol. 2007;3(1):53–7.
35. Burgers R, Liem O, Canon S, Mousa H, Benninga MA, Di Lorenzo C, et al. Effect of rectal distention on lower urinary tract function in children. J Urol. 2010;184(suppl 4):1680–5.
36. Vincent SA. Postural control of urinary incontinence: the curtsey sign. Lancet. 1966;2:631–2.

37. Kim JH, Lee JH, Jung AY, Lee JW. The prevalence and therapeutic effect of constipation in pediatric overactive bladder. Int Neurourol J. 2011;15(4):206–10.
38. Söderström U, Hoelcke M, Alenius L, Söderling A-C, Hjern A. Urinary and faecal incontinence: a population-based study. Acta Paediatr. 2004;93:386–9.
39. von Gontard A, Baeyens D, Van Hoecke E, Warzak WJ, Bachmann C. Psychological and psychiatric issues in urinary and fecal incontinence. J Urol. 2011;185(6):2303–7.
40. Hägglöf B, Andrén O, Bergström E, Marklund L, Wendelius M. Self-esteem before and after treatment in children with nocturnal enuresis and urinary incontinence. Scand J Urol Nephrol. 1997;31(Suppl 183):79–82.
41. Van Herzeele C, Dhondt K, Roels SP, Raes A, Groen LA, Hoebeke P, et al. Neuropsychological functioning related to specific characteristics of nocturnal enuresis. J Pediatr Urol. 2015;11(4):208.e1–6.

Neurogenic Bladder: Myelomeningocele, Occult Spina Bifida, and Tethered Cord

13

Pieter Dik, Laetitia M.O. de Kort, and Paul W. Veenboer

13.1 History of Spina Bifida

Hippocrates (460–370 B.C.) described the condition that we know as spina bifida [1]. The Amsterdam physician and anatomist Nicolaes Tulp was the first to describe the clinical symptoms of spina bifida in terms of skeletal deformation and was the first to coin the Latin name [2]. The Italian Giovanni Morgagni (1682–1777) described hydrocephalus in relation to spina bifida [1]. The German doctor Rudolf Virchow (1821–1902) discovered occult spina bifida. Hans Chiari (1851–1916) described in 1891 the abnormalities in the brain: the descent of the cerebellum in the fossa posterior [1]. Thanks to the improvement of neurosurgical techniques (e.g., brain shunting) in the 1960s, survival during early childhood [3] has improved drastically. In 1965 the British pediatrician Richard Smithells published that a deficiency in folic acid plays an important role in developing spina bifida [4]. During the 1970s, the American urologist Jack Lapides (1914–1995) developed clean intermittent catheterization (CIC) to treat persistent infections in the urinary tract [5]. Later, in the 1980s, CIC was widely applied to evacuate urine in neuropathic bladder patients with amazing results to prevent kidney damage [6].

P. Dik (✉)
Department of Pediatric Urology, Wilhelmina Children's Hospital, Utrecht, The Netherlands
e-mail: p.dik@umcutrecht.nl

L.M.O. de Kort • P.W. Veenboer
Department of Urology, University Medical Center Utrecht, Utrecht, The Netherlands

In recent years, it has become possible to close spina bifida prenatally. This was described in the MOMS study that was done in Philadelphia by the team of Dr. Nick Scott Adzick [7]. It became clear that brain shunts are less needed in the follow-up of this cohort although the long-term urological outcome is not clear yet and must not be overestimated at this point.

> Although the incidence of spina bifida now seems to decrease because of prenatal detection and abortion, spinal dysraphism and neuropathic bladder problems will still occur in patients who are affected with closed forms of spinal dysraphism, e.g., Currarino syndrome, lipomeningomyelocele, tethered cord syndrome, and VACTRL syndrome with anorectal malformations and sacral dysplasia or absent sacrum.

13.2 Aims of Treatment

13.2.1 Bladder

Treatment is directed to preservation of bladder and kidney function [8]. As long as bladder volume with low pressures is achieved, kidney function will be fine. Low pressures are possible by using antimuscarinic medication or in some cases operations. Intermittent catheterization is needed to ensure proper bladder evacuation. In most cases, it is possible to become dry in between catheterizations, although some incontinence may remain during transfers of straining [9].

13.2.2 Kidneys

Try to avoid feverish urinary infections, and if they occur, immediate action (broad-spectrum antibiotics) is required [10]. We think vesicoureteral reflux requires correction, especially in dilating upper tracts or recurrent pyelonephritis.

In order to estimate original kidney function, a DMSA scan can be performed when the child is still young. It has been shown that DMSA is more reliable than ultrasonography in showing renal damage in patients with spina bifida [11]. This can be repeated later in life, e.g., in puberty, for final evaluation of possible kidney damage [12].

13.2.3 Bowel

Colonic washouts have improved the quality of life in spina bifida patients [13].

From the age of 3–4 years, the technique of colon flushing is taught in order to plan the timing for evacuation of stool. Washouts can be done daily or every other day. This enables the patient to become pseudo-continent for feces. Due to irrigation of the rectum, the water together with the feces is washed out. Normal tap water can be used.

In sporadic cases, we have experienced that it is useful to make a salty water solution (NaCl 0.9%) for patients who experience pain during the colon flushing.

13.3 How to Perform Follow-Up?

13.3.1 Early After Birth

We recommend the following schedule shortly after birth:

1. Indwelling catheter until after surgery (closing of the meningomyelocele).
2. Start using oxybutynin (oral) medication three times daily (0.13 mg/kg).
3. Start using trimethoprim prophylaxis (2 mg/kg).
4. After operative closure of meningomyelocele, start teaching the parents intermittent catheterization as soon as the patient may be turned onto the back.
5. Ultrasound of the kidneys to exclude congenital abnormalities (agenesis, dysplasia, ectopia, dual systems, etc.).

In very rare cases, kidney dilation is seen shortly after birth. Generally dilatation occurs after several months in untreated patients [14]. Urodynamic examination shortly after birth is not meaningful because of spinal shock and/or as a result of the operation: the innervation of the bladder and pelvic floor can still change [8].

First urodynamic study therefore takes place after 3 months to see if a safe situation exists under the set therapy (oxybutynin and CIC). A video-urodynamic study (VUDS) is preferably carried out, also to exclude possible vesicoureteral reflux. Around that time an ultrasound study of the kidneys is performed in order to determine if there is dilation of one or both kidneys.

In the follow-up process, an urodynamic study (UDS) must be done after stopping oxybutynin for 2 days. This UDS is used for correct urodynamic diagnosis (overactivity of detrusor, hyperactivity of sphincter, dyssynergia between detrusor and sphincter complex). The first UDS is needed to evaluate whether a safe situation is achieved in the initial months [8].

13.3.2 First Years of Life

In the first 2 years, we recommend that the patient is monitored every 3 months. From the third year of life, this may be reduced to once every 6 months. From the 10th year of life, follow-up can be done annually. Ultrasound examination of the kidneys should be performed regularly.

Note that the dosage of oxybutynin needs always to be adjusted to the weight!

13.3.3 School Age

Pay attention to a CIC stoma for wheelchair-bound patients and especially for girls. At a certain moment, most girls do not want to be catheterized by varying caretakers. If an indication for a stoma exists, careful briefing about various channels including an antegrade colonic washout stoma should be given. Sometimes it is necessary to combine this surgery with bladder neck surgery and/or bladder augmentation.

13.3.4 Adolescents

The prospects for spina bifida patients continue to improve although the results must be viewed over the long term. In this respect Hunt and Woodhouse regularly advised caution in their publications [9, 15]. Adolescents tend to ignore good advice, and they are prone to postpone intermittent catheterizations especially when they can retain their urine because of successful bladder neck surgery and/or bladder augmentation surgery [16].

> Adolescents still need continuous supervision and coaching especially when they move out and parents and caretakers are far away to prevent upper tract deterioration.

13.3.5 Laboratory Tests

Laboratory tests are regularly performed: routine urinalysis and urine culture.

Creatinine in the serum is often unreliable (as a result of reduced muscle function) but is an important parameter when it is increased! [17]. Liver function should be monitored during prolonged use of trimethoprim. Prolonged use of antibiotics can cause side effects (e.g., chronic use of nitrofurantoin).

In children with an ileocystoplasty, bicarbonate should be tested (if necessary, bicarbonate should be supplied). Note that serum bicarbonate levels may suddenly be very low in cases of an infected bladder augment, probably due to hyperemia of the mucosa during infection [18].

13.4 Medication

13.4.1 Antibiotics

Antibiotic prophylaxis (trimethoprim 2 mg/kg or nitrofurantoin 2 mg/kg) may be stopped just in about 50% of the cases in the course of time [19]. Usually, bacteriuria does not lead to a true or dangerous infection because—thanks to intermittent catheterization—the infected urine is being drained away from the bladder regularly, exactly as Jack Lapides originally described [5]. However, caution is advised in patients with moderate compliance of the bladder and in patients with dilated upper urinary tract and/or vesicoureteral reflux [20]. In case of high fever during urinary infections, a broad-spectrum antibiotic should be administered intravenously.

In case of recurrent infections, it can be recommended to use a combination therapy: nitrofurantoin and trimethoprim prophylaxis alternated every other day. With this strategy, it is possible to suppress bacterial growth for many years thus avoiding prophylaxis with broad-spectrum antibiotics. However, this is our personal experience, and there is no evidence to support this.

Sometimes a bladder instillation with 2% betadine solution or chlorhexidine may be used in case of recurrent infections with resistant microorganisms, although this is not scientifically proven. Gentamycin bladder instillation is also possible, but be aware of high serum levels after repeated instillations [21].

The use of cranberries is questionable, and there is uncertainty about the right dose [22].

13.4.2 Anticholinergic Medication

Note that the dosage of oxybutynin must always be adjusted to the weight!

For children, also tolterodine and solifenacin can be used in adjusted dosages although these medications are not registered for use in children [23].

Capsaicin and related substances are as of yet not practically usable to treat neurogenic bladder [24] and cannot be used in children in the long term; oxybutynin did not seem to cause behavioral problems in one case-control study [25].

13.4.3 Combinations of Medication

In some cases, it was proven to be effective to combine oxybutynin and solifenacin or tolterodine [26].

In our experience, a combination of mirabegron and oxybutynin could also be effective in some cases. In a first study from 2016, the combination appeared to be safe and effective in children with overactive bladder [27]. Note that mirabegron is not yet registered for children!

13.4.4 Intravesical Therapy

Some children have many side effects of oral oxybutynin medication: drowsiness, dry mouth (and thereby increased risk of dental caries), heat accumulation (diminished sweat production), and fatigue. In those cases, intravesical administration of oxybutynin can be started [28]. The same dosage (as in oral) is maintained above; any overdose is not harmful. Use a standard solution 1 mg/mL. This can be applied with a syringe into the bladder with a so-called Luer-Lock bladder catheter onto which a syringe with medication is connected. In order to deliver the entire dose in the bladder reliably, some air is injected to flush the catheter lumen completely. By avoiding the first-pass effect, five times less des-ethyl-oxybutynin (DEOB) is bioavailable. DEOB is the major metabolite of oxybutynin responsible for the side effects [29]. The bioavailability of oxybutynin itself after intravesical administration is approximately three times higher compared to oral administration [30]. This may have implications for central side effects as oxybutynin is a lipophilic molecule and can penetrate the blood-brain barrier.

13.4.5 Botulin Toxin

An alternative is administration of botulinum toxin, of which onabotulinumtoxinA (Botox®) is the most commonly used form. This medication should be injected into the detrusor muscle. This is a procedure performed under general anesthesia. Botox® is an expensive drug, and its use and application are limited within hospital budgets. The duration of the effect varies between 3 and 9 months [31]. Some cases of systemic side effects (general muscle weakness) have already been described [32]. Note that the manufacturer of Botox® (Allergan) officially discourages the use of botulinum toxin in children [33].

13.5 Surgical Options

From school age (6 years), continence surgery may be suggested. This may include an ileocystoplasty, possibly (in experienced hands) a detrusorectomy [8]. A fascial sling (from the fascia of the rectus abdominis) can be applied to elevate the bladder neck, with which up until 80% (social) dryness could be achieved in one study [34].

For wheelchair-bound patients, a catheterizable stoma between umbilicus and bladder can be offered. An antegrade colonic enema stoma (ACE) can be made in the colon by cutting off the top of the appendix, attaching the open end into the skin [35].

In rare cases, a temporary vesico-vaginal fistula could be made if parents refuse to perform CIC, while the bladder is poorly compliant and high bladder pressure is present. Later in life, the fistula can be repaired when augmentation surgery is required.

13.5.1 Sling, Detrusorectomy, and Ileocystoplasty

These procedures are summarized in Fig. 13.1. Detrusorectomy is only possible in cases with a poorly compliant bladder but almost normal bladder volume [36]. This operation will be combined with bladder neck sling in most cases. Success rate for improvement of compliance is only 50% in experienced hands [37].

13.5.2 Various CIC Channels and ACE Stoma

These operations are summarized in Fig. 13.2.

Note that in case of combining the formation of a CIC stoma with an ileocystoplasty, a simple modification provides a safe long stoma with protected embedded blood supply.

In some cases, it is possible to create an ACE stoma and CIC stoma out of a long suitable appendix, just by dividing the appendix in half.

13.5.3 Complications and Solutions

Bladder rupture may occur when patients postpone CIC [18]. This condition is often missed by general pediatricians. Indeed, free abdominal fluid is present in most spina bifida patients because of the peritoneal brain shunt. Most of the bladder

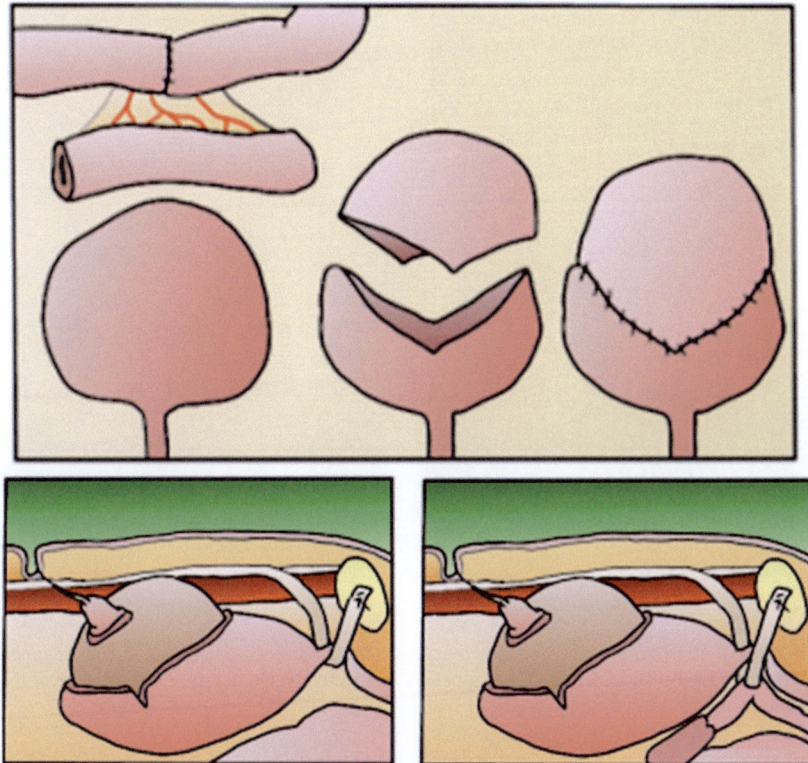

Fig. 13.1 Ileocystoplasy and continent urostomy

ruptures will heal after an indwelling catheter for several days and high-dosage broad-spectrum antibiotics.

Stomal stenosis occurs in more than 50% of the CIC channels. This could be prevented by using an indwelling ACE plug for a year or sometimes longer [38].

A stricture in a stoma canal can best be dilated using McCrea sounds: without any force, dilatation is feasible in most cases. An indwelling catheter for a few days is needed after the procedure. Sometimes it is helpful to use topical corticosteroid crème that can be administered as a layer onto the ACE stopper [38].

> Never put a catheter with an inflated balloon in a continent CIC stoma: this will destroy the tunnel, and this will lead to leakage of urine!

13.5.4 Overtreatment

In some cases, especially in occult spina bifida, it may be concluded after several years that overtreatment has taken place. In only a small minority of all spina bifida,

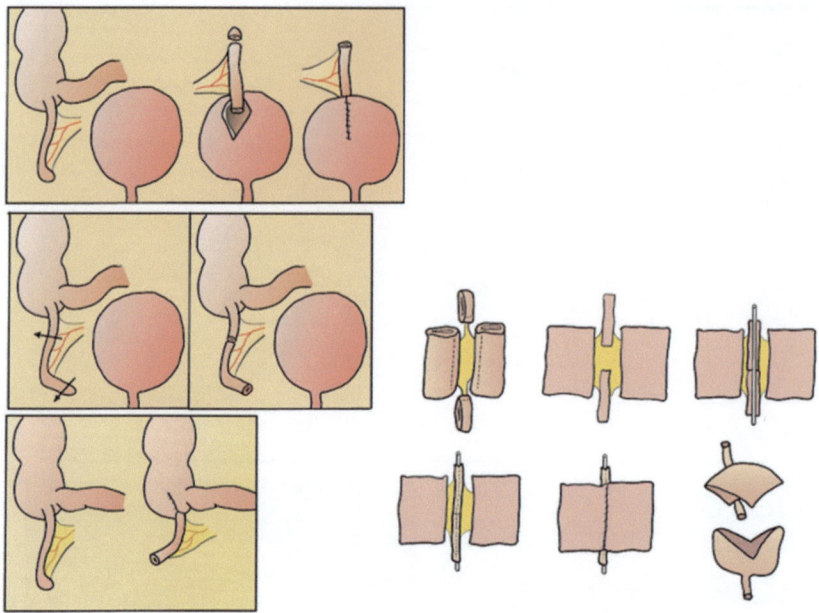

Fig. 13.2 Left: construction of a appendicovesicostomy and antegrade colonic enema-channell (ACE) by using the tip and the base of the appendix, respectively. On the right, the principe of the double Monti-tube is shown

normal voiding and continence are possible on the long term without medication or clean intermittent catheterization [39]. In the majority of patients, CIC and anticholinergics will remain necessary; in one large series of 144 patients, CIC and anticholinergics could only safely be stopped in 22/144 (15.2%), the majority of whom had a form of spina bifida occulta [6]. In another study, detrusor overactivity immediately returned after stopping antimuscarinic drugs [40].

Of particular complexity are those patients with spina bifida occulta and low sacral lesions, in which either the bladder stimulating motor neuron in S2–S3 or the bladder inhibiting Onuf nucleus is involved or both nuclei are damaged, which explains the unpredictable outcome of these spinal lesions. Our goal is to prevent possible damage to the kidneys in early life. That is why in all patients early treatment has to be started soon after birth if possible. Later the therapy can and will be adjusted based on findings with urodynamic studies.

Patients who have a safe bladder with low pressures because of a low leak point pressure run a low risk of upper tract dilatation or renal deterioration. However, also these patients may benefit to be catheterized because 1 day they will need a sling operation to become dry.

> The level of the spinal lesion will not always determine the severity of neurogenic bladder problems. Often the lesion is very asymmetrical. Therefore treatment of spina bifida always needs to be customized.

13.6 Urodynamic Studies

Urodynamic study (UDS) does not need to be repeated every year [41]. Every 2 or 3 years this is advised. And of course, UDS must be performed in changing parameters, e.g., when bladder volume suddenly decreases, incontinence occurs or worsens, or dilation of the kidneys occurs [41] – in short, when "bladder behavior" seems to change.

13.6.1 VUDS and UDS

In most cases, UDS without fluoroscopy will be sufficient for follow-up. However, in case of upper tract dilatation, video-urodynamic study (VUDS) is advocated in order to exclude or demonstrate high-grade reflux and also to estimate the bladder pressure at the moment of ureteral reflux [42]. VUDS is also useful to determine leak point pressure and the status of the bladder neck prior to bladder neck surgery or sling operation. Prior to these operations, also a new stop test is advised, meaning that the anticholinergic will be stopped shortly before the UDS. Then it can be decided whether an augmentation is also needed or that antimuscarinic therapy will be continued.

13.6.2 Pitfalls of UDS in Spinal Dysraphism

It is widely accepted that bladder pressures over 40 cm H_2O are harmful to upper tracts in the long run [43, 44]. However it must be emphasized that bladder volume has to be taken in account when bladder pressure is over 40 cm H_2O. It is clear that such a bladder pressure will not harm at a bladder volume of more than 400 mL because the patient should have emptied the bladder by that time by CIC. However, if these pressures occur at a bladder volume of less than 300 mL, one should be more cautious. This is illustrated in Fig. 13.3. But adolescents tend to postpone catheterization to dangerous limits.

In many publications, the term "poor compliance" is used. This can be confusing because in many cases the compliance is estimated on end-filling pressure. It would be more appropriate to observe bladder pressure at bladder volumes that are similar to the volumes that are measured with CIC at home. Figure 13.4 illustrates the difference between a normal compliance with high end-filling pressure and a bad compliance with high end-filling pressure. Figure 13.5 shows a typical overactive bladder that needs to be treated with medication. In Fig. 13.6, you see a typical bad compliance of scarred bladder with poor volume and high pressure in a patient that needs an ileocystoplasty.

Almost all SB patients have a small torso. Therefore the usual equation for children

$$\text{Expected bladder volume cc} = (30 \times \text{age}) + 30\,\text{cc}$$

is not applicable in patients with spina bifida: a smaller volume than expected for age may be normal.

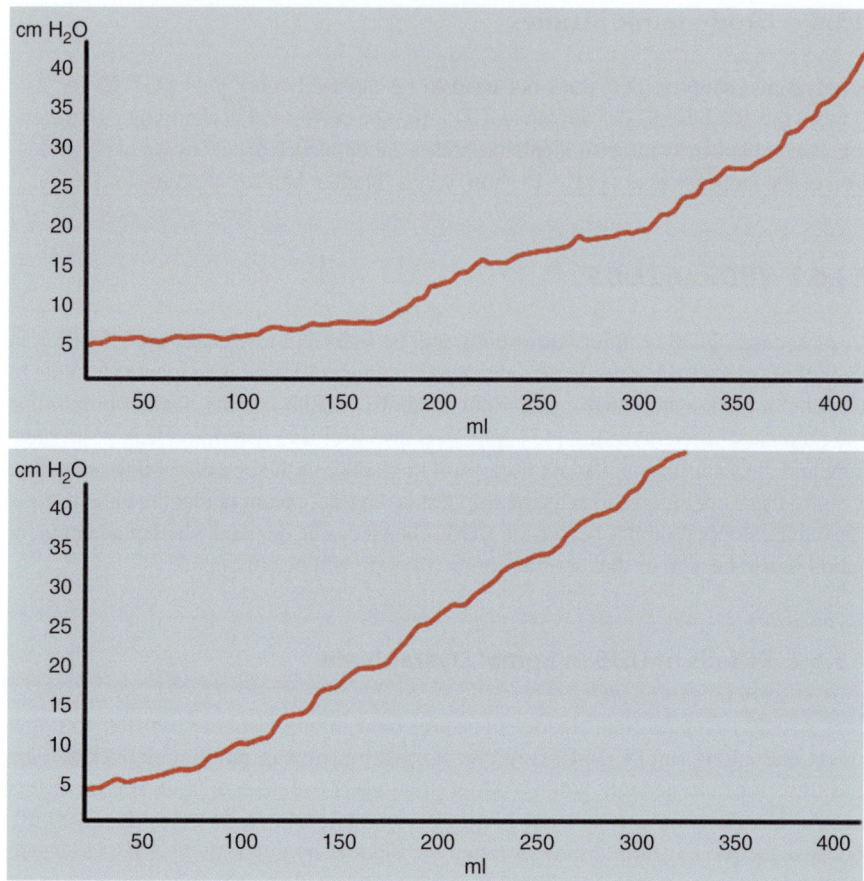

Fig. 13.3 In the upper graph, high detrusor pressures only occur at high volumes, in which low pressures can be achieved by emptying the bladder in time. In the the lower graph, there is a steady rise in pressure from the beginning of bladder filling onwards, which poses a much more dangerous situation

High pressure may occur in tethering or bladder deterioration in under treatment of infections and/or bladder contractions. Repeating of UDS after antibiotic treatment and/or higher dosage of antimuscarinics is advocated. In case of persistent high pressures, further diagnostics (e.g., MRI and consultation of a neurologist) are needed. Measurement of bladder volume at home is advised. It is very easy to estimate a bladder pressure at home, just by keeping the tube of the catheter in a upright position and measuring the length of the water column with a ruler.

13.7 Adolescents and Adults with Spina Bifida

13.7.1 Sexuality

It is very difficult to speak about this subject with an adolescent spina bifida patient. There is often a problem with sensibility, lubrication, and erections [45]. However, in a survey of young adults, it is reported that spina bifida patients have missed

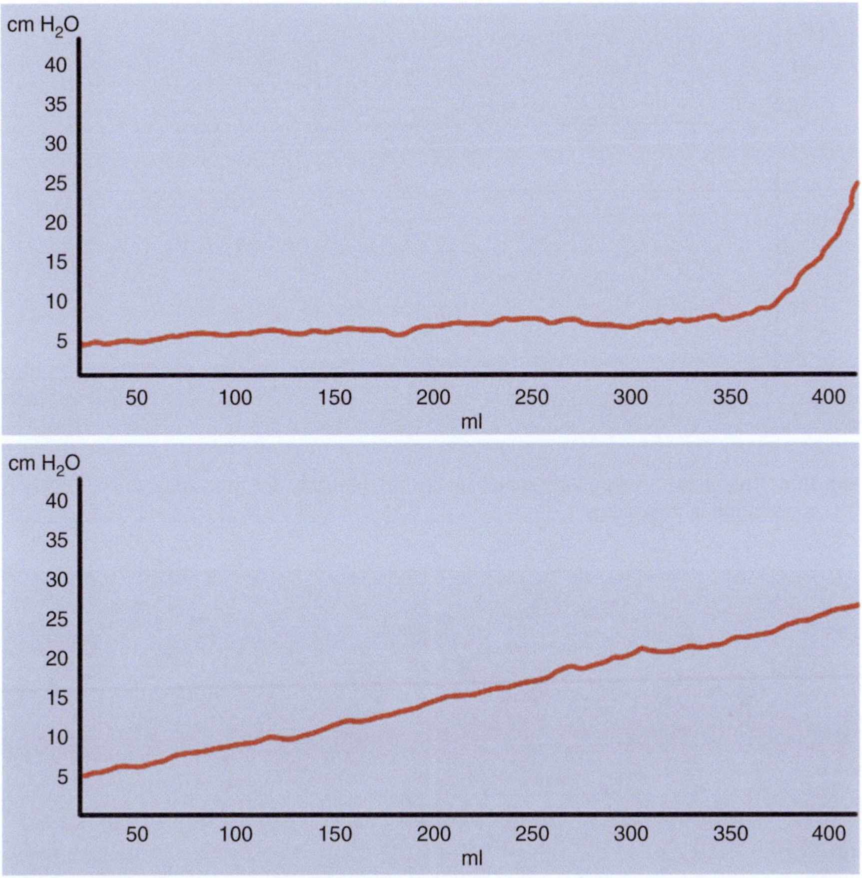

Fig. 13.4 The graph on top shows essentially a fine compliance; only at high volumes, compliance gets worse because the bladder is simply 'full'. A different situation in shown in the lower graph, in which there is a truely poor compliance

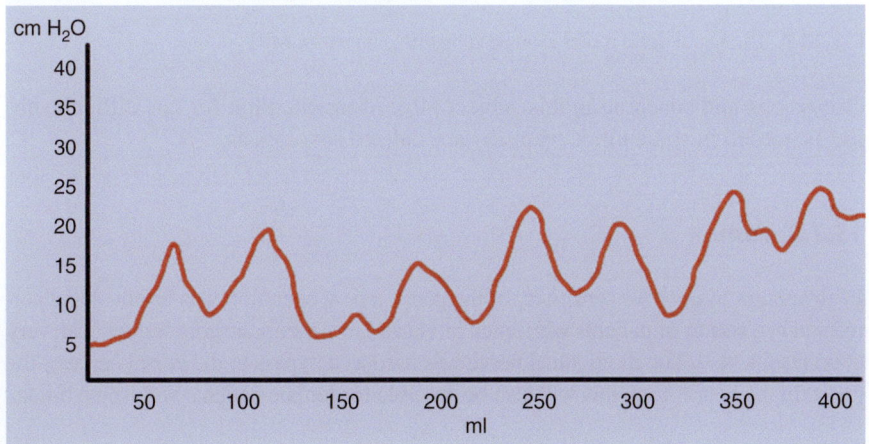

Fig. 13.5 A combination of poor compiance and overactivity

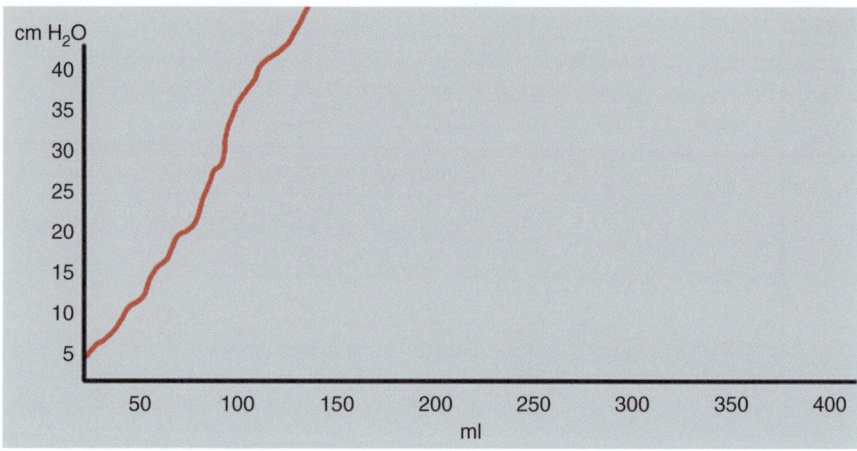

Fig. 13.6 This shows a very poorly compliant bladder, probably due to scarring; often, surgery is the only solution in these cases

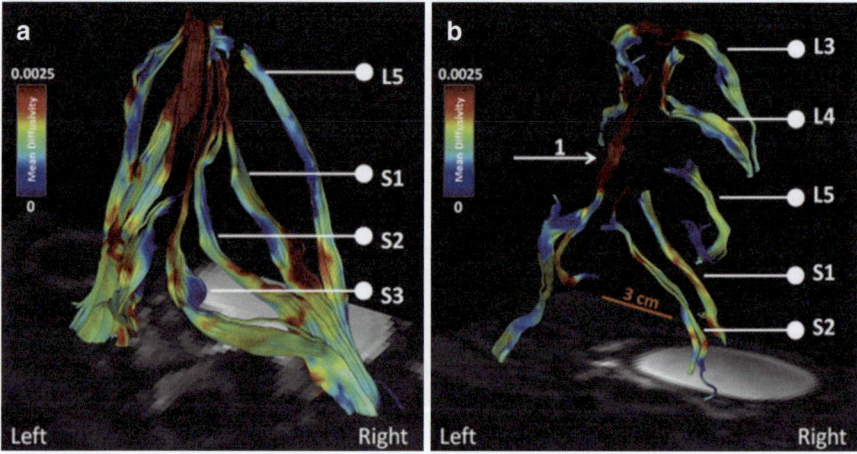

Fig. 13.7 The sacral nerve routes as imaged by diffusion tensor MRI

discussions and coaching in this subject [46]. More attention for this difficult subject is needed in spina bifida teams by specialized sexologists.

13.7.2 Tomax

In an attempt to improve sensitivity of the penis, a new operation was invented and performed in a cohort of patients with spina bifida and low traumatic cord lesions with very good results [47]. The ilioinguinal nerve was used as a bypass to the dorsal nerve of the penis. In the near future, this will also be possible for female patients with spina bifida.

13.7.3 Future Perspectives

MRI DTI of sacral nerves has shown to demonstrate the abnormal anatomy of the spinal roots in spina bifida patients as is shown in Fig. 13.7 [48]. Maybe in the (near) future, these advanced imaging techniques will make it possible to select nerves for neuroanastomoses in order to reconnect innervation to the bladder and pelvic floor or to apply selective nerve modulation and stimulation with smart implantable chips or pacemakers.

Undoubtedly therapy of spinal lesions will change in the coming years.

Conclusion

With the above policy, it might be possible to protect all spina bifida patients from terminal kidney damage. However, sometimes renal scars may still occur due to pyelonephritis in breakthrough infections, but none of the patients will need a kidney transplant or dialysis program. In case of renal scars, lifelong follow-up for blood pressure control is required.

Maintaining low bladder pressures is of the utmost importance. Continuous follow-up over many years is of great importance in the course of time. Symptoms suddenly can worsen by tethering of spinal roots and also as a result of poor therapy compliance during or after puberty.

References

1. Smith GK. The history of spina bifida, hydrocephalus, paraplegia, and incontinence. Pediatr Surg Int. 2001;17(5–6):424–32.
2. Simpson D. Nicolaes Tulp and the golden age of the Dutch Republic. ANZ J Surg. 2007;77(12):1095–101.
3. Akalan N. Myelomeningocele (open spina bifida) - surgical management. Adv Tech Stand Neurosurg. 2011;37:113–41.
4. Schorah C. Dick Smithells, folic acid, and the prevention of neural tube defects. Birth Defects Res A Clin Mol Teratol. 2009;85(4):254–9.
5. Lapides J, Diokno AC, Silber SJ, Lowe BS. Clean, intermittent self-catheterization in the treatment of urinary tract disease. J Urol. 1972;107(3):458–61.
6. Dik P, Klijn AJ, van Gool JD, de Jong-de Vos van Steenwijk CC, de Jong TP. Early start to therapy preserves kidney function in spina bifida patients. Eur Urol. 2006;49(5):908–13.
7. Adzick NS, Thom EA, Spong CY, Brock JW 3rd, Burrows PK, Johnson MP, et al. A randomized trial of prenatal versus postnatal repair of myelomeningocele. N Engl J Med. 2011;364(11):993–1004.
8. de Jong TP, Chrzan R, Klijn AJ, Dik P. Treatment of the neurogenic bladder in spina bifida. Pediatr Nephrol. 2008;23(6):889–96.
9. Woodhouse CR. Myelomeningocele in young adults. BJU Int. 2005;95(2):223–30.
10. Coulthard MG, Verber I, Jani JC, Lawson GR, Stuart CA, Sharma V, et al. Can prompt treatment of childhood UTI prevent kidney scarring? Pediatr Nephrol. 2009;24(10):2059–63.
11. Veenboer PW, Hobbelink MG, Ruud Bosch JL, Dik P, van Asbeck FW, Beek FJ, et al. Diagnostic accuracy of Tc-99m DMSA scintigraphy and renal ultrasonography for detecting renal scarring and relative function in patients with spinal dysraphism. Neurourol Urodyn. 2015;34(6):513–8.

12. Filler G, Gharib M, Casier S, Lodige P, Ehrich JH, Dave S. Prevention of chronic kidney disease in spina bifida. Int Urol Nephrol. 2012;44(3):817–27.
13. Choi EK, Shin SH, Im YJ, Kim MJ, Han SW. The effects of transanal irrigation as a stepwise bowel management program on the quality of life of children with spina bifida and their caregivers. Spinal Cord. 2013;51(5):384–8.
14. Bauer SB, Joseph DB. Management of the obstructed urinary tract associated with neurogenic bladder dysfunction. Urol Clin North Am. 1990;17(2):395–406.
15. Oakeshott P, Hunt GM, Poulton A, Reid F. Expectation of life and unexpected death in open spina bifida: a 40-year complete, non-selective, longitudinal cohort study. Dev Med Child Neurol. 2010;52(8):749–53.
16. Woodhouse CR, Neild GH, RN Y, Bauer S. Adult care of children from pediatric urology. J Urol. 2012;187(4):1164–71.
17. Ahmad I, Granitsiotis P. Urological follow-up of adult spina bifida patients. Neurourol Urodyn. 2007;26(7):978–80.
18. Husmann DA. Long-term complications following bladder augmentations in patients with spina bifida: bladder calculi, perforation of the augmented bladder and upper tract deterioration. Transl Androl Urol. 2016;5(1):3–11.
19. Zegers B, Uiterwaal C, Kimpen J, van Gool J, de Jong T, Winkler-Seinstra P, et al. Antibiotic prophylaxis for urinary tract infections in children with spina bifida on intermittent catheterization. J Urol. 2011;186(6):2365–70.
20. Robinson JL, Finlay JC, Lang ME, Bortolussi R, Canadian Paediatric Society, Community Paediatrics Committee, Infectious Diseases and Immunization Committee. Prophylactic antibiotics for children with recurrent urinary tract infections. Paediatr Child Health. 2015;20(1):45–7.
21. Defoor W, Ferguson D, Mashni S, Creelman L, Reeves D, Minevich E, et al. Safety of gentamicin bladder irrigations in complex urological cases. J Urol. 2006;175(5):1861–4.
22. Durham SH, Stamm PL, Eiland LS. Cranberry products for the prophylaxis of urinary tract infections in pediatric patients. Ann Pharmacother. 2015;49(12):1349–56.
23. Blais AS, Bergeron M, Nadeau G, Ramsay S, Bolduc S. Anticholinergic use in children: persistence and patterns of therapy. Can Urol Assoc J. 2016;10(3–4):137–40.
24. Dorsher PT, McIntosh PM. Neurogenic bladder. Adv Urol. 2012;2012:816274. https://doi.org/10.1155/2012/816274.
25. Veenboer PW, Huisman J, Chrzan RJ, Kuijper CF, Dik P, de Kort LM, et al. Behavioral effects of long-term antimuscarinic use in patients with spinal dysraphism: a case control study. J Urol. 2013;190(6):2228–32.
26. Nardulli R, Losavio E, Ranieri M, Fiore P, Megna G, Bellomo RG, et al. Combined antimuscarinics for treatment of neurogenic overactive bladder. Int J Immunopathol Pharmacol. 2012;25(1 Suppl):35S–41S.
27. Morin F, Blais AS, Nadeau G, Moore K, Genois L, Bolduc S. Dual therapy for refractory overactive bladder in children: a prospective open-label study. J Urol. 2017;197(4):1158–63.
28. Buyse G, Waldeck K, Verpoorten C, Bjork H, Casaer P, Andersson KE. Intravesical oxybutynin for neurogenic bladder dysfunction: less systemic side effects due to reduced first pass metabolism. J Urol. 1998;160(3 Pt 1):892–6.
29. Staskin DR, Salvatore S. Oxybutynin topical and transdermal formulations: an update. Drugs Today (Barc). 2010;46(6):417–25.
30. Krause P, Fuhr U, Schnitker J, Albrecht U, Stein R, Rubenwolf P. Pharmacokinetics of intravesical versus oral oxybutynin in healthy adults: results of an open label, randomized, prospective clinical study. J Urol. 2013;190(5):1791–7.
31. Scheepe JR, Blok BF, 't Hoen LA. Applicability of botulinum toxin type A in paediatric neurogenic bladder management. Curr Opin Urol. 2017;27(1):14–9.
32. Del Popolo G, Filocamo MT, Li Marzi V, Macchiarella A, Cecconi F, Lombardi G, et al. Neurogenic detrusor overactivity treated with english botulinum toxin a: 8-year experience of one single centre. Eur Urol. 2008;53(5):1013–9.

33. Highlights of prescribing information [Internet]. Available from: https://www.allergan.com/assets/pdf/botox_pi.pdf.
34. Dik P, Klijn AJ, van Gool JD, de Jong TP. Transvaginal sling suspension of bladder neck in female patients with neurogenic sphincter incontinence. J Urol. 2003;170(2 Pt 1):580,1. discussion 581-2
35. Saikaly SK, Rich MA, Swana HS. Assessment of pediatric Malone antegrade continence enema (MACE) complications: effects of variations in technique. J Pediatr Urol. 2016;12(4):246. e1–6.
36. Veenboer PW, Nadorp S, de Jong TP, Dik P, van Asbeck FW, Bosch JL, et al. Enterocystoplasty vs detrusorectomy: outcome in the adult with spina bifida. J Urol. 2013;189(3):1066–70.
37. Dik P, Tsachouridis GD, Klijn AJ, Uiterwaal CS, de Jong TP. Detrusorectomy for neuropathic bladder in patients with spinal dysraphism. J Urol. 2003;170(4 Pt 1):1351–4.
38. Polm PD, de Kort, Laetitia M. O., de Jong, Tom P. V. M., Dik P. Langetermijn follow-up van katheteriseerbare vesicostomaâ€™s bij kinderen, een vergelijking van verschillende technieken. Tijdschr Urol. 2017:1–4.
39. Veenboer PW, Bosch JL, van Asbeck FW, de Kort LM. Upper and lower urinary tract outcomes in adult myelomeningocele patients: a systematic review. PLoS One. 2012;7(10):e48399.
40. Ab E, Dik P, Klijn AJ, van Gool JD, de Jong TP. Detrusor overactivity in spina bifida: how long does it need to be treated? Neurourol Urodyn. 2004;23(7):685–8.
41. Veenboer PW, Bosch JL, Rosier PF, Dik P, van Asbeck FW, de Jong TP, et al. Cross-sectional study of determinants of upper and lower urinary tract outcomes in adults with spinal dysraphism--new recommendations for urodynamic followup guidelines? J Urol. 2014;192(2):477–82.
42. Marks BK, Goldman HB. Videourodynamics: indications and technique. Urol Clin North Am. 2014;41(3):383,91, vii-viii.
43. McGuire EJ, Woodside JR, Borden TA. Upper urinary tract deterioration in patients with myelodysplasia and detrusor hypertonia: a followup study. J Urol. 1983;129(4):823–6.
44. Snow-Lisy DC, Yerkes EB, Cheng EY. Update on urological management of spina bifida from prenatal diagnosis to adulthood. J Urol. 2015;194(2):288–96.
45. von Linstow ME, Biering-Sorensen I, Liebach A, Lind M, Seitzberg A, Hansen RB, et al. Spina bifida and sexuality. J Rehabil Med. 2014;46(9):891–7.
46. Verhoef M, Barf HA, Vroege JA, Post MW, Van Asbeck FW, Gooskens RH, et al. Sex education, relationships, and sexuality in young adults with spina bifida. Arch Phys Med Rehabil. 2005;86(5):979–87.
47. Overgoor ML, de Jong TP, Cohen-Kettenis PT, Edens MA, Kon M. Increased sexual health after restored genital sensation in male patients with spina bifida or a spinal cord injury: the TOMAX procedure. J Urol. 2013;189(2):626–32.
48. Haakma W, Dik P, ten Haken B, Froeling M, Nievelstein RA, Cuppen I, et al. Diffusion tensor magnetic resonance imaging and fiber tractography of the sacral plexus in children with spina bifida. J Urol. 2014;192(3):927–33.

Spinal Cord Injury and Iatrogenic Lesions

14

Giulio Del Popolo and Elena Tur

14.1 Introduction

Traumatic spinal cord injury is a dramatic event in the lives of men and women; it changes the motor and functional control of the body. The impact of an acquired spinal cord lesion in children and adolescents, during a delicate phase of their physiological body development, is a hard issue to manage. This represents a lifelong change for patients and their family life. Few centers in the world are dedicated to the management of this condition in pediatric patients, to address their needs and continue follow-up with the patient and family through to adulthood. Then transitional care is necessary to guarantee continuous treatment without fragmentation that could pose risks of psychological and physical complications, which need to be prevented because they are not easy to resolve.

14.2 Epidemiology

Spinal cord injury (SCI) is a traumatic condition, which can lead to sensory and motor disorganization of the normal physiology of internal organs and systems, and really changes mental and psychological issues, and social well-being as well. In children, SCI is less common than in adults and occurs in approximately 1.5–5% of cases [1, 2]. Statistical data and reviews show that the incidence of SCI increases with age [3]. The level of injury differs depending on the age category, with C2 vertebral lesions tending to occur in preteens, C4 lesions tending to occur in teenagers, and C4–C5 lesions tending to occur in adults [2]. In one series, violent etiologies (especially gunshot wounds) accounted for a significant proportion of preteen injuries (19% versus 12% in adults) [3].

G. Del Popolo (✉) • E. Tur
Neuro-Urology and Spinal Unit, Careggi University Hospital, Florence, Italy

© Springer International Publishing AG, part of Springer Nature 2018
G. Mosiello et al. (eds.), *Clinical Urodynamics in Childhood and Adolescence*,
Urodynamics, Neurourology and Pelvic Floor Dysfunctions,
https://doi.org/10.1007/978-3-319-42193-3_14

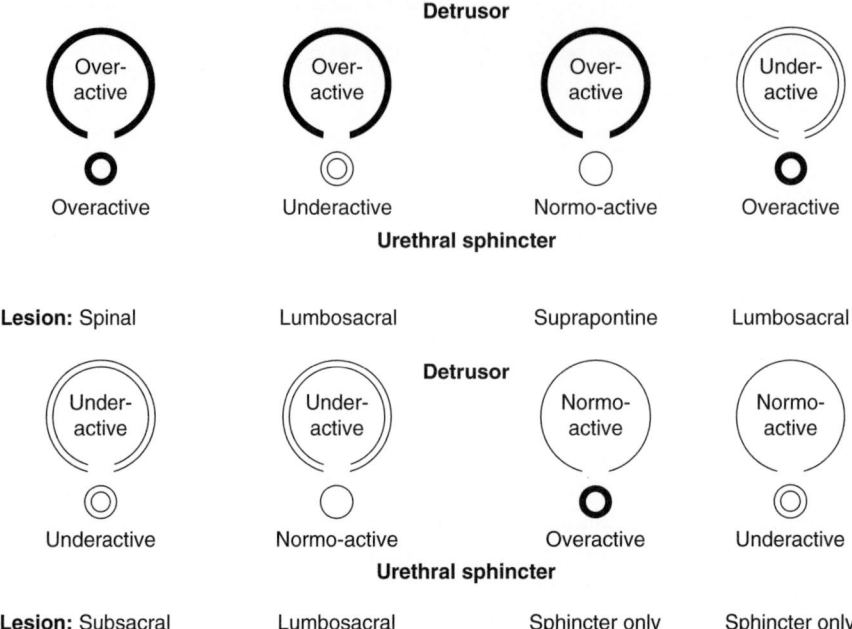

Fig. 14.1 (Source: adapted from EAU Guidelines 2015) Madersbacher classification urodynamic patterns in neuro-urological patients

There are two main mechanisms of SCI injury in pediatric patients. The motor vehicle accident mechanism is more common in young children, while in adolescents the most common mechanism is a sports injury [4]. Most studies report a large predominance of males in comparison with females [2, 4–9].

It is believed that neurological rehabilitation occurs faster in pediatric patients than in adults [9]; however, there are no accurate data to support this belief [3].

In both children and adults after SCI, bladder control is usually damaged, with typical dysfunction involving urinary retention and urinary incontinence, and a high risk of upper urinary tract infection.

On the basis of the neurological level and degree of SCI, bladder sphincter outcomes have traditionally been divided into two main urological clinical scenarios secondary to suprasacral and/or sacral lesions, but various different types of bladder sphincter dysfunction are based on urodynamic patterns as described by Madersbacher (Fig. 14.1).

14.3 Suprasacral Spinal Cord Lesions

Traumatic suprasacral SCI results in an initial period of spinal shock, during which there is detrusor acontractility (DA). After that, the interruption of nerve transmission from the pontine micturition center (PMC) to the sacral micturition center

(SMC) causes neurogenic detrusor overactivity (NDO) with detrusor sphincter dyssynergia (DSD). Clinically, patients with lesions above the cone usually suffer from incontinence secondary to NDO and urinary retention due to functional bladder outlet obstruction (BOO). Furthermore, in patients with SCI above the T5–T6 vertebral level, sudden severe hypertension can commonly occur as a manifestation of autonomic dysreflexia, which can lead to dramatic results if not properly treated [10–12] (level of evidence [LE]: 3; grade of recommendation [GR]: C).

14.4 Sacral Spinal Cord Lesions

Damage to the sacral spinal cord may present as several grades of upper and lower mononeuron lesions, which result in different urodynamic diagnoses, as well as NDO, such as in suprasacral lesions, although the most common finding is DA with subsequently urinary retention. However, particularly in individuals with partial injuries, DA may be accompanied by decreased bladder compliance [13]. The exact mechanism by which sacral parasympathetic decentralization of the bladder causes decreased compliance is still unknown.

Furthermore, if the nuclei of the pudendal nerves are injured (e.g., cauda equina), paralysis of the urethral sphincter and pelvic floor muscles will occur, often with loss of outflow resistance and stress incontinence.

Management of neurogenic lower urinary tract dysfunction (NLUTD) is an important issue in rehabilitation programs for children with SCI [14]. Impairment of bladder function results in a high risk of urinary tract deterioration, which increases morbidity [15]).

14.5 Patient Evaluation

The principal goals of managing NLUTD are preservation of upper urinary tract function and prevention of renal failure. Various approaches have been developed, and different therapies have become available over the last 30 years to achieve these goals. The most appropriate therapeutic scheme should be carried out, considering the functional classification of motor function based on clinical and urodynamic findings (Fig. 14.2).

The initial clinical assessment of patients with NLUTD should include a detailed history, systematic physical examination (Fig. 14.3), urinalysis, urinary tract imaging (e.g., ultrasound), and noninvasive urodynamic testing such as a voiding diary and postvoid residual urine (PVR) testing. In addition, most pediatric patients with SCI require a specialized assessment with an invasive urodynamic study (LE: 3; GR: B), preferably a videourodynamic study if available.

Particular attention should be paid to possible warning signs and/or symptoms (e.g., pain, infection, hematuria, and fever), which may require further investigations. However, in patients with SCI, it is often difficult to accurately report symptoms related to NLUTD complications [16–18] (LE: 3).

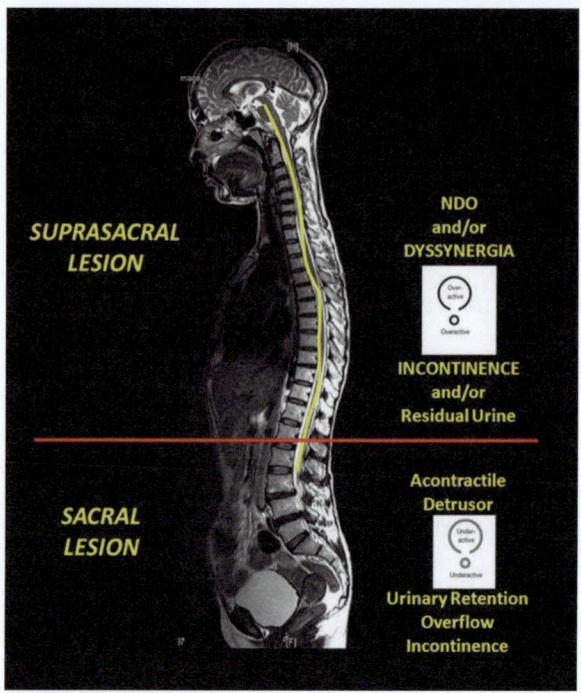

Fig. 14.2 Spinal cord lesion level and neurological bladder dysfunction with urodynamic pattern

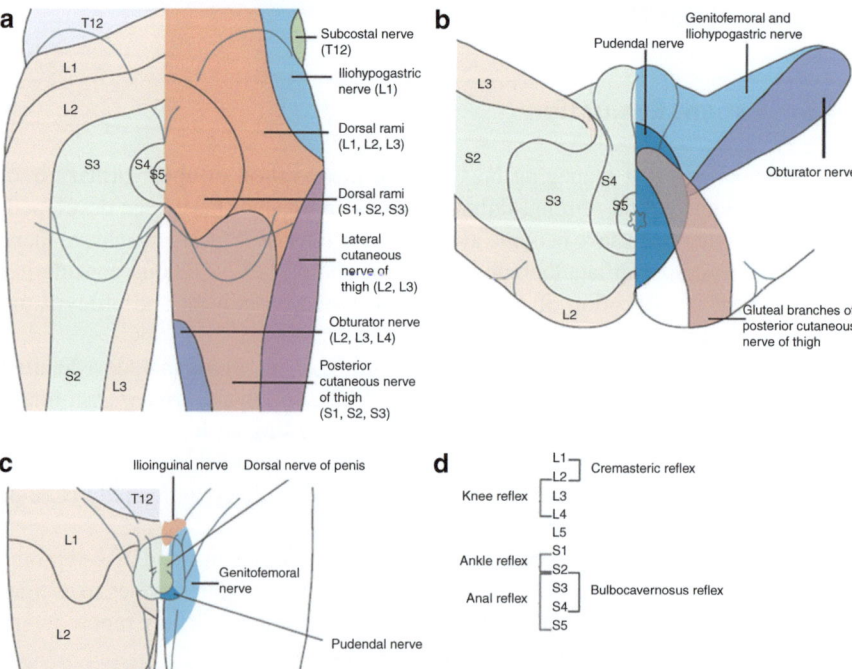

Fig. 14.3 Neurological status of a patient with neurogenic lower urinary tract dysfunction. **a** Dermatomes of spinal cord levels L2–S4

Table 14.1 Aims of treatment in neuro-urological patiens

Aim
Protection of the upper urinary tract
Improvement of urinary continence
Restoration of (parts of) lower urinary tract function
Improvement of the patient's quality of life

14.6 General Principles of Rehabilitation and Treatment

NLUTD has a strong impact on the quality of life (QoL) of SCI patients and their parents. Many aspects need to be considered when determining the treatment of choice, which also cannot be separated from the entire rehabilitation program (Table 14.1). Firstly, besides protecting the upper urinary tract and improving continence, the patient's expectations and family and social conditions should be taken into account in order to interfere as little as possible in their QoL.

In patients with high detrusor pressure during the filling phase (NDO, low detrusor compliance) or during the voiding phase (DSD, other causes of BOO), the main goal is primarily conversion of an active, aggressive high-pressure bladder into a passive low-pressure reservoir despite PVR [9, 19].

In NDO with DSD and low detrusor pressure, continence can be achieved by intermittent catheterization (IC) and pharmacotherapy (e.g., antimuscarinics). The use of medication to facilitate emptying (alpha blockers) in children with neurogenic bladder has not been well studied in the literature [20].

In NDO with severe DSD and high detrusor pressure, which are considered unsafe for preserving kidney function, both solutions can be proposed: reducing detrusor pressure (e.g., with antimuscarinics and/or botulinum toxin A [BoNT/A] injections) combined with an IC regimen or, alternatively, decreasing the bladder outlet resistance with sphincteric BoNT/A injections could be performed.

DA combined with overactivity of the sphincter may occur in sacral lesions. With this dysfunction, overflow incontinence can be controlled by self-intermittent catheterization (SIC), mostly without adjunctive pharmacotherapy. If IC is not possible, an indwelling catheter, preferable suprapubic, may be needed.

In all cases of vesicoureteral reflux presence, continuous antibiotic prophylaxis is necessary. When conservative and mini-invasive methods do not work, augmentation procedures or total bladder replacement should be performed [20].

14.7 Intermittent Catheterization

The standard therapy of SIC is an IC performed by the patient him- or herself, most frequently using an aseptic technique for managing NLUTD (LE: 1; GR: A). In children the IC is often performed by a third party, such as a parent or caregiver. The frequency of catheterization depends on many factors such as bladder volume, fluid intake, and PVR if the patient maintains spontaneous voiding without complete bladder voiding, which is recorded in a bladder diary to be combined with the

Table 14.2 Available treatments and level of evidence in neuro-urological children

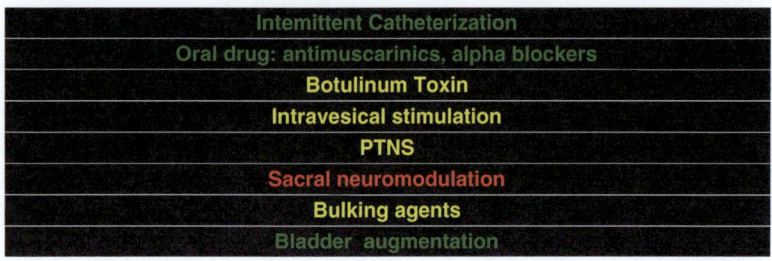

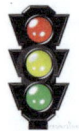

no evidence

low level of evidence

high level of evidence

urodynamic findings. Usually it is recommended that catheterization be performed 4–6 times a day during the early stage after SCI. An indwelling catheter is not recommended for routine use in long-term management.

IC should be performed in all children, especially in those with signs of possible outlet obstruction (LE: 2; GR: B). In babies without any clear sign of outlet obstruction, IC may be delayed, but babies should be monitored for urinary tract infections and upper tract changes [20].

Early initiation of IC in the newborn period makes it easier for parents to master the procedure and for children to accept it as they grow older [21, 22].

The use of IC in children with DSD eliminates residual urine and the risk of complications (LE: 3), and allows the possibility of performing surgery in the future [23, 24] (LE: 4).

14.7.1 Pharmacotherapy

Antimuscarinics (e.g., oxybutynin chloride, trospium chloride, tolterodine tartrate, and propiverine) have been documented to be effective for NDO treatment in adults (LE: 1). These medications are also used in pediatric patients.

There is no evidence of effective drug treatment for DA or neurogenic detrusor underactivity (LE: 2; GR: B). As far as alpha blockers are concerned, there have been just a few studies investigating the use of adrenergic blockade in children. Those studies reported a good response rate but lacked controls, and long-term follow-up studies are needed [25] (LE: 4; GR: C).

14.7.2 Botulinum Toxin

BoNT/A injections are an alternative treatment option for patients with NDO who are refractory to anticholinergic treatment. Detrusor injections of BoNT/A in children improve clinical symptoms and urodynamic parameters. Complete continence has been observed in approximately 65–87% of treated patients. Some studies have reported decreases in maximal detrusor pressure to at least 40 cm H_2O and increases in bladder compliance to at least 20 cm H_2O/mL. Injection of BoNT/A in therapy-resistant bladders appears to be an effective and safe treatment alternative (LE: 3; GR: C) [20] although there are no clear data on established BoNT/A dosages in children and the effectiveness of repeated injections [20].

Chemical denervation using BoNT/A injected into the external urethral sphincter has been considered a valid option to reduce the bladder outlet resistance and protect the upper urinary tract [26, 27], but it is not recommended in routine practice and should be used only as an alternative treatment.

14.8 Surgical Treatment

In cases where conservative therapy and mini-invasive treatment are ineffective, bladder augmentation should be performed. However, it works only in cases where there is competent function of the urethral sphincter. For male patients with severe DSD, bladder outlet procedures have to be performed, avoiding irreversible treatment such as sphincterotomy, since they are adult males [28].

Continent stoma could be used in cases of failure of previous bladder outlet procedures. As far as total bladder replacement is concerned, it should be done only in selected cases, considering the promising results of anticholinergic and/or mini-invasive treatment [20].

Conclusions

Early and multidisciplinary management of children affected by SCI and, more recently, a specific therapeutic strategy have shown excellent results in the rehabilitation of NLUTD, with a significant reduction in mortality related to serious urological complications, as a consequence. Furthermore, the individual clinical history, apart from neurological pathology, such as previous surgeries, should be assessed. The best solution is the most conservative and feasible treatment, according to the functional limitations of SCI patients, especially in pediatric practice. With rapidly instituted and optimal treatment, the large majority of patients can be adequately controlled without antireflux and/or major complication surgery. Treatment by a multidisciplinary team involving nurses and therapists specializing in pediatric center, such as in a spinal unit or neurourology unit, minimizes the risk of complications and optimizes the outcome for the patient. The treatment and rehabilitation programs must be tailored for each patient, taking into account the neurological and functional residual potential, combined with the social and lifelong needs of the patient. Long-term scheduled follow-up is mandatory because although neurological damage is not progressive, LUTD may evolve over time.

References

1. Patel JC, Tepas JJ, Mollitt DL, Pieper P. Pediatric cervical spine injuries: defining the disease. J Pediatr Surg. 2001;36:373–6.
2. Apple DF, Anson CA, Hunter JD, Bell RB. Spinal cord injury in youth. Clin Pediatr. 1995;34: 90–5.
3. Parent S, Mac-Thiong J-M, Roy-Beaudry M, et al. Spinal cord injury in the pediatric population: a systematic review of the literature. J Neurotrauma. 2011;28:1515–24.
4. Brown RL, Brunn MA, Garcia VF. Cervical spine injuries in children: a review of 103 patients treated consecutively at a level 1 pediatric trauma center. J Pediatr Surg. 2001;36:1107–14.
5. Bosch PP, Vogt MT, Ward WT. Pediatric spinal cord injury without radiographic abnormality (SCIWORA): the absence of occult instability and lack of indication for bracing. Spine. 2002;27:2788–800.
6. Carreon LY, Glassman SD, Campbell MJ. Pediatric spine fractures: a review of 137 hospital admissions. J Spinal Disord Tech. 2004;17:477–82.
7. Cirak B, Ziegfeld S, Knight VM, Chang D, Avellino AM, Paidas CN. Spinal injuries in children. J Pediatr Surg. 2004;39:607–12.
8. Dickman CA, Zabramski JM, Hadley MN, Rekate HL, Sonntag VK. Pediatric spinal cord injury without radiographic abnormalities: report of 26 cases and review of the literature. J Spinal Disord. 1991;4:296–305.
9. Wang MY, Hoh DJ, Leary SP, Griffith P, McComb JG. High rates of neurological improvement following severe traumatic pediatric spinal cord injury. Spine. 2004;29:1493–7.
10. Braddom RL, Rocco JF. Autonomic dysreflexia. A survey of current treatment. Am J Phys Med Rehabil. 1991;70(5):234–41.
11. Bonniaud V, Bryant D, Pilati C, Menarini M, Lamartina M, Guyatt G, Del Popolo G. Italian version of Qualiveen-30: cultural adaptation of a neurogenic urinary disorder-specific instrument. Neurourol Urodyn. 2011;30(3):354–9.
12. Silver JR. Early autonomic dysreflexia. Spinal Cord. 2000;38(4):229–33.
13. Herschorn S, Hewitt RJ. Patient perspective of long-term outcome of augmentation cystoplasty for neurogenic bladder. Urology. 1998;52:672–8.
14. Frankel HL, Coll JR, Charlifue SW, Whiteneck GG, Gardner BP, Jamous MA, et al. Long-term survival in spinal cord injury: a fifty year investigation. Spinal Cord. 1998;36:266–74.
15. Stover SL, De Lisa JA, Whiteneck GG. Spinal cord injury: clinical outcomes from the model systems. Gaithersburg, Maryland: Aspen Publishers; 1995. p. 234.
16. Jayawardena V, Midha M. Significance of bacteriuria in neurogenic bladder. J Spinal Cord Med. 2004;27(2):102–5.
17. Wyndaele JJ, Castro D, Madersbacher H, et al. Neurologic urinary and faecal incontinence. In: Abrams P, Cardozo L, Khoury S, Wein A, editors. Incontinence. 4th ed. Plymouth, UK: Health Publications; 2009. p. 793–960.
18. Witjes JA, Del Popolo G, Marberger M, Jonsson O, Kaps HP, Chapple CR. A multicenter, double-blind, randomized, parallel group study comparing polyvinyl chloride and polyvinyl chloride-free catheter materials. J Urol. 2009;182(6):2794–8.
19. Wyndaele JJ, Castro D, Madersbacher H, et al. Neurologic urinary and faecal incontinence. In: Abrams P, Cardozo L, Khoury S, Wein A, editors. Incontinence, vol. 2. Plymouth, UK: Health publications; 2005. p. 1059–62.
20. Stöhrer M, Blok B, Castro-Diaz D, Chartier-Kastler E, Del Popolo G, Kramer G, Pannek J, Radziszewski P, Wyndaele JJ. EAU guidelines on neurogenic lower urinary tract dysfunction. Eur Urol. 2009;56(1):81–8.
21. Joseph DB, Bauer SB, Colodny AH, et al. Clean intermittent catheterization in infants with neurogenic bladder. Pediatrics. 1989;84(1):72–82.
22. Lindehall B, Moller A, Hjalmas K, et al. Long-term intermittent catheterization: the experience of teenagers and young adults with myelomeningocele. J Urol. 1994;152(1):187–9.

23. Kaefer M, Pabby A, Kelly M, et al. Improved bladder function after prophylactic treatment of the high risk neurogenic bladder in newborns with myelomeningocele. J Urol. 1999;162(3 Pt 2): 1068–71.
24. HY W, Baskin LS, Kogan BA. Neurogenic bladder dysfunction due to myelomeningocele: neonatal versus childhood treatment. J Urol. 1997;157(6):2295–7.
25. Austin PF, Homsy YL, Masel JL, et al. Alpha-adrenergic blockade in children with neuropathic and nonneuropathic voiding dysfunction. J Urol. 1999;162(3 Pt 2):1064–7.
26. Franco I, Landau-Dyer L, Isom-Batz G, et al. The use of botulinum toxin a injection for the management of external sphincter dyssynergia in neurologically normal children. J Urol. 2007;178(4 Pt 2):1775–9. discussion 1779-80
27. Mokhless I, Gaafar S, Fouda K, et al. Botulinum a toxin urethral sphincter injection in children with nonneurogenic neurogenic bladder. J Urol. 2006;176(4Pt2):1767–70. Discussion 1770
28. Groen J, Pannek J, Castro Diaz D, Del Popolo G, Gross T, Hamid R, Karsenty G, Kessler TM, Schneider M, 't Hoen L, Blok B. Summary of European Association of Urology (EAU) Guidelines on Neuro-Urology. Eur Urol. 2016;69(2):324–33.

Cerebral Palsy and Other Encephalopathies

15

Stuart Bauer

15.1 Background

Cerebral palsy is a nonprogressive neurologic disturbance due to a presumed anoxic injury to the fetal or infant brain during this critical time in development that results in disorders of movement and posture causing limitations in activities of affected individuals. It is the most common physical disability in childhood, affecting approximately 3.3 per 1000 8-year-old children in the United States with variable degrees of disability. Its prevalence varies by region and is more common in black and white children than in those of Hispanic descent and 1.2 times more common in boys than girls [1]. It is seen in premature, low birth weight infants who were subjected to perinatal infection, seizures, or intracranial hemorrhage. Sensation, perception, cognition, communication, and behavior may also be affected [2]. In addition, physical impairments ranging from gross or fine motor development to altered muscle tone and gait abnormalities are often apparent [3]. The Gross Motor Function Classification System (2007; GMFCS–E & R; http://motorgrowth.canchild.ca/en/GMFCS/resources/GMFCS-ER.pdf) is based on self-initiated movement, with emphasis on sitting, transferring, and mobility. This five-level scale ranges from 1 (walks without limitations) to 5 (transported in a manual wheelchair) has specific descriptions with relevant age band categories for each level of disability.

S. Bauer
Department of Urology, Boston Children's Hospital, Boston, MA, USA
e-mail: stuart.bauer@childrens.harvard.edu

© Springer International Publishing AG, part of Springer Nature 2018
G. Mosiello et al. (eds.), *Clinical Urodynamics in Childhood and Adolescence*,
Urodynamics, Neurourology and Pelvic Floor Dysfunctions,
https://doi.org/10.1007/978-3-319-42193-3_15

15.2 Causative Factors for Incontinence

Affected children will often achieve urinary continence, albeit at an age later than their age-adjusted normal peers [4, 5]. Not infrequently, daytime continence is achieved first, followed by nighttime continence within the next year, but this is clearly dependent on either the ability to get to a bathroom facility quickly enough or signal that there is a need to empty the bladder. Overall, 14% [6] to 34% [7] of children are continent of urine before 5 years of age. The median age for achieving continence in those with high intellectual capacity and diplegia or hemiplegia varies from 3.6 to 4.1 years. For those with low intellectual capacity and tetraplegia, this milestone is achieved much later (10.1–13.2 years) [4]. Most studies do not correlate mobility (or GMFCS level) with achievement of continence [6, 8, 9]. In 97 children evaluated with a standardized dysfunction voiding symptom survey, investigators found 25% of those who were able to walk had lower urinary tract (LUT) dysfunction compared with 75% in those who were unable to do so ($P < 0.001$) [6] . LUT symptoms become more prevalent as the children age, from 11% in children under age 5 to 30% in those over 30 years [6, 9] .

15.3 Symptomatology

The incidence of urinary symptoms in children with cerebral palsy varies by the specifics of the investigation, namely, the breadth and numbers of patients evaluated and in what settings—a clinic versus a school—that houses a large number of handicapped children. Thus, the range of symptomatology is quite varied—16% [9] to 94% [10] . Despite the fact that males are slightly more likely to have cerebral palsy, girls are more prone than boys to have LUT symptoms [6, 8]. Daytime urinary incontinence is the most common symptom, occurring in 23–94% of affected youths, with an overall prevalence of 35–45% [4, 7, 9–12]. Urgency and frequency are also part of this constellation of symptoms [9, 12]. Monosymptomatic enuresis is seen in as little as 3% [7], but it has been reported in up to 13% [6, 12], again depending on age of the patient. The occurrence of urinary tract infection (UTI) is also variable, being noted in 5–57% [6, 8, 10, 13]. When using Rome III criteria, constipation can be detected in 33–66% of affected youngsters [6, 10, 12]. Upper urinary tract deterioration, defined primarily as hydronephrosis, is uncommon, appearing in less than 5%, but with a range of 0.5–12% [6, 9, 10, 13]. Other parameters of "deterioration" that have been reported include asymmetric renal size, vesicoureteral reflux, and microlithiasis [6, 9, 10]. Factors that raise the risk of upper urinary tract deterioration include increasing age, clinical symptoms of detrusor sphincter dyssynergia (urinary retention, interrupted uroflow patterns, hesitancy), and recurrent UTI [10].

15.4 Pathogenesis

The cause of LUT symptoms in children with cerebral palsy seems to be related to abnormal bladder function rather than to decreased mobility or an inability to communicate, that many of these children suffer from. The type of dysfunction involving the lower urinary tract, when it does occur, is related to which areas of the central nervous system that were affected by the insult: cerebral cortex involvement leads to detrusor overactivity; lesions at or below the pontine mesencephalic center may produce detrusor sphincter dyssynergy; and when the sacral spinal cord is affected, this can cause detrusor areflexia and incontinence from paralysis of the pelvic nerves [3]. When urodynamic testing has been undertaken in those with symptoms, normal LUT function has been found in only one third [6]. Detrusor overactivity is noted in approximately 30% [9, 10, 14]. Detrusor underactivity is documented in 6% [9]. Smaller than expected normal bladder capacity has been detected in 42–93% [6, 8, 10]. This may be related to the presence of detrusor overactivity leading to early evacuation of urine [12]. Sphincter dyssynergy is found in approximately 12% [10, 12, 14]. It should be noted that the incidence of these abnormal urodynamic parameters is related to selection bias involved in investigating patients with symptoms of unresolved incontinence or recurrent UTI. The true prevalence of abnormal urodynamic LUT function is unknown but probably much less than of what has been quoted as a considerable number of vertebral palsied individuals who have normal continence and no UTIs. However, some investigators have noted abnormal urodynamics in the absence of clinical LUT symptoms and recommend testing in everyone [15, 16].

Elevated residual urine volume [greater than 25 mL] has been found to occur in 13% [6]. Uroflow patterns may be very variable with a bell-shaped curve noted in 63%, a staccato pattern in 17%, an intermittent pattern in 13%, a plateau-shaped curve in 3%, and a tower-shaped pattern in 3% [9]. Obviously, this variability is related to many factors such as the degree of spasticity noted in each individual, the presence of detrusor over- or underactivity, and how much they may strain to empty. No one has correlated upper urinary tract deterioration with the type of LUT function these patients exhibit on urodynamic evaluation nor with uroflow patterns and/or residual urine volume may they have. Frequency and urge incontinence often persist into adulthood [17, 18].

15.5 Management

The management of the urinary tract in affected individuals varies considerably, depending on the presentation, severity of symptoms, and one's proclivity for full evaluation. In infancy, it is probably not necessary to image the urinary tract unless there is a suspicion that an abnormality is likely, based on family history or prenatal ultrasonography. Most often babies have normal voiding and bowel habits. It is only after toilet training is attempted that symptoms of incontinence or subtle signs of dysfunction may surface. It is important at this stage for parents or caregivers not to become frustrated with the potentially slow pace of continence achievement, which depends on many factors including cognitive and language development. Ensuring the child well hydrated and on an appropriate bowel regimen are the first measures to institute. As the child matures, scheduling regular visits to the bathroom and encouraging him/her to void and have daily or every other day bowel movements should eventually lead to a successful outcome.

Regardless of the degree of success in toilet training, urinary tract imaging or residual urine measurements are not needed. It is only when considering medical intervention that obtaining a KUB, or pelvic ultrasound, to determine the degree of constipation (or assessment of rectal fullness) and residual urine measurements are necessary beforehand and afterward, to ensure medical therapy has not altered the ability to empty.

Management of urinary tract pathology such as lithiasis, vesicoureteral reflux, and/or hydronephrosis is based on the same principles employed for treating those conditions in children without spastic diplegia.

No specific surveillance measures are needed in this population, especially since the neurologic condition is not a dynamic disease process. If the individual is able to remain continent and empty the bladder at regular intervals with no new onset of incontinence, they can be followed expectantly, especially if there has been no deterioration in upper or lower urinary tract function. However, assessment of affected adults reveals frequency, and urge incontinence may persist into adulthood, so careful observation is necessary [17, 18].

15.6 Specific Recommendations

Given the fact that affected children often have LUT symptoms, upper urinary tract deterioration is rare. Therefore, recommendations for evaluation must be cautiously promulgated. Most patients can be managed initially with minimal investigation and conservative treatment. In those with frequency, urgency, and/or incontinence, initial investigation should include a urinalysis and culture to rule out UTI and, if possible, a minimally invasive uroflow and/or a bladder ultrasound scan to measure residual urine volume. Conservative measures, such as adequate hydration, stringent timed voiding (or toileting), and making sure the individual has regular and complete bowel movements and is not suffering from constipation, have helped reduce symptoms substantially. Once considered an initial mainstay of treatment, antimuscarinic therapy is now only employed following implementation of an effective bowel management program that routinely empties the colon and rectum and ensures that residual urines can be feasibly measured after this class of drugs is instituted. This is partly due to their potential adverse effects.

If these routine standards of care have been initiated and if the judicious addition of anticholinergic medication has not resulted in resolution of symptoms, further investigation with urodynamic studies can be undertaken. Recurrent, nonfebrile urinary tract infection may be further investigated with renal and bladder ultrasonography, looking for the presence of hydronephrosis, renal parenchymal thinning, nephrolithiasis, discrepancy in size between the two kidneys, and distal ureteral dilation. If any of these parameters are present or the individual has a febrile urinary infection, then lower urinary tract imaging (voiding or nuclear cystography) is undertaken to rule out vesicoureteral reflux or bladder outlet obstruction. Increased bladder wall thickness (greater than 6 mm in a bladder that is filled to at least 60% of its expected capacity) on imaging may signify detrusor overactivity or detrusor sphincter dyssynergy that then warrants urodynamic investigation. In addition, children with other factors known to be associated with the potential for upper urinary tract deterioration (urinary retention, interrupted urinary stream, hesitancy) should also undergo urodynamic testing.

15.7 Conditions of the Brain (Tumors, Infarcts, Encephalopathies)

15.7.1 Presentation

The most common finding in children with neurogenic bladder dysfunction resulting from CNS tumors is urinary incontinence and/or urinary retention [19, 20]. Other less often presenting symptoms include UTI, straining or difficulty voiding, hydronephrosis, or urinary urgency [19, 20]. In some children, development of bladder symptoms may herald progression or recurrence of the disease [19] .

15.7.2 Pathogenesis

Urodynamic studies of children with neurogenic bladder resulting from CNS tumors demonstrate poor compliance, inability to void, high voiding pressures, detrusor overactivity, and elevated postvoid residual urine volume. Electromyographic assessment of external urethral sphincter function (EMG) revealed either the presence or absence of motor unit action potentials [19, 20]. When there was electrical activity in the sphincter, sacral reflex testing was either positive or negative and either synergic or dyssynergic when the bladder emptied. There is no specific correlation between tumor location and any specific urodynamic parameter. Nor is there a difference in urodynamic findings in patients with intracranial versus extracranial tumors or in those with suprasacral versus sacral involvement [20].

There is little literature related to neurogenic dysfunction that arises from other brain conditions such as encephalopathies or infarcts in children. Fortunately, the incidence of this condition is very low, 2 per 1000 neonates [21]. One study notes that voided volume and rate of consciousness with voiding are significantly lower in newborns with hypoxic ischemic encephalopathy (HIE) than in those without HIE [22]. Those with HIE have significantly higher postvoid residual urine volumes and voiding frequencies, but the exact etiology is uncertain [22]. In reviewing our experience of urodynamic testing in older children with HIE who were not toilet trained, most have smaller than normal (for age) capacity bladders—due to detrusor overactivity—and normal sphincter EMG reactivity and bladder sphincter synergy (Bauer, personal assessment).

15.7.3 Specific Recommendations

Variations in the types of storage and voiding function may occur independent of tumor location. As a consequence, routine urologic investigation including renal ultrasonography and urodynamic studies in all children with CNS tumors is recommended when the individual child has or develops urinary incontinence and urinary infection or there is a need to know how the tumor is affecting LUT function, despite the absence of symptoms, or as a reason to change or add further antitumor treatment [19, 20]. Children with an encephalopathy who are not fully toilet trained or who have had recurrent UTI may be at risk of having bladder and/or urethral sphincter dysfunction. After careful screening to make sure they are not constipated, further investigation is appropriate. Those who are symptomatic should undergo renal and bladder ultrasonography and urodynamic investigation, especially if they do not empty their bladder when voiding.

15.8 Conditions of the Spinal Cord and Brain

15.8.1 Transverse Myelitis

15.8.1.1 Presentation

Transverse myelitis is a clinical syndrome caused by an immune-mediated inflammatory process that affects the spinal cord [23, 24]. Approximately 1400 new cases are diagnosed in the United States annually, 28% of which are children [25]. The peak incidence is between 10 and 30 years of age [25]. Males and females are equally affected [23]. The diagnosis must be considered in the presence of sensory, motor, or autonomic dysfunction of the spinal cord, bilateral neurologic signs and/or symptoms, a clearly defined sensory level, and inflammation in the spinal cord as noted by cerebrospinal fluid pleocytosis or an increased T2 signal on MRI [25, 26] (Fig. 15.1).

In 60–75% of children with upper respiratory illness or gastroenteritis, immunizations for mumps, measles or varicella, mycoplasma pneumonia, herpes, or *listeria monocytogenes* may be an antecedent. *Campylobacter jejuni* in

Fig. 15.1 T2-weighted magnetic resonance sagittal image of the spine of an 8-year-old boy who presented with lower extremity weakness and urinary retention. Increased signal intensity of the spinal cord is noted from T3 to T8

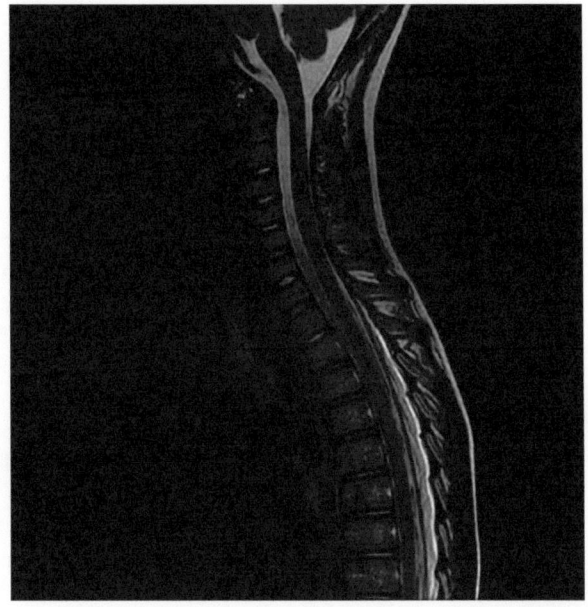

association with antiganglioside antibodies has been implicated as a cause in one study [24].

Transverse myelitis is heralded by the sudden onset of lower back pain or lower extremity muscle weakness that rapidly progresses to paralysis and often to urinary retention [27]. Bladder dysfunction may occur simultaneously with the motor dysfunction but commonly follows it [23]. Bowel dysfunction can also occur at presentation [23]. In the acute stage, there may be a varying period of spinal shock that may persist up to 6 weeks after onset [28]; however, this often gradually progresses to lower extremity spasticity and detrusor overactivity. The segment of the spinal cord affected by the disease determines the motor deficit [23]. During the acute phase of the disease, treatment options include steroids, plasma exchange, and intravenous immunoglobulin G (IgG) [23]. Recovery usually commences within 2 weeks to 3 months after onset of symptoms, the most significant return of function occurring within the first 6 months [23]; sometimes, improvement continues up to 2 years after the event [25]. LUT function is often the last to recover, if at all [24, 29].

15.8.1.2 Pathogenesis
The LUT is affected in as much as 86% of children [26]. More than 95% of affected children with urinary tract symptoms have retention of urine during the acute phase of the illness [23, 30, 31, 32, 33]. Urodynamic investigation during the acute phase reveals detrusor areflexia or underactivity in close to 70% [32], detrusor overactivity in 13%, decreased compliance in 30%, and detrusor dyssynergy in 20% [32]. After resolution of spinal shock, the urodynamic patterns

identifiable are detrusor overactivity (59–90%), decreased compliance (47%), bladder sphincter dyssynergy (17–80%), and detrusor leak point pressure greater than 40 cm H_2O (12–33%). Detrusor underactivity is noted rarely after resolution of the acute phase [32, 34, 35].

Approximately one third of children will be able to void spontaneously after the acute phase [23, 35], but some children (57–73%) will require CIC to empty their bladder [23, 35]. Antimuscarinics are needed to manage symptoms of detrusor overactivity in 14–64% [23, 34, 35]. For children with persistent incontinence despite CIC and antimuscarinics, owing to small capacity, poor compliance, or unremitting overactivity, intradetrusor injections of botulinum toxin and bladder augmentation have been helpful [35]. Up to 77% may have persistent bowel dysfunction; consequently, most require active bowel management [35].

Although some reports have not correlated recovery of LUT function with recovery of motor function [34, 35], others have demonstrated an association [23, 32, 36]. One study found children with full motor recovery were likely to have full recovery of LUT function—normal voiding with continence and no need for antimuscarinic medication. It was also noted that partial recovery of motor function is associated with partial recovery of LUT function, meaning that children can void spontaneously but require antimuscarinics for incontinence. Children with no motor recovery or those who were wheelchair dependent were likely to require CIC and possibly antimuscarinics [23].

UTI [23], VUR [35], hydroureteronephrosis [35], chronic renal insufficiency [35], bladder calculi [32], and bladder diverticula [32] have been noted infrequently in children with transverse myelitis. If CIC is initiated late in the disease process, there is an increased risk of decreased bladder compliance and upper urinary tract deterioration [35], with 5% demonstrating hydronephrosis and/or VUR in affected children [35]. Neither neurologic deficits nor urinary symptoms are able to predict the risk of upper urinary tract deterioration, and ambulatory status does not correlate with urodynamic findings [35].

15.8.1.3 Specific Recommendations

Urodynamic studies and a baseline renal and bladder ultrasound are suggested once the acute phase of the neurologic injury has stabilized, to identify those who may have detrusor sphincter dyssynergy (DSD). Children with bladder underactivity and/or DSD will benefit from the early introduction of CIC and antimuscarinic therapy, respectively [35]. Urodynamic studies should be repeated after resolution of the acute phase (approximately 6 months) to guide therapy for incontinence and preservation of the upper urinary tract. Voiding or radionuclide cystography is indicated in the presence of detrusor sphincter dyssynergy or recurrent UTI. Because these children are at risk for upper urinary tract deterioration, annual follow-up including renal ultrasonography is recommended as outlined in Table 15.1. Urodynamic studies are advisable if there is a change in LUT symptoms or in sonographic imaging.

Table 15.1 Summary: International Children's Continence Society recommendations for the diagnostic evaluation and follow-up of congenital neuropathic bladder dysfunction in children

Condition	Type of investigation	Indications
1. Cerebral palsy		
Spastic diplegia	Renal/bladder ultrasound	Lower urinary tract symptoms persisting beyond toilet training
	Uroflowmetry/postvoid residual	Wetting despite timed voiding
	KUB	Wetting despite timed voiding
	Voiding cystourethrography	Upper urinary tract abnormalities Recurrent urinary infection
	Urodynamic studies: Cystometrogram/sphincter EMG	Signs suggestive of dyssynergy Incomplete emptying on uroflowmetry
2. Central nervous system		
Tumors	Uroflowmetry/postvoid residual	Lower urinary tract symptoms
	Urodynamic studies: Cystometrogram/sphincter EMG	Spinal cord involvement in disease
3. Transverse myelitis		
	Urodynamic studies: Cystometrogram/sphincter EMG	Lower urinary tract symptoms Persisting beyond 6 weeks
	Urodynamic studies: Cystometrogram/sphincter EMG	Lower urinary tract symptoms Persisting beyond 6 months

References

1. Kirby RS, Wingate MS, Van Naarden BK, Doernberg NS, Arneson CL, Benedict RE, Mulvihill B, Durkin MS, Fitzgerald RT, Maenner MJ, Patz JA, Yeargin-Allsopp M. Prevalence and functioning of children with cerebral palsy in four areas of the United States in 2006: a report from the Autism and Developmental Disabilities Monitoring Network. Res Dev Disabil. 2011;32(2):462–9.
2. Richards CL, Malouin F. Cerebral palsy: definition, assessment and rehabilitation. Handb Clin Neurol. 2013;111:183–95.
3. Wang M-H, Harvey J, Baskin L. Management of neurogenic bladder in patients with cerebral palsy. J Pediatr Rehabil Med. 2008;1:123–5.
4. Roijen LE, Postema K, Limbeek VJ, et al. Development of bladder control in children and adolescents with cerebral palsy. Dev Med Child Neurol. 2001;43:103.
5. Ozturk M, Oktem F, Kisloglu N, Demirci M, Altuntas I, Kutluhan S, Dogan M. Bladder and bowel control in children with cerebral palsy. Croat Med J. 2006;47:264–70.
6. Silva JAF, Alvares RA, Barboza AL, Monteiro RTM. Lower urinary tract dysfunction in children with Cerebral Palsy. Neururol Urodyn. 2009;28:959–63.
7. Richardson I, Palmer LS. Clinical and urodynamic spectrum of bladder function in Cerebral Palsy. J Urol. 2009;182:1945–8.
8. Ersoz M, Kaya K, Erol SK, Kulakli F, Akyuz M, Ozel S. Noninvasive evaluation of lower urinary tract function in children with Cerebral Palsy. Am J Phys Med Rehabil. 2009;88:735–41.
9. Murphy KP, Boutin SA, Ide KR. Cerebral Palsy, neurogenic bladder and outcomes of lifetime care. Dev Med Child Neurol. 2012;54:945–50.
10. Gündoğdu G, Kömür M, Avlan D, Sarı FB, Delibaş A, Taşdelen B, Naycı A, Okuyaz C. Relationship of bladder dysfunction with upper urinary tract deterioration in cerebral palsy. J Pediatr Urol. 2013;9(5):659–64.

11. Reid CJD, Borzyskowski M. Lower urinary tract dysfunction in cerebral palsy. Arch Dis Child. 1993;68:739–42.
12. Karaman M, Kaya C, Caskurlu T, Guney S, Ergenekon E. Urodynamic findings in children with cerebral palsy. Int J Urol. 2005;15:717–20.
13. Silva JAF, Gonsalves MDC, Saverio AP, Oliveira IC, Carrerette FB, Damio R. Lower urinary tract dysfunction and ultrasound assessment of bladder wall thickness in children with Cerebral Palsy. Urology. 2010;76:942–5.
14. Decter RM, Bauer SB, Khoshbin S, et al. Urodynamic assessment of children with cerebral palsy. J Urol. 1987;138:1110.
15. Houle AM, Vernet O, Jednak R, Pippi Salle JL, Farmer JP. Bladder function before and after selective dorsal rhizotomy in children with cerebral palsy. J Urol. 1998;160(3 Pt 2):1088–91.
16. Bross S, Honeck P, Kwon ST, Badawi JK, Trojan L, Alken P. Correlation between motor function and lower urinary tract dysfunction in patients with infantile cerebral palsy. Neurourol Urodyn. 2007;26(2):222–7.
17. Mayo ME. Lower urinary tract dysfunction in cerebral palsy. J Urol. 1992;147(2):419–20.
18. Yokoyama O, Nagano K, Hirata A, et al. Clinical evaluation for voiding dysfunction in patients with cerebral palsy. Nippon Hinyokika Gakkai Zasshi. 1989;80:591–5.
19. Soler D, Borzyskowski M. Lower urinary tract dysfunction in children with central nervous system tumours. Arch Dis Child. 1998;79(4):344–7.
20. Nguyen HT, Sencan A, Silva A, Carvas FA, Bauer SB. Urodynamic studies are recommended in children with central nervous system tumors regardless of location. J Urol. 2010;184:2516–20.
21. Pierrat V, Haouari N, Liska A, et al. Prevalence, causes and outcomes at 2 years of age of newborn encephalopathy: population based study. Arch Dis Child Fetal Neonatal Ed. 2005;90:257–61.
22. Wen JG, Yang L, Xing L, Wang YL, Jin CN, Zhang Q. A study on voiding pattern of newborns with hypoxic ischemic encephalopathy. Urology. 2012;80(1):196–9.
23. DaJusta DG, Wosnitzer MS, Barone JG. Persistent motor deficits predict long-term bladder dysfunction in children following acute transverse myelitis. J Urol. 2008;180:1774–7.
24. Kalra V, Sharma S, Sahu J, Sankhyan N, Chaudhry R, Dhawan B, Mridula B. Childhood acute transverse myelitis: clinical profile, outcome, and association with antiganglioside antibodies. J Child Neurol. 2009;24(4):466–71.
25. Krishnan C, Kaplin Aansverse I, Deshpande DM, Pardo CA, Kerr DA. Transverse myelitis: pathogenesis, diagnosis, and treatment. Front Biosci. 2004;9:1483.
26. Suthar R, Sankhyan N, Sahu JK, Khandelwal NK, Singhi S, Singhi P. Acute transverse myelitis in childhood: a single centre experience from North India. Eur J Paediatr Neurol. 2016;20(3):352–60. https://doi.org/10.1016/j.ejpn.2016.01.013. Epub 2016 Feb 13
27. Knebusch M, Strassburg HM, Reiners K. Acute transverse myelitis in childhood: nine cases and review of the literature. Dev Med Child Neurol. 1998;40:631.
28. Guttmann L. Spinal shock. In: Vinken PJ, Bruyn GW, editors. Handbook of clinical neurology, vol. 26. Injuries of the spine and spinal cord, Part II. Amsterdam: North Holland; 1976. p. 243–62.
29. Cheng W, Chiu R, Tam P. Residual bladder dysfunction 2 to 10 years after acute transverse myelitis. J Paediatr Child Health. 1999;35(5):476–8.
30. Pidcock FS, Krishnan C, Crawford TO, Salorio CF, Trovato M, Kerr DA. Acute transverse myelitis in childhood: center-based analysis of 47 cases. Neurology. 2007;68(18):1474–80.
31. Gatti JM, Perez-Brayfield M, Kirsch AJ, Smith EA, Massad HC, Broecker BH. Acute urinary retention in children. J Urol. 2001;165(3):918–21.
32. Kalita J, Kapoor R, Misra UK. Bladder dysfunction in acute Transverse Myelitis: Magnetic resonance imaging and neurophysiological and urodynamic correlations. J Neurol Neurosurg Psychiatry. 2002;73:154–9.

33. Miyazawa R, Ikeuchi Y, Tomomasa T, Ushiku H, Ogawa T, Morikawa A. Determinants of prognosis of acute transverse myelitis in children. Pediatr Int. 2003;45(5):512–6. Review. PMID: 14521523
34. Ganesan V, Borzyskowski M. Characteristics and course of urinary tract dysfunction after acute transverse myelitis in childhood. Dev Med Child Neurol. 2001;43:473–5.
35. Tanaka ST, Stone AR, Kurzrock EA. Transverse myelitis in children: long-term urological outcomes. J Urol. 2006;175(5):1865–8. discussion 1868
36. Dunne K, Hopkins IJ, Sheild LK. Acute transverse myelopathy in childhood. Dev Med Child Neurol. 1986;28:198.

Urinary Incontinence in Children and Adolescents with Mental and Physical Disabilities: Comorbidities and Barriers

16

Mario Patricolo and June Rogers

Continence is one of those clinical conditions that one seldom thinks about if he/she does not have a problem. It acquires massive proportions if one does. Urinary and fecal incontinence, chronic constipation with fecal soiling, are devastating conditions for the patient and require complex management, involving also relatives of affected individuals. The abovementioned conditions, including the ones of neurogenic etiopathogenesis, can be associated to the insurgence and persistence of chronic kidney disease (CKD) and to renal/intestinal failure. Patients with disabilities represent a particularly challenging group, and when growing into adolescents and young adults, they belong to an indeed difficult and unique age group. Moreover, bladder and bowel management needs to be tailored in view of several associated systemic and localized comorbidities, including psychological issues. Currently the published literature on this subject is limited. Many groups have not focused on these nonglamorous aspects of bladder and bowel care. The management of bladder and bowel dysfunction is complex. The challenge becomes more difficult if associated with disabilities and during the transition between childhood and adulthood. Adolescents and young adults affected by bladder and bowel issues, such as incontinence, constipation, dysfunctional voiding, fecal soiling, and neurogenic bladder and neurogenic bowel, don't receive adequate care in hospitals and satisfactory home care, in many geographical areas, and not only in developing countries. The challenges become enormous if adolescents and young adults are also disabled with unique comorbidities associated and/or leading to bladder and bowel problems. In

M. Patricolo (✉)
Al Noor Hospital, Abu Dhabi, UAE

J. Rogers
Manchester Disabled Living, Manchester, UK

© Springer International Publishing AG, part of Springer Nature 2018
G. Mosiello et al. (eds.), *Clinical Urodynamics in Childhood and Adolescence*, Urodynamics, Neurourology and Pelvic Floor Dysfunctions,
https://doi.org/10.1007/978-3-319-42193-3_16

the presence of obvious physical (motility/sensitivity) and psychological (neurodevelopmental delays, autism, etc.) additional limitations, tailored management needs to be defined. Children with lower IQ associated with physical disability and/or syndromes have an increased risk of incontinence, which can persist into adulthood if not treated adequately. Although the association of attention deficit hyperactivity disorder, (ADHD), and incontinence has been shown in many studies, further research is needed on this condition and on other specific disorders, such as autism.

In this chapter we highlight the need and importance of identifying comorbidities associated with bladder and bowel problems in children and during the delicate transitional phase of adolescence, in individuals affected by disabilities, and to suggest adequate solution to overcome barriers and provide long-term surveillance. Currently, in Europe, there are virtually no integrated pathways for children and adolescents "per se" with bladder/bowel problems—never mind those with additional needs. Incontinence in the context of disability is a particular problem. Leaking urine is frequently assumed by professionals, patients, and relatives to be and inevitable aspect of the disability, and, subsequently, it is not investigated promptly and properly. Parents sometimes receive unclear messages from healthcare providers, regarding expectations on continence in children with functional or intellectual disabilities. As a consequence, training and education are left too late or are not pursued at all. Also limitations in time available for each outpatient's consultations are particularly influential in cases with complex disabilities that, by definition, require more time of an individual affected by isolated continence issues. School problems are more evident in children with disabilities. Bullying and lack of adequate accessibility and of special need assistance can lead to the choice of containment devices or clean intermittent catheterization, rather than the regular use of toilet. This negative pattern is also made easier by the lack of clarity in *who needs to do what* to help the disable child or adolescent with incontinence. Is it the teacher? Is it a special need assistant? Is it the family? Is it the continence advisor or the school nurse? The transition phase between childhood and adulthood is at higher risk of loss at follow-up in children with disability than in those without. We need also to be mindful of the fact that some of these youngsters do not actually present with frank urological or gastroenterological conditions or symptoms such as frequency, urgency, wetting, soiling, or continuous incontinence; they are apparently clean and dry and toilet trained, and it is not until they have a major issue such as UTI, urinary retention, renal dilatation, or reduced renal function that underlying bladder and bowel problems are picked up. The above mentioned unique pattern of presentation, highlights the importance of accurate history taking in clarifying the condition and allowing to identify abnormal voiding and defecation patterns, irregular bowel movements (e.g., once per week), etc. Many of these children (particularly those with autism or other psychological or behavioral disorders) "hold on" with very infrequent voiding and are therefore at high risks of developing dysfunctional voiding with large residuals. It is also noticeable that poor awareness of treatment options promotes a feeling in many sufferers that nothing can be done or that surgery will be the inevitable result. We intend to inspire healthcare providers to observe and acknowledge that people with disabilities can be made aware of the numerous available treatment options and that they have potential for continence training, protection of bladder and bowel function, of renal integrity and that their continence issues are not necessarily leading to invasive and complex procedures to be resolved.

Comorbidities in children, adolescents, and young adults associated with disturbances are late diagnosis due to difficult verbalization, assumption that the urinary or fecal problems are simply part of the disability picture, reduced dexterity and posture issues—renal failure, associated metabolic (e.g., Fanconi's disease) conditions and psychological conditions (depression, psychosis), short bowel syndrome, gastrostomy—feeding, swallowing difficulties affecting fluid intake and diet, dietary intolerances, paradoxical or allergic reaction to essential medication (anticholinergic, alpha-blockers, laxatives, etc.), forgetfulness regarding medication intake or deliberate avoidance, lack of clinical knowledge and experience with these conditions, at a primary care level, lack of trained home care and school nursing, etc.

We identified 359 causes of incontinence (reported by the Symptom Checker http://symptoms.rightdiagnosis.com/cosymptoms/bladder-incontinence-all.htm for those conditions associated with incontinence, in all ages). The most relevant conditions for pediatric and adolescent age are meningomyelocele (MMC), Down syndrome, and mucopolysaccharidosis such as Sanfilippo syndrome, Beckwith-Wiedemann syndrome, diabetes/obesity, cerebral palsy, ADHD, autism, chromosome 11 deletion, depression, spastic paraplegia associated or not to congenital syndromes, and obsessive compulsive disorders. All of the above mentioned conditions are present, with associated comorbidities influencing bowel and bladder function and outcomes of the treatment provided for them.

In a previous study, the review of the literature showed the higher incidence of lower urinary tract symptoms in children with physical and learning difficulties. In particular, we suggested that boys with Down's syndrome frequently present with bladder outflow obstruction (see below), secondary to detrusor sphincter dyssynergia, with high risk for renal parenchyma damage and renal function loss, as well as CKD. Other studies highlighted that individuals with moderate to severe learning disabilities present with risk factors for developing post-void residual higher than the control population and that a third of all cases with cerebral palsy in young age have significant post-void residual. From the review of a long series of messages posted by patients and/or their relatives on social network groups, it was concluded that in Europe and North America as well as in Eastern Countries, Africa and South Asia, the provision of home care for continence issues is limited, and also the institution of the "continence advisor" is not as developed and efficient for children, adolescents, and young adults as opposed to what it is for adults. Moreover the availability of essential medication and equipment for home care and for bowel and bladder management is limited in many areas of the world where there are high rates of disabilities associated with incontinence. The situation becomes as severe as a "Cry for Help" in those cases affected by CP, tetraplegia, or a combination of various debilitating conditions, frequently present in adolescents and young adults. Late diagnosis only when the symptoms and signs become severe (pyelonephritis, enterocolitis, tethered cord and related symptoms, etc.), the difficulty of verbalizing problems, limits in performing self-clean intermittent catheterization and bowel washouts, lack of knowledge at primary care level, when "dry" is confused with "normal bladder" and confusing definitions of constipation, multi-persons care of the disable individual, especially in the Middle East and Southern European Countries and Africa, and lack of Multispecialistic Integrated Care Pathways and dedicated guidelines, tailored to the limitations experienced by the disabled teenager and young adult, are outstanding issues reducing the efficacy of continence, bowel and bladder issues management, at present.

We are going to describe in details below, a few conditions frequently found in children and adolescents, which suffers of associated comorbidities, influencing continence and bladder/bowel function:

Mucopolysaccharidosis type 3
Cerebral palsy
Attention deficit hyperactivity disorder
Autism
Trisomy 21

Mucopolysaccharidosis type 3 (MPS3): also known as Sanfilippo disease is a lysosomal storage disorder caused by missing or defective enzymes. There are three types of MPS3, each one due to the alteration of a different enzyme needed to completely break down the heparin sulfate sugar chain. MPS3 affects 1:85.000 live births. It affects male and female with a 1:1 ratio, and it is always progressive and life-limiting. The lack of the enzymes fails to break the heparin sulfate down, which is an essential component of the connective tissue, causing the accumulation of glycosaminoglycan in nearly all cell types. The symptoms start between 2 and 4 years of age, and the disease is rarely diagnosed only in adulthood. MPS3 is associated with severe neurological symptoms: progressive dementia, aggressive behavior, hyperactivity, seizures, and severe sleep disorders. Also bone abnormalities, skin diseases, scoliosis, and respiratory obstruction are associated to MPS3. Some individuals will die in teenager years, but a significant number of patients will survive into their 30s, 40s, and even 50s. The most prominent feature of Sanfilippo disease is degeneration of the central nervous system (CNS). As a consequence of the rapid deterioration of CNS function, children are in phase 1 or phase 2 of the disease, but adolescents and young adults are frequently in the third phase of the disease, and in these ages, nursing care takes precedence among all clinical priorities. The bone, muscle, and joint disease progresses, with progressive loss of dexterity and ambulation. Feeding ability also deteriorates, and gastrostomy tube (GT) insertion is performed to allow GT feeds. Incontinence in the late stages of phase 2 and during phase 3, as well as fecal soiling also made more severe by episodes of loose stools, becomes severe and difficult to manage. Scoliosis is also severe in most cases; overflow fecal incontinence due to "obstipation" (sluggish bowel peristalsis) develops; dementia deteriorates; and tissue healing becomes poor. Those whose degree of dementia and physical deterioration is not too severe may be violent, depressed, and self-isolating, and catalepsy may occur when under emotional stress or when incontinence worsens. No treatment is available for the underlying cause of the disease. Intrathecal enzyme replacement is being studied at present, and gene therapy is also subject of active research. Substitute reduction therapy, glycosaminoglycan production, has been used in MPS3. In early years MPS3 patients are hyperactive and accident prone, but when spasticity establishes, dexterity and ambulation are lost. Physiotherapy and hydrotherapy and all the available neurorehabilitation techniques are mandatory. Some MPS3 cases can be toilet trained, but this achievement is sadly only temporary. In fact, as soon as the neurological disease progresses, they will lose sensation of being wet or soiled, and the vesical innervation and bladder/bowel sphincter innervation are compromised inducing neurogenic bladder and bowel. Patients affected by MPS3 need special school nursing and 1:1 support. The requirement for direct nursing care rises to 2:1 when somatic paralysis and dementia become more severe. The home and school environment requires adapting to the patient's condition. A few hospices have recently expanded the service to provide appropriate respite service to young adults. For Sanfilippo disease cases, the transition from pediatric to adult services can be very problematic and needs direct and good communication among teams. An MPS Society exists, and resources and information can be gathered on their website: www.mpssociety.org.uk.

Cerebral palsy (CP): CP is defined as persistent nonprogressive but not unchanging disorder of the brain, caused by prenatal, perinatal, and postnatal damage during the first year of life. In CP neurological damage and other factors (posture, dexterity limitation, communication issues, impairment of cognitive function, care issues, etc.) can lead to the inability of achieving continence or delays in toilet training. Prevalence of urinary incontinence in CP cases varies between 36% and 73%. Due to the fact that different groups of CP cases present different outcomes, it has been assumed that low mental capacity cases and/or more severe spasticity manifestation is causative factors in delaying dryness in CP cases. There is a dramatic difference in the capacity of achieving dryness in earlier age in those cases with high intellectual capacity and hemiplegia (3.6–4.1 years) than in those with low intellectual capacity and tetraplegia (10.1–13.2 years). Children with spastic tetraplegia and low intellectual capacity have a small probability of becoming dry before the age of eight (39%). This imposes different strategies in different degrees of mental development and physical limitations in CP cases. Most importantly the expectation of patients, relatives, and carers, including school teachers, school nurses, and special need assistant, has to be adjusted, based on the above data, to avoid frustration and misunderstanding of the definition of good outcome, in CP and continence achievement. Nevertheless, with adequate adjustments to age-related expectation in cases with intermediate severity of CP, dryness from urine and cleanliness from stools with toilet attendance can be achieved.

Autism: autism is a mental condition usually present from early childhood, characterized by great difficulty in communicating and forming relationships with other people and in using language and abstract concepts. Autism and other learning disabilities are associated in delays of toilet training or in acquiring continence to urine and stools, all together. Children with autism have a higher risk of nocturnal enuresis and day time wetting (30 vs. 0–25% vs. 4.7% in a series of 40 children with autism) of cases, compared to control cases. Children affected by autism also present a more frequent occurrence of lower urinary tract symptoms, in particular urgency and postponement. Psychological issues and comorbid psychological disorders occur in higher rate in children with autism. All autistic children should be investigated for urinary incontinence or LUTS as well as bowel problems. Delayed milestone of toilet training may occur despite the Patients may present preserved or only mildly reduced cognitive ability. Acquisition of bowel control, in these cases, seems to be more complex than acquisition of bladder control, and there are frequently fears of sitting on the toilet. Children with autism may remain resistant to many different treatment approaches and continue to refuse to eliminate on the toilet. They present with rigid adherence to routine and have an extreme dislike for change. Like in the case of parauresis, this behavior has been suggested to be based on anxiety. Particular approaches have been suggested to reduce toilet fears and rigidity of adherence to a specific habit. One is the "transfer of stimulus control" which means to shift the child from pamper to pamper on a special sit similar to the toilet and then bringing the seat progressively closer to the toilet and put finally the child on the toilet. The technique described by L. Smith et al. is tedious and requires time and patience, but is effective, being based on "fading and reward" technique of slowly removing the diaper and slowly moving to the toilet while being rewarded for any progress achieved. The loss of repeated rituals will be harder for children with more severe degrees of autism and learning disabilities as opposed to the milder forms. Specialized multidisciplinary teams and strict parental compliance are instrumental for the success of these approaches to continence issues in disability.

ADHD (A – attention; D – deficit; H – hyperactivity; D – disorder): ADHD is a brain disorder marked by an ongoing pattern of inattention and/or hyperactivity-impulsivity that interferes with functioning or development. ADHD and incontinence are both frequent in children and can be associated with each other with significant frequency. Most studies in the literature focused on the association of ADHD and NE, but some have also considered fecal incontinence and day time urinary incontinence. Pediatric cases of day time urinary incontinence (DTUI) have actually a greater risk for ADHD than those with NE. Children with fecal incontinence have the highest overall comorbidity of psychological disorders, but not necessarily entering the profile of ADHD. Moreover, the genetic features of ADHD, bedwetting, and day time urinary incontinence are different. It is possible to speculate that genetic factors are not responsible for the association which could be functional or acquired. The association between ADHD and NE and DUI and fecal incontinence makes positive outcomes more difficult to achieve, partially because of the prioritization of the treatment of one condition than the other, rather than applying a multidisciplinary integrated pathway, to treat both conditions at the same time. A combined, pediatric, psychological, and pediatric urological pathway should be in place, for these children.

Down's syndrome: Trisomy 21, otherwise called Down's syndrome (DS), represents the most common syndrome in individuals with learning difficulties.

These cases frequently present comorbidities influencing both bowel and bladder function (gastrointestinal comorbidities: Hirschsprung's disease, duodenal anomalies, renal anomalies, bladder outlet functional obstruction, cognitive impairment, etc.). DS is the most common chromosomal abnormality, and individuals with DS have increased risk of congenital conditions including cardiac and gastrointestinal defects, as well as metabolic and renal diseases. However, renal and urinary tract anomalies have received less attention than other congenital malformations in DS. In the 1960, Berg et al. first noted the coincidence of renal anomalies and DS with 3.5% of autopsy cases having renal malformations and later studies showing a higher incidence of up to 21% [1]. Hypospadias and urethral abnormalities (such as posterior urethral valves—PUVs) have also been noted in this population. The incidence of hypospadias has been calculated as appearing in approximately 0.3% of all live births, with the incidence in boys with DS being approx. 6.5%—almost 20 times increased risk [2]. The overall prevalence of renal and urinary tract anomalies (RUTAs) in the DS population is four to five times higher than in the general population, including the increased risk of PUVs [3]. Dysfunctional voiding (DV), a condition in which the sphincter does not relax, while the bladder tries to expel the urine by contracting, is at higher risk in DS than in general population. The etiology of this condition in DS is not clear, but it may be partly related to overtraining of the pelvic floor in an attempt to encourage the individual to stay dry, leading to DV. Dysfunctional voiding leads to functional obstruction due to associated urinary retention with increased bladder pressures. Another contributing factor is the presence of abnormalities such as undiagnosed posterior urethral valves [4]. Hicks et al. [5] carried out a study to verify the hypothesis that boys with DS have bladder outflow obstruction secondary to detrusor sphincter dyssynergia (DSD). They identified high potential for renal injury: 50% of boys studied required urinary diversion for dilated upper tracts following bladder outflow obstruction, 77% had bladder dysfunction, and 68% had history of wetting. They concluded that the high risk is not fully appreciated, and it was important that all children and young people with DS, particularly those with wetting problems, have detailed history and a bladder scan. This problem has also been reported in adult patients and, although most common in boys, has been reported in a female with DS [6, 7]. The issue for this group of individuals is that history taking may be difficult due to impaired cognitive function and that the existence of some problems may be masked or neglected resulting in a delay in diagnosis. Voiding impairment is a common problem in this group and could be a contributory factor to the development of a DV. As a result of the relatively high incidence of urinary problems in individuals with DS, regular review and symptom investigation should be carried out to help facilitate early diagnosis and prompt treatment intervention in order to prevent upper urinary tract deterioration. It has been said that gastrointestinal abnormalities, both structural and functional, affect up to 77% of all individuals with DS [8]. Hirschsprung's disease (congenital megacolon) and anorectal malformations, including imperforate anus, are more common in DS than in the general populations, and if these are not well managed and treated appropriately early in childhood, they may lead to chronic problems in adulthood.

An audit of adults with DS attending a hospital clinic identified a wide range of problems [9]. These included celiac disease which was likely in 12%, constipation in 19%, and unexplained diarrhea in 19%. They recommended that specially designed protocols should be developed to help identify and manage these problems. Constipation may also be a particular problem in those with learning and physical difficulties for a number of reasons, including poor mobility and altered muscle tone. As the onset of constipation can be quite insidious and difficult to detect, it may not be recognized by those individuals who have reduced ability to perceive and report their symptoms. Often the first sign that constipation may be present is that the child or young person starts to soil due to underlying fecal impaction. It is important not to presume therefore that the development of fecal soiling is due to the person developing a behavioral issue or "incontinence" and to ensure that they are fully investigated for the presence of any underlying constipation.

Conclusions

The group of patients with physical and learning disabilities (PLDs) are more likely than others to have problems with continence. PLDs are challenging conditions which require a continuum of care and integrated care pathways from the younger age to adulthood and old age. PLDs influence the onset, the persistence, the worsening of urinary and fecal incontinence, retentive constipation, and soiling and also influencing and reducing the chances of adequate treatment and favorable outcomes. People with PLDs have the right to the same quality of service as everyone else, but they don't always get it. Sometimes, instead of receiving the regular services, such as pelvic floor rehabilitation, electrotherapy, and neuromodulation, medication, etc., they are given containment material (diapers) or started only on clean intermittent catheterization. There is a great deal that can be done to help and support people with learning disabilities to manage continence issues and also to facilitate the situation for those who take care of them. People with PLDs are also associated to the term: "complex needs"; this term is defined as: "Those needs arising both from learning disability and from other difficulties such as physical disability, sensory impairment, mental health problems, challenging behavior and autism." Despite many of the above persons cannot reach satisfactory continence without complex healthcare support, a relevant number of people with complex needs are capable of managing their own continence, with or without support. The management of continence and associated comorbidities in disabled people means delivering the correct support in ways that are tailored to suit the specific needs of the condition and also individual needs of the specific patient and his/her circumstances. This has to occur while upholding dignity, privacy, and human rights. As the bowel and bladder are socially primary indicators of "good health," achievement of satisfactory continence in these patients is an indicator of health status.

The main issues in managing children adolescents and young adults with incontinence and associated comorbidities are the perception that incontinence is not a physical problem, a culture of self-blame, difficult access to continence services, low threshold for the patient and the relatives to accept that incontinence is inevitable in the picture of disability, lack of age-specific services, poor continuum of care in the absence of standardized integrated care pathways, from primary care to specialized services (especially in developing countries and areas of need), and limits imposed in school and work environment.

Increased awareness for healthcare providers, patients, relatives, or carers and standardization of terminology, standardized integrated care pathways, focus on case-finding, and the will and ability of healthcare providers at all levels, to tailor care to individual needs of disable people, are the solutions available in our hands and in front of our eyes, needed to guarantee adequate quality of life, dignity, and independence to children, adolescents, and young adults affected by PLDs and incontinence.

References

1. Ariel, et al. The urinary system in Down syndrome: a study of 124 autopsy cases. Pediatr Pathol. 1991;11:879.
2. Lang D, et al. Hypospadias and Urethral Abnormalities in Down syndrome. Clin Pediatr. 1987;26:40–2.
3. Kupferman JC, Druschel CM, Kupchik GS. Increased prevalence of renal and urinary tract anomalies in children with Down syndrome. Pediatrics. 2009;124(4):e615–21. Epub 2009 Sep 14
4. Seki & Shahab (2011) Dysfunctional voiding of non-neurogenic neurogenic bladder: a urological disorder associated with down syndrome in genetics and etiology of down syndrome. Ed Prof Subrata Dey.
5. Hicks JA, Carson C, Malone PS. Is there an association between functional bladder outlet obstruction and Down's syndrome? J Pediatr Urol. 2007;3(5):369–74.
6. Culty T, et al. Posterior urethral valves in adult with Down syndrome. Urology. 2006;67(2):424. e1–2.
7. Kai N, et al. A female case with Down syndrome and non-neurogenic neurogenic bladder. Int J Urol. 2007;14:867–8.
8. Moore SW. Down's syndrome and the enteric nervous system. Pediatr Surg Int. 2008;24(8):873–83.
9. Wallace RA. Clinical audit of gastrointestinal conditions occurring among adults with Down syndrome attending a specialist clinic. J Intellect Develop Disabil. 2007;32(1):45–50.

Monosymptomatic Enuresis

17

Eliane Garcez da Fonseca

17.1 Definitions

Enuresis is defined as an intermittent urinary incontinence that occurs exclusively during sleeping periods after the age of 5 years, when the volitional control of micturition is expected [1]. The condition can be both a social and psychological distress for the child, and it requires effort and attention from the parents [2]. Its high prevalence and psychosocial effects validate the importance of the subject.

Monosymptomatic enuresis (MNE) is a subgroup of enuresis. MNE occurs without any other lower urinary tract (LUT) symptoms (nocturia excluded) and bladder dysfunction. Children with MNE can comfortably control the urine when awake. Children with enuresis and any LUT symptoms are said to suffer from *non-monosymptomatic enuresis* [1]. This classification is of utmost importance to guide the need for further investigation and best treatment option.

In accordance to its onset, enuresis can be also classified as primary or secondary enuresis. The term secondary enuresis should be reserved for those children who have had a previous dry period, which exceeds 6 months. If this is not the case, the term primary enuresis should be used. Primary enuresis occurs in 75–90% of children with enuresis, whereas secondary enuresis occurs in 10–25% and is associated with behavioral comorbidities that necessitate investigation [1].

E.G. da Fonseca
The University of the State of Rio de Janeiro, Souza Marques Medical School, Rio de Janeiro, RJ, Brazil
e-mail: fonsecaeg@gmail.com

© Springer International Publishing AG, part of Springer Nature 2018
G. Mosiello et al. (eds.), *Clinical Urodynamics in Childhood and Adolescence*, Urodynamics, Neurourology and Pelvic Floor Dysfunctions,
https://doi.org/10.1007/978-3-319-42193-3_17

17.2 Epidemiology

Studies in different countries show a prevalence of enuresis of around 10% among children and adolescents and of 10–15% at the age of 7 years [3, 4]. It has an annual spontaneous resolution rate of approximately 10–15%, but not all cases resolve spontaneously. Nocturnal enuresis persists in up to 3% of adolescents and 1% of untreated adults [5, 6]. It is more common in boys than in girls. Family history is often positive in these children. If one parent is enuretic, the risk that the child develops the condition is of 44%; if both parents are enuretic, the risk rises to 77% [7]. This inheritance is important in the different types of enuresis, and there is no good correlation between phenotype (MNE or NMNE) and genotype [8].

Currently, there are changing views regarding how many children with enuresis are truly monosymptomatic. The first epidemiological studies on enuresis often fail to identify the presence of LUTS and to differentiate between monosymptomatic and non-monosymptomatic nocturnal enuresis, showing an overestimated MNE prevalence [9]. In the last decade, the greater awareness about the importance of bladder function alongside ICCC's LUTS standardization [10] has highlighted this issue, resulting in an increase in the identification of children with LUTS and NMNE. Daytime incontinence was found to be associated with nocturnal enuresis [11–15], and MNE was found to represent less than half of all children with nocturnal enuresis [14, 16–18]. Many of these children were previously considered to have MNE due to a superficial evaluation [9, 11]. A detailed evaluation is very important for a good treatment result and will be further explored in the clinical evaluation section of this chapter.

17.3 Pathology

Monosymptomatic enuresis is a multifactorial condition. Three major pathogenic mechanisms are well accepted as crucial, with a varying degree of influence in each child: nocturnal polyuria, detrusor overactivity, and an increased arousal threshold or sleep disorder.

Nocturnal polyuria is related to a lack of the normal nocturnal increase in vasopressin secretion and, as a result, an exaggerated urine production [19]. Other renal circadian rhythms, such as solute handling and glomerular filtration rate, might also be disturbed [20, 21]. Although nocturnal polyuria is common in children with MNE, not all of them have polyuria [22], and not all patients with polyuria have vasopressin deficiency [23].

Bladder overactivity is clinically evident in children with NMNE, but it also has a subclinical role in an MNE subgroup with detrusor contractions and decrease in bladder capacity. This means that the bladder tends to contract before it is full, or to become full before morning, or even both. Bladder dysfunction is related to inappropriate central nervous system control of the detrusor muscle [24, 25].

Neither polyuria mechanism nor nocturnal detrusor overactivity explains why children do not awake when the bladder is full. An **increased arousal threshold** is considered to be the reason for enuretic children difficulties to wake up despite the signals from the bladder. This disorder in the arousal mechanisms could be secondary to a disturbance in the area around locus coeruleus [26]. Yeung et al. demonstrated, by polysomnography and continuous cystometry, an interaction between bladder overactivity and cortical arousability, which was defined as a "bladder–brain dialogue." The authors suggested that the transition from light sleep to awakening was suppressed by long-term overstimulation caused by signals from the bladder to the brain [27]. In addition, sleep fragmentation caused by increased cortical arousals was demonstrated in children with refractory nocturnal enuresis, using video polysomnography [28]. It is clear from the literature that fragmented sleep is less restorative than consolidated sleep and leads to sleepiness-related daytime impairment [29]. Sleep fragmentation can lead to sleep deprivation in children with nocturnal enuresis, influencing the endocrine, metabolic, immune, inflammatory, and cardiovascular regulation. A substantial increase in diuresis, a higher heart rate, and higher blood pressure with suppressed plasma levels of all sodium-retaining hormones have been demonstrated [30].

Enuresis may also be caused by obstructive sleep apneas due to adenotonsillar hypertrophy. It is considered to be a symptom of sleep-disordered breathing. There are two, nonexclusive, possible explanations for this: first, the constant arousal stimuli from the obstructed airways cause paradoxically high arousal thresholds, and, second, the negative intrathoracic pressure causes polyuria via increased secretion of the atrial natriuretic peptide [26, 31].

Comorbid conditions also have a central role in the pathogenesis and treatment of enuresis. Among these conditions, constipation and neuropsychiatric disorders, such as attention-deficit hyperactivity disorder, are common comorbidities.

Epidemiological studies show that 20–30% of all children with enuresis present clinically relevant behavioral problems at rates, which are two to four times higher than in children with no enuresis. Psychological disorders are more frequent in children with secondary enuresis (up to 75%) and non-monosymptomatic subgroups. The children with monosymptomatic nocturnal enuresis are the subgroup with the lowest comorbidity rates. Attention-deficit hyperactivity disorder (ADHD) is the most specific comorbid disorder with enuresis, with a comorbidity rate of 28.3%. ODD and conduct disorders as well as emotional disorders, such as depressive and anxiety disorders, can also coexist with enuresis. These comorbidities have a negative effect on compliance and outcome if not addressed and left untreated [32].

Constipation associated with nocturnal enuresis, especially non-monosymptomatic constipation, is quite frequent. The gastrointestinal and genitourinary tracts have the same embryological origin, the same innervation (sacropelvic plexus), and the same anatomical location. Different studies have shown the improvement and resolution of enuresis with the proper treatment of constipation [33, 34].

17.4 Psychosocial Impact of Enuresis

Enuresis and delayed bladder control are common sources of psychosocial problems for both parents and children. Nocturnal enuresis is associated with poor school performance and can cause loss of self-esteem, social isolation, stress, and family violence during childhood and adolescence. In addition to work overload with pajamas, bedlinen, and mattresses because of nocturnal urinary loss, there is also a significant monetary cost associated with diapers, a new mattress, and a new sofa, to name but a few.

The results of researches carried out in different countries have shown violence against enuretic children. The conviction that a child wets the bed on purpose increases the risk of punishment [2, 35]. The reported rates of punishment vary in the different cultures. Fonseca et al., in a population-based study with 296 children and adolescents, found out that 53.3% of enuretics felt excluded or had been ridiculed because of bedwetting and that 46.7% had been punished. It is noteworthy that 42.9% of those punished for bedwetting were children of parents who also often wet their beds when children. Although most enuretics felt excluded, were ridiculed, and had already been physically punished for bedwetting, only one received treatment for bedwetting [14]. Can et al. studied the physical abuse of children with enuresis and found that 42.1% of enuretic children were spanked, 12.8% were beaten, and 40.6% of children were medically neglected [36]. Karaman et al. found at least one punishment method was applied to 291 (58.1%) of children with NE. Punishment methods of parents were detected as child's condemnation (257 patients, 51.3%), child's craving deprivation (120 patients, 23.9%), child's humiliation in the presence of other children (113 patients, 22.6%), and child's reprimand threat of punishment (203 patients, 40.5%) [35]. Alpaslan AH et al. reported a case of death as a result of physical violence during toilet training [37].

The reasons for the non-treatment were fourfold: (1) enuresis was not considered a problem to take the child to the doctor; (2) those responsible did not know there were treatments for bedwetting; (3) the child itself was found guilty of bedwetting; and (4) socioeconomic difficulties [14]. These data highlight the psychosocial impact of enuresis, lack of knowledge on the subject, and scarce access to treatment.

17.5 Clinical Assessment

Enuresis is a symptom and may be a condition of intermittent incontinence that occurs exclusively during sleeping periods. As a symptom, it should always be assessed. The complaint of "wetting the bed" should always be valued and initially investigated by history and physical examination. This initial evaluation has to identify both the enuretic child due to underlying medical conditions and the child with relevant comorbid conditions, as well as to indicate whether further investigations are needed (Table 17.1) and what the best treatment option is.

A good history taking is the mainstay of the enuretic child evaluation. This should include a detailed bladder- and bowel-oriented history and also questions about psychological or neuropsychiatric comorbidities, upper airway obstruction, and systemic diseases. The following topics should be included:

1. **Bedwetting features**: Is it a primary or secondary enuresis? How often does it occur? How many nights in a week or month? How many incontinence episodes per night? Does the child also have nocturia? Is there any difficulty to wake up?

Table 17.1 Warning findings that indicate the need of additional investigation before enuresis treatment

During history taking:
– Daytime urinary incontinence
– Continuous urinary incontinence
– Straining, weak stream, or drip
– Urgency, holding maneuvers
– Urinary tract infection
– Constipation and/or fecal incontinence
– Low concentrated urine, polyuria
– Excessive thirst, need to drink during the night
– Nausea, weight loss, fatigue
– History of gestational diabetes and neonatal asphyxia
During physical examination:
– Neurocutaneous stigmata in the back (lumbosacral region)
– Intergluteous groove: short or asymmetric
– Abnormality in the neurological examination
– Orthopedic changes of lower limbs and/or spine
– Abdominal mass palpation
– Growth deficit
Initial investigation:
– Glucosuria
– Proteinuria
– Leukocyturia or nitrite test positive
– Hematuria
– Bladder wall thickness, post void residual urine, hydronephrosis, and kidney cysts found on kidney and urinary tract ultrasound

More than one enuretic episode per night indicates detrusor overactivity. Frequent bedwetting indicates detrusor overactivity and a poor prognostic [6, 11]. Nocturia indicates that the child is not extremely difficult to arouse from sleep. Comorbid conditions are more common in children who were previously dry than in those with primary MNE. In addition, it is relevant to ask about previous treatment. Has the child been treated for bedwetting? What is the treatment being used? Has it been done correctly? What are the results?

2. **Lower urinary tract symptoms (LUTS):** Relevant LUTS are: voiding frequency smaller than or equal to three or greater than or equal to 8×/day, current or previous daytime incontinence, urgency, hesitancy, straining, intermittency (interrupted micturition), holding maneuvers, weak stream, feeling of incomplete emptying, post-micturition dribble and genital or LUT pain. The child with monosymptomatic nocturnal enuresis—the focus of this chapter—does not show other lower urinary tract symptom and his or her physical examination is normal. Concomitant daytime bladder symptoms mean that the child has NMNE. Urgency, usually accompanied by frequency and nocturia, with or without urinary incontinence, in the absence of urinary tract infection (UTI) or other obvious pathology is indicative of overactive bladder (OAB). It is important to distinguish children

who void with a weak or interrupted stream and must use abdominal pressure to pass urine. The latter must be sent to a specialized center without delay because these signals are suggestive of anatomical bladder outlet obstruction. The history of recurrent urinary tract infection (UTI) and vesicoureteral reflux should also alert to the possibility of lower urinary tract dysfunction. UTI and recurrent bacteriuria often have residual urine. If the child presents continuous incontinence, i.e., drip loss between the normal voiding 24 h/day, it is mostly always caused by ectopic ureter.

The systematic search for lower urinary tract symptoms during anamnesis should always be emphasized. Parents often do not spontaneously report, due to their ignorance, or consider them to be normal. Other times, parents consider the urgency and incontinence as a result of the child's laziness, which would rather play until the last minute instead of going to the bathroom as soon as he or she feels the urge to.

3. **Constipation and fecal incontinence** should always be investigated. Constipation often leads to detrusor overactivity and/or residual urine. Constipation is often overlooked, and if it is not treated, it may be difficult to get the child dry. Constipation manifests by difficulty in defecation, stool frequency of less than three times per week, pain and abdomen bloating, painful defecation, fecal soiling, hard consistency of stool, and history of large diameter stools which may obstruct the toilet. ROME IV criteria are widely accepted in the diagnosis of constipation (Table 17.2) [38], and the use of Bristol stool scale facilitates the identification of the appearance of the stool [39]. Aspects 1 and 2 are characteristic of intestinal constipation.
4. **Behavioral and psychosocial problems** should be investigated: Problems at home or school. What is the impact of bedwetting? If the child shows significant difficulty to socialize, it is necessary to consider the possibility of psychiatric illness.
5. **Upper airway obstruction:** Children with heavy snoring or nocturnal apneas should be seen by an otorhinolaryngologist for a possible surgical correction.
6. **Diabetes mellitus or diabetes insipidus** should be suspected in case of a history of weight loss, thirst, polyuria, and secondary enuresis. Short stature, fatigue, polyuria, and dehydration suggest **underlying kidney disease**. Although these diagnoses correspond to a small percentage of cases of enuresis, they are important in order to discard them.

Table 17.2 Roma IV diagnose criteria of functional constipation

Diagnostic criteria must include 1 month of at least two of the following in children of a developmental age of at least 4 years:
1. Two or fewer defecations in the toilet per week
2. At least one episode of fecal incontinence per week
3. History of retentive posturing or excessive volitional stool retention
4. History of painful or hard bowel movements
5. Presence of a large fecal mass in the rectum
6. History of large diameter stools which may obstruct the toilet
After appropriate evaluation, the symptoms cannot be fully explained by another medical condition.

7. In the **history of pregnancy, labor, and birth**, risk factors should be investigated for perinatal anoxia, including prematurity, cyanosis, respiratory distress, congenital infections, and sepsis. These conditions are associated with lower urinary tract dysfunction, often without any other apparent neurological signs. History of gestational diabetes relates to sacral agenesis and neurogenic bladder. History of delayed psychomotor development may indicate a dysfunction of the central nervous system (CNS) which also affects the urinary tract. This is often not perceived or valued.
8. **Family history** of enuresis, incontinence, or kidney disease should be investigated.

Physical examination should focus on weight, height, blood pressure, abdominal mass palpation, genitalia, neurological examination, orthopedic changes of lower limbs and/or spine, and inspection of the lumbosacral region for cutaneous stigmas—hair tufts, cutaneous appendices, hemangiomas, hypo- or hyperchromic spots, dimples, lipoma, and intergluteous groove, short, or asymmetric. These signals in the lumbosacral region suggest a possible occult dysraphism and neurogenic bladder secondary to this. This is because of common embryonic origin of the skin and CNS.

After history taking and physical examination have excluded any of the aforementioned changes, the child can be classified as having monosymptomatic nocturnal enuresis and treated at primary level. This will be addressed below.

17.6 Additional Examination

17.6.1 Bladder Diary

Notes of frequency and of urine output are recommended in nocturnal enuresis to exclude the possibility of reduced bladder capacity. The highest urinated volume (excluding first morning urine) should be compared to the estimated bladder capacity (EBC) for the age. The latter shall be calculated by the following formula: $BC = 30 \times age + 30$ or $BC = (age + 1) \times 30$. The bladder capacity is considered low when it is smaller than or equal to 65% of the estimated value, and is considered increased when greater than or equal to 130% of the estimated value [1, 10]. Frequent, small voiding and urgency indicate reduced bladder capacity and detrusor overactivity. Infrequent voiding and holding maneuvers indicate voiding postponement.

In non-monosymptomatic nocturnal enuresis and enuresis resistant to first-line treatment, the record of urine volume is essential. The diary should also include a note of fluid intake and the presence of other urinary symptoms, such as urgency, incontinence, and hesitation. This intake note can contribute to the diagnosis of polydipsia. The full bladder diary consists of a seven-night recording of incontinence episodes and nighttime urine measurements to evaluate volume enuresis and 48 h daytime frequency and chart volume (which do not need to be recorded on two consecutive days) to evaluate for LUT dysfunction [1].

Nocturnal urine output excludes the last voiding before sleep but includes the first voiding in the morning. In enuretic children, urine voided during sleep should be collected in diapers and the change of diaper weight be measured. **Nocturnal polyuria** is a term relevant mainly in children suffering from enuresis and is defined as a nocturnal urine output exceeding 130% of estimated bladder capacity for the child's age [1].

The ability of the child and family to fill the bladder diary gives a good indication of their future compliance to the treatment.

17.6.2 Bowel Diary

A 7-day bowel diary is advisable to help to diagnose constipation and should include the Bristol stool form scale.

17.6.3 Urine Dipstick Test

Urine dipstick test is used to search the presence of glucose, leukocytes, protein, erythrocytes and bacteria in urine. Diabetes should be considered in the presence of glycosuria, and kidney disease, in the presence of proteinuria.

17.6.4 Ultrasound

Ultrasound measurement of bladder wall thickness, post void residual urine, and rectal diameter can be useful to indicate voiding dysfunction and occult constipation [40, 41]. Hydronephrosis and kidney cysts can eventually be found, although usually no abnormalities are seen in patients with MNE.

17.6.5 Blood Tests, X-Rays, and Invasive Urodynamics

There is no indication of blood tests, X-rays, and invasive urodynamic in patients with monosymptomatic nocturnal enuresis. In case the previously mentioned evaluations are changed, evaluation should be individualized. Uroflowmetry and measurement of residual urine can be helpful when voiding dysfunction or bladder outlet obstruction is suspected.

17.7 Treatment

Enuresis tends to disappear spontaneously as the child grows, with 15% of resolution rate by year, but a significant proportion of patients continue to wet the beds into adolescence or adulthood. Many adults with LUTS were enuretic children.

17.7.1 General Measures

The treatment of nocturnal enuresis always needs to start with a clear explanation of the condition and its mechanisms to the parents and patients. It is imperative to clarify the fact that enuresis is involuntary and that the child does not lose urine intentionally. Thus, neither patient nor his or her parents are to blame. Knowing that enuresis has a high frequency as well as the enuresis history of the parents and/or family helps to reassure the child, to lessen his or her embarrassment and to strengthen self-esteem.

It is necessary to provide guidance on the importance of the regular trip to the bathroom. The child should void regularly every second or third hour, and its postponement should be avoided. Yet, fluid intake needs to be sufficient during the day and reduced at night. At least half of the day's fluid intake needs to be before the afternoon. The diet should be low in caffeine and rich in fiber, and the excess of sodium should be avoided. If there is constipation, this needs to be treated with diet, regular trip to the bathroom (preferably after meals), developing the habit of going straight to the bathroom upon the first sensation of rectal filling (not postponing), and osmotic laxatives and enemas, if necessary.

17.7.2 Active Treatment

The active treatment for nocturnal enuresis shall be offered to children over the age of 6 who feel disturbed by the condition and are willing to undergo treatment. The International Children's Continence Society (ICCS) recommends using the alarm as the first nondrug option and desmopressin as the first drug option for medical treatment for monosymptomatic enuresis [42]. The cases of reduced bladder capacity can better respond to treatment with alarm. The cases of nocturnal polyuria can better respond to desmopressin. The therapeutic options should be presented to the child and family with their pros and cons so that they can decide upon the best treatment for them.

17.7.3 Alarm

The use of the alarm in the treatment of enuresis has an evidence level IA and results in continence in up to 70% of cases. It is believed to act by the arousal response and/or the increase in bladder capacity. Its use is safe and with great healing potential but requires time, commitment, and motivation of both child and family. The alarm consists of a moisture sensor to be placed in the underwear connected to an audible or vibrating alarm. Moisture detection causes the alarm to go off. Parents need to participate actively, helping to wake up the child in the first 2 weeks. The child ought to maintain the continued use of the alarm and go to the bathroom whenever the alarm goes off. In the case of enuresis, the child ought to complete urination in the toilet, changing his pajamas and resetting the alarm. The child's difficulty to wake up to the alarm in the first 2 weeks of use shall be anticipated at the time the treatment is indicated so that parents do not give up on the treatment by thinking it has not worked. The result is not immediate, and the use shall be discontinued after 2–3 months without response. Difficulties relate to the discomfort often caused to brothers and family. Some children can turn off the alarm after some time, so it is important for parents to make sure that the child wakes up whenever the alarm goes off.

17.7.4 Desmopressin

Desmopressin is an analogue of the antidiuretic hormone (ADH). Desmopressin works by mimicking the action of ADH, which causes the urine to become concentrated in a smaller volume overnight, which allows the majority of children to sleep through the night without needing to pass urine. It is a therapy with level of evidence IA. Around 30% of patients show a complete response whereas 40% of patients a partial one. The curative potential is low. The best result is obtained in children with nocturnal polyuria and normal bladder capacity. Reduced bladder capacity indicates poor response.

Desmopressin is an easy-to-use medication with a quick effect and can be used in children older than 5 years. It is given either as oral tablets or in MELT (MELT oral lyophilisate) presentation. But MELT is not yet available in all countries. The nasal spray is not recommended for bedwetting owing to an increased incidence of serious side effects. Younger children often prefer MELT since it avoids the swallowing of tablets. Desmopressin in either form should be taken before bedtime.

Given its antidiuretic effect, the use cannot be associated with an excessive fluid intake because of the risk of water intoxication and hyponatremia. Children should restrict their fluid intake from 1 h before taking the medicine to 8 h afterward so as to avoid this serious side effect. If the family needs a general recommendation about fluid intake, a good rule is an evening intake of 200 mL (6 oz) or less and then no intake until the next morning [42]. Desmopressin should be avoided in children who have fluid control problems, such as in heart failure, and if the child is likely to find difficulty in complying with fluid restriction requirements.

Desmopressin tablets should be taken at least 1 h before going to sleep, since the maximum renal concentrating effect and minimal diuresis are attained after 1–2 h. Oral MELT tablets should be taken 30–60 min before bedtime. The ordinary dose of the tablets and MELT formulation is 0.2–0.4 mg and 120–240 mcg, respectively. This dose is not influenced by body weight or age. The beginning of the desmopressin effect is perceived immediately. If after 2 weeks there is no effect, treatment shall be discontinued. In children with a good response to treatment, this can be maintained with daily administration or be used in special situations, such as trips and nights away from home, according to the family's choice. In the first option, medication-free intervals are required every 3 months in order to verify if medication is still needed. If during this period the child presented enuresis, treatment may be restarted for another 3 months [43].

17.7.5 Enuresis Resistant to First-Line Treatment

The child who does not respond to treatment with desmopressin and/or alarm should be evaluated by a specialist. History needs to be remade, and it is necessary to check whether previous treatment was done correctly. Constipation and severe respiratory obstruction shall be excluded. The evaluation of these patients shall include voiding diary, measurement of nighttime urine production, ultrasound of the urinary tract, and uroflowmetry [42, 44].

The first-line treatment of resistant enuresis includes the possibility of alarm association with desmopressin, constipation treatment, and correction of airway obstruction. The second-line treatment includes the use of anticholinergics, with or without desmopressin. The anticholinergics should not be used with the child who presents UTI and residual urine >20 mL once or >10 mL in more than one examination. Constipation should also be ruled out before the anticholinergic treatment is started. The third-line treatment includes the use of imipramine, with or without desmopressin. There is a risk of overdosage and cardiotoxicity when imipramine is used. Imipramine should only be considered if the child has no history of syncope or palpitations, and there are no cases of sudden cardiac death or unstable arrhythmias in the family. If there is any doubt, an ECG should be performed to exclude long QT syndrome. There are reports of cardiotoxicity and death by accidental ingestion of younger siblings. The family should be informed to keep the pills securely locked [42, 44].

References

1. Austin PF, Bauer SB, Bower W, et al. The standardization of terminology of lower urinary tract function in children and adolescents: update report from the Standardization Committee of the International Children's Continence Society. J Urol. 2014;191(6):1863–5.
2. Soares AH, Moreira MC, Monteiro LM, et al. A enurese em crianças e seus significados para suas famílias: abordagem qualitativa sobre uma intervenção profissional em saúde. Rev Bras Saude Mater Infant. 2005;5:301–11.
3. Bower WF, Moore KH, Shepherd RB, et al. The epidemiology of childhood enuresis in Australia. Br J Urol. 1996;78:602–6.
4. von Gontard A, Heron J, Joinson C. Family history of nocturnal enuresis and urinary incontinence: results from a large epidemiological study. J Urol. 2011;185:2303–7.
5. Hjalmas K, Arnold T, Bower W, et al. Nocturnal enuresis: an international evidence based management strategy. J Urol. 2004;171:2545–61.
6. Yeung CK, Sreedhar B, Sihoe JD, et al. Differences in characteristics of nocturnal enuresis between children and adolescents: a critical appraisal from a large epidemiological study. BJU Int. 2006;97:1069–73.
7. Gimpel GA, Warzak WJ, Kuhn BR, et al. Clinical perspectives in primary nocturnal enuresis. Clin Pediatr. 1998;37(1):23–9.
8. Loeys B, Hoebeke P, Raes A, et al. Does monosymptomatic enuresis exist? A molecular genetic exploration of 32 families with enuresis/incontinence. BJU Int. 2002;90:76–83.
9. Van Herzeele C, Vande Walle J. Incontinence and psychological problems in children: a common central nervous pathway? Pediatr Nephrol. 2016;31(5):689–92.
10. Nevéus T, von Gontard A, Hoebeke P, et al. The standardization of terminology of lower urinary tract function in children and adolescents: report from the Standardization Committee of the International Children's Continence Society. J Urol. 2006;176(1):314–24.

11. Fonseca EMGO, Monteiro LMC. Clinical diagnosis of bladder dysfunction in enuretic children and adolescents. J Pediatr. 2004;80(2):147–53.
12. Soderstrom U, Hoelcke M, Alenius L, et al. Urinary and faecal incontinence: a population-based study. Acta Paediatr. 2004;93:386–9.
13. Sureshkumar P, Jones M, Cumming R, et al. A population based study of 2,856 school-age children with urinary incontinence. J Urol. 2009;181:808–16.
14. Fonseca EG, Bordallo AP, Garcia PK, et al. Lower urinary tract symptoms in enuretic and nonenuretic children. J Urol. 2009;182:1978–83.
15. Swithinbank LV, Heron J, von Gontard A, et al. The natural history of daytime urinary incontinence in children: a large British cohort. Acta Paeiat. 2010;99:1031–6.
16. Kajiwara M, Inoue K, Usui A, et al. The micturition habits and prevalence of daytime urinary incontinence in Japanese primary school children. J Urol. 2004;171:403–7.
17. Mota DM, VictoraII CG, HallaII PC. Investigation of voiding dysfunction in a population-based sample of children aged 3 to 9 years. J Pediatr. 2005;81(3):225–32.
18. Kyrklund K, Taskinen S, Rintala RJ, et al. Lower urinary tract symptoms from childhood to adulthood: a population based study of 594 finnish individuals 4 to 26 years old. J Urol. 2012;188:588–93.
19. Rittig S, Knudsen UB, Nørgaard JP, Pedersen EB, Djurhuus JC. Abnormal diurnal rhythm of plasma Vasopressin and urinary output in patients with enuresis. Am J Phys. 1989;256:F664–71.
20. De Guchtenaere A, Vande Walle C, Van Sintjan P, Raes A, Donckerwolcke R, Van Laecke E, Hoebeke P, Vande Walle J. Nocturnal polyuria is related to absent circadian rhythm of glomerular filtration rate. J Urol. 2007;178:2626–9.
21. Dossche L, Raes A, Hoebeke P, De Bruyne P, VandeWalle J. Circadian rhythm of glomerular filtration and solute handling related to nocturnal enuresis. J Urol. 2016;195:162–7.
22. Rasmussen PV, Kirk J, Borup K, Nørgaard JP, Djurhuus JC. Enuresis nocturna can be provoked in normal healthy children by increasing the nocturnal urine output. Scand J Urol Nephrol. 1996;30:57–61.
23. Hunsballe JM, Hansen TK, Rittig S, Nørgaard JP, Pedersen EB, Djurhuus JC. Polyuric and non-polyuric bedwetting—pathogenetic differences in nocturnal enuresis. Scand J Urol Nephrol. 1995;S173:77–9.
24. Schmidt F, Jorgesen TM, Djurhuus JC. The relationship between the bladder, the kidneys and CNS. Scand J Urol Nephrol Suppl. 1995;173:51–2.
25. Nevéus T, Tuvemo T, Lackgren G, et al. Bladder capacity and renal concentrating ability in enuresis: pathogenic implications. J Urol. 2001;165:2022–5.
26. Nevéus T. Nocturnal enuresis—theoretic background and practical guidelines. Pediatr Nephrol. 2011;26(8):1207–14.
27. Yeung CK, Diao M, Sreedhar B. Cortical arousals in children with severe enuresis. N Engl J Med. 2008;358:2414–5.
28. Dhondt K, van Herzeele C, Roels SP, et al. Sleep fragmentation and periodic limb movements in children with monosymptomatic nocturnal enuresis and polyuria. Pediatr Nephrol. 2015;30:1157–62.
29. Stepanski EJ. The effect of sleep fragmentation on daytime function. Sleep. 2002;25(3):268–76.
30. Mahler B, Kamperis K, Schroeder M, et al. Sleep deprivation induces excess diuresis and natriuresis in healthy children. Am J Physiol Ren Physiol. 2012;302:F236–43.
31. Umlauf MG, Chasens ER. Sleep disordered breathing and nocturnal polyuria: nocturia and enuresis. Sleep Med Rev. 2003;7:403–11.
32. von Gontard A, Baeyens D, Hoecke EV, et al. Psychological and psychiatric issues in urinary and fecal incontinence. J Urol. 2011;185:1432–7.
33. Loeninge-Baucke V. Urinary incontinence and urinary tract infection and their resolution with treatment of chronic constipation of childhood. Pediatric. 1997;100:228–32.
34. Borch L, Hagstroem S, Bower WF, et al. Bladder and bowel dysfunction and the resolution of urinary incontinence with successful management of bowel symptoms in children. Acta Paediatr. 2013;102(5):e215–20.

35. Alpaslan AH, Coskun KS, Yesil AA, et al. Child death as a result of physical violence during toilet training. J Forensic Legal Med. 2014;28:39–41.
36. Can G, Topbas M, Okten A, et al. Child abuse as a result of enuresis. Pediatr Int. 2004;46(1):64–6.
37. Karaman MI, Koca O, Kucuk EV, et al. Methods and rates of punishment implemented by families to enuretic children in Turkey. Int Braz J Urol. 2013;39(3):402–7.
38. Hyams JS, Di Lorenzo C, Saps M, et al. Childhood functional gastrointestinal disorders: child/adolescent. Gastroenterology. 2016;150:1456–68.
39. Lewis SJ, Heaton KW. Stool form scale as a useful guide to intestinal transit time. Scand J Gastroenterol. 1997;32(9):920–4.
40. Bright E, Oelke M, Tubaro A, et al. Ultrasound estimated bladder weight and measurement of bladder wall thickness—useful noninvasive methods for assessing the lower urinary tract? J Urol. 2010;184:1847–54.
41. Joensson IM, Siggard C, Rittg S, et al. Transabdominal ultrasound of rectum as a diagnostic tool in childhood constipation. J Urol. 2008;179:1997–2002.
42. Nevéus T, Eggert P, Evans J, et al. Evaluation of and treatment for monosymptomatic enuresis: a standardization document from the International Children's Continence Society. J Urol. 2010;183:441–7.
43. Lottmann H, Baydala L, Eggert P, et al. Long-term desmopressin response in primary nocturnal enuresis: open-label, multinational study. Int J Clin Pract. 2009;63(1):35–45.
44. Nevéus T. The evaluation and treatment of therapy-resistant enuresis: A review. Ups J Med Sci. 2006;111(1):61–72.

Nonmonosymptomatic Nocturnal Enuresis

18

Kwang Myung Kim

18.1 Definition

Nonmonosymptomatic nocturnal enuresis (NMNE) is defined as the presence of diurnal voiding symptoms—such as urgency, frequency, urge incontinence, infrequent voiding, and straining—in a patient with nocturnal enuresis. In contrast, patients with monosymptomatic enuresis (MNE) have no diurnal voiding symptoms [1, 2].

18.2 Epidemiology

In enuresis patients aged 7 years the incidence of NMNE is about 20–30%. In the British Avon Longitudinal Study, nocturnal enuresis was found in about 15% of 8242 7½-year-old children. Among them, 31.5% were classified as having NMNE and 68.5% as having MNE [3]. As patients grow older, the incidence of NMNE decreases. There is a strong possibility that NMNE patients have not only voiding dysfunction but also bowel problems such as constipation or stool incontinence. These comorbid symptoms are referred to as bladder and bowel dysfunction (BBD). Patients with diurnal voiding symptoms frequently have an associated psychiatric problem such as attention deficit hyperactivity disorder (ADHD) and offensive behavior [4].

K.M. Kim, M.D. (✉)
Department of Pediatric Urology, Seoul National University Children's Hospital, Seoul, Republic of Korea
e-mail: kwang@plaza.snu.ac.kr

18.3 Pathophysiology

The etiology of nocturnal enuresis can be summarized as (1) awakening disorder; (2) nocturnal polyuria; and (3) decreased functional bladder volume [5]. All three pathophysiological problems are related to developmental delay of central regulation of nocturnal voiding. Diurnal symptoms are also thought to result from developmental delay in which the central regulation of the voiding reflex arc is inadequate. If the patient has an overactive bladder, irritating symptoms of frequency and urgency arise and lead to decreased functional bladder capacity and desmopressin-resistant nocturnal enuresis. Urge incontinence develops when the patient's sphincteric activity is not strong enough to prevent leakage. In some patients, strong and chronic sphincteric contraction leads to dysfunctional voiding, straining during voiding, infrequent voiding, and increased residual volume.

Bowel dysfunction influences bladder function. Constipation causes irritating bladder symptoms by influencing the micturition reflexing arc and decreasing bladder capacity through mechanical volume effects.

Diurnal voiding symptoms are frequently associated with psychiatric comorbidity. Although the reason why ADHD patients have frequent nocturnal enuresis is not well established, treatment of this psychiatric problem before treatment of nocturnal enuresis results in a high rate of successful treatment of nocturnal enuresis.

18.4 Pretreatment Patient Examination

For history taking regarding diurnal voiding symptom, we must check the voiding frequency per day, the severity of urgency, and the daily frequency and volume of urge incontinence. Completion of a 2-day voided volume chart is usually used for measuring the severity of these symptoms. Visual analog scaling of urgency and completion of a "Dry Pie" chart of urge incontinence are also helpful [6]. In addition, the constipation and stool incontinence history should be checked. The Rome III classification [7] and the Bristol Stool Form Scale [8] are helpful for objective documentation of bowel problems. A history of cystitis or recurrent cystitis symptoms such as dysuria and suprapubic pain suggest the presence of NMNE rather than NME.

Physical examination must include the whole abdomen, external genitalia, and lower back area. In particular, careful inspection of the sacral area to exclude signs of spina bifida or a lipomyelomeningocele should be performed. Uroflowmetry and an ultrasonic postvoiding residual urine examination are mandatory. If there is a severely abnormal finding, a formal urodynamic study can be performed for further examination. Sometimes genitourinary tract ultrasonography is needed to check for a genitourinary tract anomaly and measurement of the bladder wall thickness and rectal diameter for constipation.

18.5 Treatment

The first goal of treatment of NMNE must be treatment of diurnal voiding symptoms. Without treatment of diurnal voiding symptoms, nocturnal enuresis frequently does not respond to conventional treatment, which includes desmopressin drug therapy and bedwetting alarm therapy.

Before treatment of diurnal voiding symptoms, we have to treat any underlying disease aggravating diurnal voiding symptoms. Constipation and stool incontinence should be treated before starting treatment of enuresis [9]. If the patient has a psychiatric problem such as ADHD, a psychiatric consultation must be arranged for the child to receive appropriate treatment of this underlying disease.

Desmopressin drug therapy and bedwetting alarm therapy are most commonly used for treating nocturnal enuresis irrespective of whether there are diurnal symptoms. In nonmonosymptomatic enuresis, however, an anticholinergic agent must be added for the treatment of diurnal voiding symptoms such as frequency, urgency, and urge incontinence. If the patient has dysfunctional voiding, an alpha blocker or biofeedback treatment is recommended for efficient voiding.

Care must be taken during anticholinergic drug therapy because the side effects of anticholinergics include aggravation of constipation and a dry mouth. In addition, caffeine-containing beverages are prohibited so as not to increase overactive bladder contraction.

Desmopressin monotherapy for NMNE results in a high rate of failure of treatment [10], and anticholinergic monotherapy for MNE also results in a low rate of treatment success [11].

Desmopressin drug therapy or bedwetting alarm therapy can be started with anticholinergic drug therapy initially or when the patient has persistent enuresis despite treatment of voiding dysfunction and bowel dysfunction.

Recently, transcutaneous electrical nerve stimulation (TENS) has been attempted to treat enuresis [12], daytime incontinence [13, 14], and bowel dysfunction [15]. Although there was no strict classification of enuresis as MNE or NMNE in these studies, TENS seems to be one treatment modality for NMNE.

References

1. Neveus T, von Gontard A, Hoebeke P, Hjalmas K, Bauer S, Bower W, et al. The standardization of terminology of lower urinary tract function in children and adolescents: report from the standardization committee of the International Children's Continence Society. J Urol. 2006;176:314–24.
2. Franco I, von Gontard A, De Gennaro M. International Childrens's Continence Society. Evaluation and treatment of nonmonosymptomatic nocturnal enuresis: a standardization document from the International Children's Continence Society. J Pediatr Urol. 2013;9:234–43.
3. Butler R, Heron J, The Alspac Study Team. Exploring the differences between mono- and polysymptomatic nocturnal enuresis. Scand J Urol Nephrol. 2006;40:313–9.

4. Joinson C, Heron J, Butler U, von Gontard A. Psychological differences between children with and without soiling problems. Pediatrics. 2006;117:1575–84.
5. Neveus T, Eggert P, Evans J, International Children's Continence Society, et al. Evaluation of and treatment for monosymptomatic enuresis: a standardization document from the International Children's Continence Society. J Urol. 2010;183:441–7.
6. Bower WF, Moore KH, Adams RD. A noble clinical evaluation of childhood incontinence and urinary urgency. J Urol. 2001;166:2411–5.
7. Rasquin A, Di LC, Forbes D, Guiraldes E, Hyams JS, Staiano A, et al. Childhood functional gastrointestinal disorders: child/adolescent. Gastroenterology. 2006;130:1527–37.
8. Lewis SJ, Heaton KW. Stool form scale as a useful guide to intestinal transit time. Scand J Gastroenterol. 1997;32:920–4.
9. Roth EB, Austin PF. Evaluation and treatment of nonmonosymptomatic enuresis. Pediatr Rev. 2014;35:430–6.
10. Lovering JS, Tallett SE, McKendry JB. Oxybutynin efficacy in the treatment of primary enuresis. Pediatrics. 1988;82:104–6.
11. Glazener CM, Evans JH, Peto RE. Drugs for nocturnal enuresis in children (other than desmopressin and tricyclics). Cochrane Database Syst Rev. 2003;4:CD002238.
12. Kajbafzadeh AM, Lida Sharifi-Rad L, Mozafarpour S, Ladi-Seyedian S. Efficacy of transcutaneous interferential electrical stimulation in treatment of children with primary nocturnal enuresis: a randomized clinical trial. Pediatr Nephrol. 2015;30:1139–45.
13. Hagstroem S, Mahler B, Madsen B, Djurhuus JC, Rittig S. Transcutaneous electrical nerve stimulation for refractory daytime urinary urge Incontinence. J Urol. 2009;182:2072–8.
14. Lordêlo P, Teles A, Veiga ML, et al. Transcutaneous electrical nerve stimulation in children with overactive bladders: a randomized clinical trial. J Urol. 2010;184:683–9. Incontinence. J Urol. 2009
15. Veiga ML, Lordêlo P, Farias T, Barroso U Jr. Evaluation of constipation after parasacral transcutaneous electrical nerve stimulation in children with lower urinary tract dysfunction—a pilot study. J Pediatr Urol. 2013;9:622–6.

Overactive Bladder

19

Lorenzo Masieri, Chiara Cini, and Maria Taverna

19.1 Introduction

Detrusor overactivity is the most common voiding dysfunction in children. This condition is also known as overactive bladder (OAB), urge syndrome, hyperactive bladder syndrome, persistent infantile bladder, or detrusor hypertonia [1]. Idiopathic OAB is defined by the International Continence Society (ICS) as a complex symptom of urinary urgency, which may or may not be associated with urgency urinary incontinence, urinary frequency, and nocturia in the absence of pathological or metabolic factors [2]. As the OAB symptomatology is concerned, the International Children's Continence Society (ICCS) states that Urgency incontinence is often also present, as the increased voiding frequency, but these symptoms are not necessary prerequisites for the use of the term OAB [3]. The OAB in children is characterized by involuntary detrusor contractions and urethral instability [4]. The etiology has been variously ascribed to maturation delay, prolongation of infantile bladder behavior, or shortening of acquired toilet-training habits [5]. Early diagnosis and appropriate treatment could affect upper urinary tract function and drainage and ultimate bladder functions.

L. Masieri (✉) • C. Cini • M. Taverna
Division of Pediatric Urology, Meyer Pediatric Hospital, Florence, Italy
e-mail: lorenzo.masieri@meyer.it

19.2 Epidemiology

OAB is a common problem in the pediatric population. The reported prevalence in healthy children in the age group of 5–13 years ranges from 16.6% to 17.8% and decreases with age [6, 7]. In incontinent children OAB accounts for 21–58% of cases [8]. In a US population survey of 1192 individuals aged 1.5–27 years, diurnal accidents occurred in 13% of children aged 4 years, 7% of children aged 5 years, 10% of children aged 6 years, and 5% of children aged 7 years [9]. Urge symptoms seem to peak in children aged 6–9 years and to diminish with the puberty, with a spontaneous resolution rate for daytime wetting of 14% per year [10]. Hellstrom et al., assessing the prevalence of urinary incontinence in 7-year-old Swedish children, found that diurnal incontinence was more common in girls (6.7%) than in boys (3.8%) [11].

19.3 Etiology

Overactive bladder is a multifactorial problem not completely understood. In children, OAB may arise from various etiologies, including neurogenic, anatomic, inflammatory, and idiopathic causes. Moreover:

- Neurogenic etiologies include myelomeningocele, cerebral palsy, spinal cord injury, sacral agenesis, and imperforate anus. Twenty-two percent of children with a lumbosacral myelomeningocele have uninhibited bladder contractions [12].
- The most common anatomic abnormality associated with OAB is posterior urethral valves (24%) [13].
- Inflammatory processes in the bladder wall (e.g., urinary tract infections), enuresis, constipation, fecal incontinence, and delayed toilet training are considered risk factors associated with OAB irritating receptors in the submucosa and detrusor muscle [14].
- Idiopathic OAB is thought to be secondary to delayed maturation of the reticulospinal pathways and inhibitory centers in the midbrain and cerebral cortex. Development of continence and voluntary voiding involves maturation of the nervous system and behavioral learning. Normally by the age of 5 years, unless organic causes are present, the child is able to void at will and to postpone voiding in a socially acceptable manner [15, 16]. The delay in bladder-sphincter coordination during voiding causes a persistent isometric contraction of the detrusor and incomplete relaxation of the sphincter leading the bladder muscle to hypertrophy and to a gradual decrease in functional bladder capacity and increased bladder instability.
- A finding that confirms a central process and a genetic mode of transmission for voiding dysfunction is the Ochoa urofacial syndrome [17].

19.4 Pathophysiology

The symptoms of OAB are believed to be caused by detrusor contractions during the filling phase, which causes urgency. These contractions are countered by voluntary tightening of the pelvic floor muscles to postpone voiding and to minimize wetting. The voiding phase is essentially normal but may be associated with a powerful detrusor contraction. A neurogenic origin following any disorder that involves the higher centers or the nerve pathways responsible for the control of urination can be hypothesized. There are various efferent and afferent neural pathway reflexes, as well as central and peripheral neurotransmitters involved in urinary storage and bladder emptying. Serotonergic activity facilitates urine storage. Dopaminergic pathways may exert inhibitory (Dl receptors) or facilitatory (D2 receptors) effects on voiding. Acetylcholine is the predominant peripheral neurotransmitter responsible for bladder contraction [18]. ATP may have a prominent role in bladder contractions in patients with overactive bladder. The role of these neurotransmitters can be better understood with functional magnetic resonance imaging and positron emission tomography [19]. Stimulation of the hypogastric plexus originating from spinal levels T-10 through L-2 results in detrusor muscle relaxation and intrinsic sphincter contraction, inhibiting micturition. Stimulation of passive sympathetic nerves originating from spinal levels S-2 through S-4 has the opposite effect. Functional magnetic resonance imaging and positron emission tomography indicate that bladder fullness is associated with increased activity in the anterior mesencephalon pons and medulla (micturition center) and in the cortical centers, primarily in the anterior and posterior cingulate gyrus which is associated with behavior control [20]. The inability to activate this cingulate gyrus and suppress autonomic activities leads to hyperreflexia. Inactivity in the cingulate gyrus might explain the overactive bladder found in familial settings and the association of voiding dysfunction in patients with behavioral, learning, and psychiatric disorders [21].

19.4.1 The Role of Constipation

There is a close association between constipation and overactive bladder [22]. The mainstay in the management of overactive bladder is the correction of constipation and fecal retention. Some theories suggest that the increased fecal mass stored in the rectum and sigmoid may exert some type of pressure on the bladder wall decreasing functional bladder capacity. Miyazato et al. found that rectal distention leads to decreased amplitude and duration of bladder contraction, and it can almost abolish bladder activity [23]. It is possible that stretch receptors in the bladder wall stimulated by the extrinsic fecal mass trigger detrusor contractions and sustain a vicious cycle of continued contractions. Moreover colonic contractions may be triggering bladder contractions via shared neural pathways in the pelvis or spinal cord. Ustinova reported that acute colitis triggers bladder hyperactivity in rats, providing experimental evidence for cross talk between pelvic viscera [24]. The correction of constipation must be pursued using several techniques with a high-fiber diet and increased fluid intake or some kind of stool softener and/or cathartic. Commonly used methods to evaluate constipation are the Bristol stool form scale and the Leech method to assess the level of stools within the intestine by plain radiography [25]. The recent introduction of medications such as tegaserod for the management of the irritable bowel syndrome may have a role in the future management of overactive bladder dysfunction [26].

19.5 Clinical Presentation

Signs and symptoms of overactive bladder in children can vary in their typical presentation. According to the International Children's Continence Society definition [3], the core symptom of OAB in children is urgency, and they will be seen clutching the penis or squatting and sitting on their heels in an attempt to prevent incontinence. It may occur with urge incontinence, urinary frequency, and nocturnal enuresis. Many children have no sense that they are wetting when they have accidents. Other children just have an increased sense to void and voiding quite frequently. Many of the signs and symptoms of OAB are due to faulty perceptions of bladder signals and habitual nonphysiological responses to such signals [27]. The definition of urinary frequency in a child is who has a normal fluid intake is not well established. However, many believe that a child who voids more than seven times per day has urinary frequency. Depending on fluid intake and urine production, children may experience more episodes of incontinence later in the day as a consequence of fatigue and an impaired ability to concentrate. The perpetual tonic activity of the external sphincter can lead to tightening, fibrosis, and incomplete relaxation of the external sphincter with turbulent urine flow and resultant urethral discomfort, typically called bulbar urethritis. In some girls we also see dysuria, vaginal pain, and gross hematuria. The onset can be slow and insidious, with a gradual increase in the strength of the urge to void or quite sudden with episodes of incontinence in children who were normally dry in a short period.

19.6 Comorbidities

Comorbidities, like UTIs, bowel dysfunctions, endocrinological disorders, psychiatric issues, and chromosome abnormalities, have to be treated simultaneously with the incontinence problems. Some of the consequences of OAB result from the child's voluntary attempts to maintain continence during the involuntary detrusor contractions with coping mechanisms to produce perineal compression. This may lead to functional and morphologic changes in the bladder, which can increase the risk of urinary tract infections (UTIs) and vesicoureteral reflux. Frequent voluntary contractions of the pelvic floor muscles may also lead to postponement of defecation. More than 50% of children with lower urinary tract symptoms evaluated in a tertiary referral center fulfilled diagnostic criteria for functional defecation disorders [28]. In children who have problems with incontinence, the incidence of behavioral and psychiatric disorders is three times higher than in the general population.

19.6.1 OAB and Obesity

Currently, obesity is a common and growing problem worldwide. The prevalence of childhood obesity has doubled in the past few decades in the United States and Taiwan [29, 30]. There are few studies evaluating the effects of obesity on LUTS and voiding function in children. Previous reports stated that children with elimination disorders have higher obesity rates (62–86%) than the normal population [31]. Obesity was an independent risk factor for pediatric OAB symptoms [32]. Obese children are at a higher risk of nocturnal enuresis when compared to children of normal weight; obese girls are at a higher risk of daytime incontinence [33, 34]. Obesity is linked to OAB symptoms through lifestyle factors (excessive eating and drinking) and its association with hyperglycemia, which can cause diuresis and lower urinary tract symptoms. Obesity also exposes the pelvic floor to elevated intra-abdominal and intravesical pressure, which may compromise the functional bladder capacity.

19.7 Diagnosis

The evaluation of pediatric OAB begins with history taking, physical examination, and laboratory investigation (urinalysis) to exclude underlying pathological or metabolic disorders that may mimic or cause OAB. Differential diagnoses for OAB include dysfunctional voiding and voiding postponement [35]. Frequency/volume charts and bladder diaries are essential tools providing information of diagnostic and therapeutic value for the child and his family. They will allow the child's caregivers to document maximal and average voided volumes, voiding frequency, incontinence episodes, bowel movements, fluid intake, and urine production [36]. Invasive testing is performed for specific indications such as a history of vesicoureteral reflux, febrile UTI, stress incontinence or suspected obstruction (weak urine stream or straining), or underlying neurologic etiology.

19.7.1 History

The history takes into account perinatal issues, developmental milestones, current mental status, school performance, events at the time of toilet training, patterns of bladder and bowel emptying regimens, and features of incontinent episodes. A review of fluid intake (including kind of fluid) is important to note. In girls, voiding habits should be reviewed to teach proper positioning during voiding to eliminate vaginal reflux voiding as a source of incontinence [35].

19.7.2 Physical Examination

Physical examination findings are usually within normal limits in children who have idiopathic OAB. Some children with urinary incontinence can have perineal excoriation. A neurological examination should be performed to rule out an underlying neurologic etiology. The examination includes an assessment of perineal sensation and perineal reflexes supplied by sacral segments S1–S4, evaluation of anal sphincter tone, and evaluation of the buttocks, legs, and feet for signs of occult neurospinal dysraphisms of the lumbosacral area. The position and caliber of the urethral meatus should be inspected. The abdominal examination should include assessment for a distended bladder and a full sigmoid/descending colon (suggestive of constipation). Symptoms of pediatric OAB and urinary incontinence may lead to embarrassment in the child. The child may be inappropriately labeled as having a psychological problem and refrain from social activities [27].

19.8 Prognosis

The natural history of OAB in children is unknown. Data on the optimal duration of therapy are limited. OAB in children is not believed to be a chronic condition; however, little long-term information is available. Curran reported an average time to resolution of OAB symptoms of 2.7 years. Age and gender were not significant predictors of resolution, although symptom resolution was more likely in girls than in boys [37]. Childhood incontinence in girls has been noted to be a risk factor for urge symptoms and severe incontinence in adult women [38].

19.9 Management

19.9.1 Conservative Management

Treatment modalities should be tailored to the individual child and specific condition. The non-pharmacological treatment options (urotherapy) remain the basic intervention. Standard urotherapy includes educating children and parents about LUT anatomy and function, providing information, and demystification [39]. Urotherapy involves the active management of bowel dysfunction, implementation of fluid intake, and regular visits to the toilet through the use of a timer watch or wetting alarm during the day [40]. The cognitive registration of urge symptoms and the need to use the toilet immediately without the use of holding maneuvers is the main goal of treatment [41]. Specific urotherapy includes various forms of biofeedback pelvic floor muscle relaxation techniques, neuromodulation, and intermittent catheterization. Additional interventions of urotherapy involve cognitive behavioral therapy and psychotherapy. Despite the low level of evidence, the grade of recommendation is high, because urotherapy alone leads to least adverse effects and has proven to be clinically useful for many children.

19.9.2 Pharmacologic Treatment

Pharmacotherapy is second-line treatment and should always be combined with urotherapy. It is initiated if behavioral therapy fails or symptoms are severe. The first-line drug for OAB has been anticholinergics which block M2/M3 receptors in the bladder suppressing bladder contractility [42]. Oxybutynin IR and oxybutynin ER are the only antimuscarinics approved by the FDA for the treatment of overactive bladder symptoms in children at recommended daily dose of 0.3–0.6 mg/kg/d (maximum 15 mg/d in total). When only partial improvement was noted on a single medication, another drug (an additional anticholinergic, imipramine or desmopressin) can be added to the regimen [37]. In some countries, propiverine has been approved for use in children at 0.4–0.8 mg/kg/d in two divided doses and trospium for older children (age 12 years). Other substances such as tolterodine and solifenacin can be administered if other drugs fail, but have to be prescribed off-label.

Alpha-blockers are quite effective for OAB, especially in patients with primary bladder neck dysfunction [43] or external sphincter dyssynergia reducing bladder outlet resistance and avoiding obstruction-related detrusor overactivity, but are still considered "off-label" [42]. A link with anxiety disorders and significant voiding dysfunctions has been reported in the literature. Many of these patients seem to respond favorably to the introduction of imipramine or 5-HT reuptake inhibitors although they do not carry a diagnosis of psychiatric disorders. The introduction of newer anticholinergics that show high levels in the bladder and possibly bind to muscarinic receptors in the bladder mucosa may have a greater role in OAB management in the future.

19.9.3 Biofeedback Therapy

Biofeedback techniques allow to train pelvic floor muscle relaxation viewing abdominal muscle activity, perineal muscle direction of movement, and visualization of electromyographic activity from muscles within the pelvic girdle. This can be combined with displaying of real-time uroflow or interactive computer games in which children attempt to move an icon of their choice, within the predetermined ranges that have been set [44, 45]. Each session lasts approximately 45 minutes with a trained nurse performing the biofeedback therapy. Biofeedback therapy is limited by the ability of the child to cooperate with the healthcare provider running the session. Children younger than 5 years with significant learning disabilities, behavior problems, and other neurological problems are not candidates for biofeedback [46].

19.9.4 Neuromodulation

Neuromodulation has been used to treat a variety of childhood LUT dysfunctions, mainly OAB and neurogenic bladder dysfunction; the mode of application includes transcutaneous, intravesical, endoanal, anogenital, posterior tibial nerve, and sacral nerve implantation.

19.9.4.1 Sacral Nerve Modulation

Sacral neuromodulation delivered via implantable electrodes offers efficacy in improving neurogenic bladder dysfunction. Up to date, case series reported benefits in pediatric OAB, dysfunctional elimination syndrome, and Fowler syndrome [47]. Selective stimulation of the sacral and pudendal nerves has led to significant improvement in overactive bladder in patients who have had stimulators implanted. The role of spinal stimulation in children is still to be clearly defined [48].

19.9.4.2 Peripheral Nerve Stimulation

Electrical tibial nerve stimulation is based on the traditional Chinese practice of using acupuncture points over the common peroneal posterior tibial nerves to inhibit bladder activity. A limited number of reports of its use in children have indicated efficacy [48, 49]. The use of TENS involving the S3 region with surface electrodes made this technique applicable in children. The mechanism for neuromodulation is not well understood. The hypothesis is that the electrical current directly affects the central nervous system by artificially activating neural structures and facilitating both neural plasticity and normative afferent and efferent activity innervating the low urinary tract [50].

19.9.5 Cognitive Therapy

Cognitive therapy encompasses a whole variety of techniques such as "self-monitoring" (observation and registration), organization of activities, and "labeling" (using positive suggestive statements). Behavioral therapy focuses on observable behavior, aiming at modifying it with a variety of techniques using positive or negative reinforcement.

19.9.6 Psychotherapy

If a comorbid disorder is suspected through a questionnaire, a psychological or psychiatric assessment is recommended. If a clinically relevant disorder is present, counseling is always indicated. If the disorder is incapacitating, psychotherapy and/or pharmacotherapy is recommended [51].

19.9.7 Botulinum Toxin A

Botulinum toxin (BTX) is a potent neurotoxin that inhibits acetylcholine release at the presynaptic junction and reduces sensory purinergic receptors in the bladder. Clinical effects begin within 5–7 days after injection and are reversible within

6 months. Doses vary between 5 and 12 IU/kg body weight with a maximal dose of 300–360 IU BTX, in 20–50 injection sites [52]. Studies in spinal cord-injured adults and children with spina bifida have proved effective to decrease detrusor hyperactivity with multiple injections throughout the floor of the bladder. BTX has been used off-label to manage children with neuropathic bladder and treatment-resistant non-neurogenic bladder dysfunction [53]. Evidence had shown that efficacy is maintained with repeated injections [54]. The level of evidence for using botulinum toxin A is low; it may be considered in children with OAB or UI only if all other treatment options have failed.

Conclusions

Detrusor overactivity is ubiquitous in a considerable number of conditions that affect a child's lower urinary tract. It is becoming apparent that the vesicocentric theories that were proposed in the past for overactive bladder must make way in favor of a more corticocentric way of thinking. Currently anticholinergics seem only able to treat symptoms; norepinephrine and 5-HT are critical in the modulation of voiding processes. Treatment with this group of drugs must be further investigated. The use of stimulation modalities, whether peripheral or central, needs continued exploration in the future. Functional disorders characterized by detrusor overactivity are more readily managed when the diagnosis is made early, reducing the psychological trauma the wetting may pose on the social development of the child and preventing further problems in adulthood.

References

1. Sarica K, Yagci F, Erturhan S, Yurtseven C. Conservative management of overactive bladder in children: evaluation of clinical and urodynamic results. J Pediatr Urol. 2006;2:34–9.
2. Abrams P, Cardozo L, Fall M, et al. The standardisation of terminology of lower urinary tract function: report from the standardisation sub-committee of the international continence society. Neurourol Urodyn. 2002;21:167–78.
3. Neveus T, von Gontard A, Hoebeke P, et al. The standardization of terminology of lower urinary tract function in children and adolescents: report from the standardisation Committee of the International Children's continence society. J Urol. 2006;176:314–24.
4. Bauer SB. Special considerations of the overactive bladder in children. Urology. 2002;60: 43–8; discussion 49.
5. Fernandes E, Vernier R, Gonzalez R. The unstable bladder in children. J Pediatr. 1991;118:831–7.
6. Nijman RJM, Bower W, Butler U. Diagnosis and management of urinary incontinence and encopresis in children. Inc. 2005;2:965.
7. Chung JM, Lee SD, Kang DI, et al. Prevalence and associated factors of overactive bladder in Korean children 5-13 years old: a nationwide multicenter study. Urology. 2009;73:63–9. https://doi.org/10.1016/j.urology.2008.06.063.
8. Hoebeke P, Van Laecke E, Van Camp C, et al. One thousand video-urodynamic studies in children with non-neurogenic bladder sphincter dysfunction. BJU Int. 2001;87:575–80.
9. Bloom DA, Seeley WW, Ritchey ML, McGuire EJ. Toilet habits and continence in children: an opportunity sampling in search of normal parameters. J Urol. 1993;149:1087–90.

10. Himsl KK, Hurwitz RS. Pediatric urinary incontinence. Urol Clin North Am. 1991;18:283–93.
11. Hellström AL, Hanson E, Hansson S, et al. Micturition habits and incontinence in 7-year-old Swedish school entrants. Eur J Pediatr. 1990;149:434–7.
12. Dator DP, Hatchett L, Dyro FM, et al. Urodynamic dysfunction in walking myelodysplastic children. J Urol. 1992;148:362–5.
13. Peters CA, Bolkier M, Bauer SB, et al. The urodynamic consequences of posterior urethral valves. J Urol. 1990;144:122–6.
14. Kass EJ, Diokno AC, Montealegre A. Enuresis: principles of management and result of treatment. J Urol. 1979;121(6):794.
15. Nørgaard JP, van Gool JD, Hjälmås K, et al. Standardization and definitions in lower urinary tract dysfunction in children. International Children's continence society. Br J Urol. 1998;81(Suppl 3):1–16.
16. Hjälmås K. Functional daytime incontinence: definitions and epidemiology. Scand J Urol Nephrol Suppl. 1992;141:39–44; discussion 45–6.
17. Ochoa B. The urofacial (Ochoa) syndrome revisited. J Urol. 1992;148:580–3.
18. Van Arsdelen K, Wein A. Physiology of micturition. Clin Neuro-Urology. 1991:56–9.
19. Kuhtz-Buschbeck JP, van der Horst C, Pott C, et al. Cortical representation of the urge to void: a functional magnetic resonance imaging study. J Urol. 2005;174:1477–81.
20. Griffiths D, Derbyshire S, Stenger A, Resnick N. Brain control of normal and overactive bladder. J Urol. 2005;174:1862–7. https://doi.org/10.1097/01.ju.0000177450.34451.97.
21. Franco I. Overactive bladder in children. Part 1: pathophysiology. J Urol. 2007;178:761–768; discussion 768. https://doi.org/10.1016/j.juro.2007.05.014.
22. Loening-Baucke V. Urinary incontinence and urinary tract infection and their resolution with treatment of chronic constipation of childhood. Pediatrics. 1997;100:228–32.
23. Miyazato M, Sugaya K, Nishijima S, et al. Rectal distention inhibits bladder activity via glycinergic and GABAergic mechanisms in rats. J Urol. 2004;171:1353–6.
24. Ustinova EE, Gutkin DW, Pezzone MA. Sensitization of pelvic nerve afferents and mast cell infiltration in the urinary bladder following chronic colonic irritation is mediated by neuropeptides. Am J Physiol Renal Physiol. 2007;292:F123–30.
25. Riegler G, Esposito I. Bristol scale stool form. A still valid help in medical practice and clinical research. Tech Coloproctol. 2001;5:163–4.
26. Evans BW, Clark WK, Moore DJ, Whorwell PJ. Tegaserod for the treatment of irritable bowel syndrome and chronic constipation. Cochrane Database Syst Rev. 2007;14:CD003960.
27. van Gool JD, de Jonge GA. Urge syndrome and urge incontinence. Arch Dis Child. 1989;64:1629–34.
28. Burgers R, de Jong TPVM, Visser M, et al. Functional defecation disorders in children with lower urinary tract symptoms. J Urol. 2013;189:1886–91.
29. Ogden CL, Carroll MD, Curtin LR, et al. Prevalence of high body mass index in US children and adolescents, 2007-2008. JAMA. 2010;303:242–9.
30. Chen LJ, Fox KR, Haase A, Wang JM. Obesity, fitness and health in Taiwanese children and adolescents. Eur J Clin Nutr. 2006;60:1367–75. https://doi.org/10.1038/sj.ejcn.1602466.
31. Erdem E, Lin A, Kogan BA, Feustel PJ. Association of elimination dysfunction and body mass index. J Pediatr Urol. 2006;2:364–7. https://doi.org/10.1016/j.jpurol.2006.05.002.
32. Chang S-J, Chiang I-N, Lin C-D, et al. Obese children at higher risk for having overactive bladder symptoms: a community-based study. Neurourol Urodyn. 2015;34:123–7. https://doi.org/10.1002/nau.22532.
33. Weintraub Y, Singer S, Alexander D, et al. Enuresis--an unattended comorbidity of childhood obesity. Int J Obes. 2013;37:75–8. https://doi.org/10.1038/ijo.2012.108.
34. Schwartz B, Wyman JF, Thomas W, Schwarzenberg SJ. Urinary incontinence in obese adolescent girls. J Pediatr Urol. 2009;5:445–50. https://doi.org/10.1016/j.jpurol.2009.07.005.
35. Lettgen B, von Gontard A, Olbing H, et al. Urge incontinence and voiding postponement in children: somatic and psychosocial factors. Acta Paediatr. 2002;91:978–84; discussion 895–6.
36. Hoebeke P, Bower W, Combs A, et al. Diagnostic evaluation of children with daytime incontinence. J Urol. 2010;183:699–703. https://doi.org/10.1016/j.juro.2009.10.038.

37. Curran MJ, Kaefer M, Peters C, et al. The overactive bladder in childhood: long-term results with conservative management. J Urol. 2000;163:574–7.
38. Fitzgerald MP, Thom DH, Wassel-Fyr C, et al. Childhood urinary symptoms predict adult overactive bladder symptoms. J Urol. 2006;175:989–93.
39. Austin PF, Bauer SB, Bower W, et al. The standardization of terminology of lower urinary tract function in children and adolescents: update report from the standardization Committee of the International Children's continence society. J Urol. 2014;191:1863–1865.e13.
40. Hagstroem S, Rittig N, Kamperis K, et al. Treatment outcome of day-time urinary incontinence in children. Scand J Urol Nephrol. 2008;42:528–33.
41. Vijverberg MAW, Stortelder E, de Kort LMO, et al. Long-term follow-up of incontinence and urge complaints after intensive urotherapy in childhood (75 patients followed up for 16.2-21.8 years). Urology. 2011;78:1391–6.
42. Austin PF, Homsy YL, Masel JL, et al. Alpha-adrenergic blockade in children with neuropathic and nonneuropathic voiding dysfunction. J Urol. 1999;162:1064–7.
43. Donohoe JM, Combs AJ, Glassberg KI. Primary bladder neck dysfunction in children and adolescents II: results of treatment with alpha-adrenergic antagonists. J Urol. 2005;173:212–6.
44. Shei Dei Yang S, Wang CC. Outpatient biofeedback relaxation of the pelvic floor in treating pediatric dysfunctional voiding: a short-course program is effective. Urol Int. 2005;74:118–22. https://doi.org/10.1159/000083281.
45. Herndon CD, Decambre M, McKenna PH. Interactive computer games for treatment of pelvic floor dysfunction. J Urol. 2001;166:1893–8.
46. Hoekx L, Wyndaele JJ, Vermandel A. The role of bladder biofeedback in the treatment of children with refractory nocturnal enuresis associated with idiopathic detrusor instability and small bladder capacity. J Urol. 1998;160:858–60.
47. Groen L-A, Hoebeke P, Loret N, et al. Sacral neuromodulation with an implantable pulse generator in children with lower urinary tract symptoms: 15-year experience. J Urol. 2012;188:1313–7. https://doi.org/10.1016/j.juro.2012.06.039.
48. Hoebeke P, Renson C, Petillon L, et al. Percutaneous electrical nerve stimulation in children with therapy resistant nonneuropathic bladder sphincter dysfunction: a pilot study. J Urol. 2002;168:2605–2607; discussion 2607–8. https://doi.org/10.1097/01.ju.0000037424.62620.f9.
49. Barroso U, Tourinho R, Lordêlo P, et al. Electrical stimulation for lower urinary tract dysfunction in children: a systematic review of the literature. Neurourol Urodyn. 2011;30:1429–36. https://doi.org/10.1002/nau.21140.
50. Patidar N, Mittal V, Kumar M, et al. Transcutaneous posterior tibial nerve stimulation in pediatric overactive bladder: a preliminary report. J Pediatr Urol. 2015;11:351.e1–6. https://doi.org/10.1016/j.jpurol.2015.04.040.
51. von Gontard A, Baeyens D, Van Hoecke E, et al. Psychological and psychiatric issues in urinary and fecal incontinence. J Urol. 2011;185:1432–6. https://doi.org/10.1016/j.juro.2010.11.051.
52. Hoebeke P, De Caestecker K, Vande Walle J, et al. The effect of botulinum-a toxin in incontinent children with therapy resistant overactive detrusor. J Urol. 2006;176:321–8. https://doi.org/10.1016/S0022-5347(06)00301-6.
53. Hassouna T, Gleason JM, Lorenzo AJ. Botulinum toxin A's expanding role in the management of pediatric lower urinary tract dysfunction. Curr Urol Rep. 2014;15:426. https://doi.org/10.1007/s11934-014-0426-1.
54. Game X, Mouracade P, Chartier-Kastler E, et al. Botulinum toxin-a (Botox) intradetrusor injections in children with neurogenic detrusor overactivity/neurogenic overactive bladder: a systematic literature review. J Pediatr Urol. 2009;5:156–64. https://doi.org/10.1016/j.jpurol.2009.01.005.
55. Barroso UJ, Viterbo W, Bittencourt J, et al. Posterior tibial nerve stimulation vs parasacral transcutaneous neuromodulation for overactive bladder in children. J Urol. 2013;190:673–7. https://doi.org/10.1016/j.juro.2013.02.034.

Daytime Lower Urinary Tract Conditions

20

Marleen van den Heijkant

20.1 Introduction

The prevalence of daytime lower urinary tract (LUT) conditions in children shows an increasing incidence and affects around 17% of school-aged children [1]. In the current pediatric urology outpatients' clinic, this patient group includes 40% of all patients [2].

The International Children's Continence Society (ICCS) updated their report on the standardization of terminology of lower urinary tract (LUT) function in children and adolescents in 2017, and "daytime lower urinary tract conditions" is the current term used [3, 4]. In this patient group, any possible (anatomical) uropathy or neurogenic bladder should be excluded. The children with wetting during nighttime have enuresis.

The etiology and clinical presentation of children with daytime LUT conditions will be described in this chapter. The ICCS stresses the close relationship of bowel emptying issues with bladder function and therefore labels this relationship as bladder and bowel dysfunction (BBD). The term dysfunctional elimination syndrome connotes an anomaly or condition and is therefore abandoned [3].

BBD is a term, which covers LUT dysfunction as well as bowel dysfunction. Various functional disorders of the detrusor-sphincter complex may exist during the early development of normal mechanisms of micturition control [5]. In a Swedish study, normal daytime control of bladder function is reached at 4 years of age, while nighttime control is usually achieved between 5 years and 7 years of age [6]. An American study reported a mean age of daytime urinary control at 2.4 ± 0.6 years [7]. Hoebeke et al. state in one of the ICCS standardization documents that in contrast to the adult population, where urinary incontinence is always considered a

M. van den Heijkant, F.E.B.U., F.E.A.P.U. (✉)
Department of Urology, UZ Leuven, Gasthuisberg, Leuven, Belgium
e-mail: marleen.vandenheijkant@uzleuven.be

pathological condition, urinary incontinence in children has to be evaluated within the context of patient developmental age an early urological history [8].

The reference point for LUT symptoms is >5 years of age as this age is used by the DSM-5 and International Classification of Diseases-10 (ICD-10) to characterize urinary incontinence disorders. Moreover, a minimum of one episode per month and a minimum duration of 3 months should be used to term it as a condition [9, 10]. In 30–40% of the children with daytime incontinence, behavioral disorders are found [11].

Children with daytime LUT dysfunction can be divided into children with storage (or filling phase) dysfunction as well as voiding (emptying phase) dysfunction. The ICCS stresses that this classification is not evidence based and there may be overlap between these conditions [3]. Certain symptoms may evolve over time.

20.2 Diagnostic Investigations

Diagnostic assessment consists of noninvasive screening and starts with medical history taking from both the parents and the child with bladder and defecation diary, Bristol stool chart [12–14]. The ICCS developed a standardization document for children with daytime incontinence [8], and the use of a validated standardized questionnaire is recommended in order to guarantee a structured approach [15, 16].

Clinical examination with genital inspection should follow during the first visit. In boys, inspection of the penis should rule out anatomical abnormalities like hypospadias, phimosis, buried penis, and meatus stenosis after circumcision, In girls, inspection of the introitus can reveal labial fusion [17], and the position and direction of the urethral meatus can be assessed [18, 19]. Observation of the lumbosacral spine and neurological examination of the lower extremities can help to exclude neuropathy.

Urine analysis can rule out a urinary tract infection, proteinuria, and in case of urinary frequency, calciuria should be excluded [20].

Uroflowmetry with or without electromyography (EMG) recording combined with abdominal ultrasonography is a noninvasive tool to assess urodynamics. Postvoid residuals can be measured, as well as fecal impaction with rectum diameter [21], and bladder wall thickness can be assessed, which can be measured with a full and empty bladder [22]. However for bladder wall thickness, reference values are still lacking [3]. The upper urinary tract will be evaluated, to rule out secondary hydronephrosis with or without kidney anomalies or secondary kidney damage.

Only in selected cases resistant to initial treatment, failed treatment, or suspicion of neurological problems, invasive (video) urodynamic investigation could be considered [5]. In case of obstruction in boys, a cystoscopy under general anesthesia could follow to rule out or treat posterior urethral valves (PUV), syringocele, congenital obstructive posterior urethral membrane (COPUM), or Moormann's ring. In case of suspicion of a neurogenic bladder, MRI of the lumbosacral spine and medulla can exclude or demonstrate an occult neurologic lesion like tethered cord, lipoma, or other rare conditions, which can result in a neurogenic bladder [5].

20.3 Storage (Filling Phase) Dysfunction

Storage symptoms include an increased or decreased voiding frequency (<3 or >8 times a day) and daytime urinary incontinence, which can exist intermittent or continuous, the latter mostly associated with a congenital anomaly or iatrogenic origin (as described in Chap. 21). Urgency is the acute need to void, often due to bladder overactivity [3].

20.3.1 Overactive Bladder (OAB)

Children with OAB have the urgency to void, usually combined with frequency (>8 times a day) and nocturia with or without urinary incontinence. Children with OAB usually have detrusor overactivity, which can only be confirmed by cystometry during an invasive urodynamic investigation [3]. Chapter 19 further describes this condition. Children often show holding maneuvers (called the "curtsy sign") to prevent micturition or leaking [23]. In boys with urinary incontinence and overactive bladder resistant to medical therapy and a urodynamically proved bladder outlet obstruction (BOO), urethral obstruction could be excluded or treated by cystoscopy [24].

20.3.2 Underactive Bladder

In this condition, children void with an increased abdominal pressure to start, maintain, or complete voiding, which is called straining [3]. The bladder diary of these children may reveal a low frequency of voiding with a normal fluid intake but can also show frequency in case of incomplete emptying of the bladder. Uroflowmetry usually shows an interrupted or plateau-shaped flow pattern, and additional invasive urodynamics can demonstrate detrusor underactivity and can in this way rule out bladder outlet obstruction. Underactive bladder is seen in around 7% of children with dysfunctional voiding. In this subgroup, the female to male ratio is 5:1 [25].

20.3.3 Voiding Postponement

Children with voiding postponement habitually postpone voiding during the day. The bladder diary shows a low voiding frequency during the day [3]. The child can show holding maneuvers to postpone voiding and suppress urgency. Methods commonly seen are standing on tiptoe, forcefully crossing the legs, or squatting with a hand or heel pressed into the perineum (Vincent's curtsy) [23].

This behavior can be assessed by medical history taking. With a full bladder, sudden feeling of urgency as well as urinary incontinence may be expressed. Usually these children show a reduced fluid intake in their bladder diaries as an adaption to reduce the urinary incontinence [4]. This condition is more often seen in children with psychological comorbidity or behavioral disturbances [11]. These children are at risk on the long term to develop an underactive bladder with weak or even absent detrusor contraction.

20.3.4 Bladder and Bowel Dysfunction

Severe BBD can be seen in children where neurologic abnormality is excluded. This severe condition shows changes in the upper urinary tract like hydronephrosis with or without vesicoureteral reflux (VUR) and renal scarring and is often called "Hinman-Allen syndrome," which is labeled by the ICCS as a historical term [3, 26–28]. This syndrome is also called nonneurogenic dysfunctional voiding in literature [29, 30].

20.4 Voiding (Emptying) Phase Dysfunctions

Voiding or emptying phase dysfunction means dysfunction in the interaction with the urinary sphincter and pelvic floor during detrusor contraction and contains several symptoms. Children with hesitancy have difficulties to start voiding. Children with straining complain of making strong efforts to start voiding often with an increased abdominal pressure. A weak or intermittent stream can be observed and confirmed by uroflowmetry. Dysuria is a burning sensation or discomfort during voiding. Dysuria at the start of voiding suggests usually a urethral problem, whereas terminal dysuria suggests a bladder problem [3].

20.4.1 Dysfunctional Voiding (DV)

Children with DV habitually contract the urethral sphincter or pelvic floor during voiding [3] and could be accompanied by feelings of incomplete emptying, and an acute urinary retention may develop. A neurogenic bladder should be excluded. Uroflowmetry combined with electromyography recording (EMG) demonstrates a staccato flow pattern, with or without interruption. In girls, LUT dysfunction is common and can be accompanied by urinary tract infections (UTI). In girls with dysfunctional voiding (DV) and UTI or underactive bladder, meatus anomalies could be found [24]. A few publications in literature describe an anterior deflected urinary stream or meatus stenosis in girls, which could result in the inability to void in an ideal toileting position. During micturition, these girls void over the rim of the toilet or wet their buttocks and legs during micturition. Surgical correction of these meatus deformities in girls may add to success rates in dysfunctional voiding [18, 19].

20.4.2 Vaginal Reflux

Vaginal reflux or vaginal voiding can be seen in toilet-trained girls when they stand up after voiding [3, 31]. They express daytime urinary incontinence in small amounts shortly after voiding, also called post-micturition dribble. Usually they void with adducted legs, and as a consequence, urine is entrapped inside the introitus. Girls can complain of dysuria as urine passes over the irritated skin. Sometimes, even labial adhesions due to local inflammation or irritation can be seen with physical examination. This voiding pattern can be visualized during voiding cystourethrogram, with refluxing urine appearing within the vagina during voiding. Treatment is based on changing voiding habits emphasizing abduction of the legs and forward leaning posture during voiding [3].

20.4.3 Giggle Incontinence

Giggle incontinence is a rare syndrome seen in girls. This form of urinary incontinence is expressed by extensive bladder emptying or urinary leakage during or immediately after laughter [3, 4]. These girls usually have large volume voids with a bladder diary. Bladder function is normal when there is no laughter. Although the etiology is not clear yet, Feldman et al. suggest a mechanism mediated by the central nervous system similar to that of cataplexy, in which an emotional event causes muscle hypotonia [25]. A few case series suggest a central nervous system etiology as well reporting effectiveness of methylphenidate [32, 33]. Chandra et al. suggest that the condition is related to detrusor instability and therefore advocates the use of anticholinergic medication [34]. In one case series, biofeedback to train to contract the external sphincter was effective in nine girls with giggle incontinence [35].

20.4.4 Bladder Outlet Obstruction (BOO)

A low velocity urinary flow during voiding is called bladder outlet obstruction and can be accompanied by residuals. A BOO can be mechanical as well as functional. Initially a flow-EMG can be performed to make this distinction, however with a strained pelvic floor; further distinction can be made with invasive urodynamic investigation. In case of a mechanical obstruction, an increased detrusor pressure, a reduced urinary flow rate, and a relaxed pelvic floor can be seen in a pressure-flow study. After a pressure-flow study, a cystoscopy under general anesthesia could reveal the source and level of obstruction. In boys, a cystoscopy may reveal posterior urethral valves (PUV) or other reasons of urethral obstruction, like congenital obstructive posterior urethral membrane (COPUM), Moormann's ring, or syringocele. Boys with a syringocele may present with post-micturition dribble; involuntary leakage of urine immediately after voiding has finished. In case of a meatus stenosis (for example, after circumcision), boys can complain of spraying or splitting of the urinary stream. Spraying and post-micturition dribble can also be seen in boys with a status after hypospadias correction, with or without development of a urethral diverticulum as a (usually long term) postoperative complication of hypospadias surgery. Symptoms like a feeling of incomplete emptying may exist, and an acute urinary retention could develop meaning that the child has the sensation of an inability to void despite having a full bladder [3].

20.4.5 Valve-Bladder Syndrome

The majority of boys with posterior urethral valves develop progressive impairment of detrusor contractility during micturition many years after treatment of the posterior urethral valves [36–39]. In a selection of children, overnight catheter drainage in conjunction with daytime clean intermittent catheterization can reduce diuresis and urinary tract infections and improve urinary continence [40].

20.4.6 Extraordinary Daytime Only Urinary Frequency

This condition refers to toilet-trained children who have urinary frequency of small volumes of less than 50% of the expected bladder capacity according to age during the day without having urinary incontinence or nocturia [3]. In these cases, conditions like polydipsia, diabetes mellitus, nephrogenic diabetes insipidus, daytime polyuria, UTI, viral syndrome, and hypercalciuria should be excluded [3, 20].

20.4.7 Bladder Neck Dysfunction

In children with bladder neck dysfunction, the bladder neck opens late or insufficiently and results in a reduced urinary flow despite an adequate detrusor contraction [3, 25, 41, 42]. Children can complain of hesitancy, frequency, urgency, weak urinary stream, and dysuria and could have a sense of incomplete emptying. This condition can only be observed during invasive videourodynamics. Alternatively, it could be diagnosed during uroflowmetry with EMG recording, but EMG lag time has not been validated yet [3]. The treatment of bladder neck dysfunction is not well known yet, but a few studies show positive results with the treatment of alpha-blockers [43, 44].

> **Conclusions**
> Daytime lower urinary tract symptoms contains a wide spectrum of conditions, usually possible to diagnose with noninvasive urodynamic tools. Some conditions may involve over time; however for some conditions, early recognition, long-term follow-up and management are important to ensure good voiding behavior.

References

1. Sureshkumar P, Jones M, Cumming R, Craig J. A population based study of 2856 school-age children with urinary incontinence. J Urol. 2009;181(2):808–15.
2. Farhat W, Bägli DJ, Capolicchio G, et al. The dysfunctional voiding scoring system: quantitative standardization of dysfunctional voiding symptoms in children. J Urol. 2000;164:1011–5.

3. Chang SJ, Van Laecke E, Bauer SB, et al. Treatment of daytime urinary incontinence: A standardization document from the International Children's Continence Society. Neurourol Urodyn. 2017;36(1):43–50.
4. Nevéus T, von Gontard A, Hoebeke P, et al. The standardization of terminology of lower urinary tract function in children and adolescents: report from the standardisation Committee of the International Children's continence society. J Urol. 2006;176(1):314–24.
5. Tekgül S, Dogan HS, Kočvara R, Nijman JM, Radmayr C, Stein R, Silay MS, Quaedackers J, Undre S. European Urology guidelines on Paediatric Urology; 2017.
6. Jansson UB, Hanson M, Sillén U, Hellström AL. Voiding pattern and acquisition of bladder control from birth to age 6 years-a longitudinal study. J Urol. 2005;174(1):289–93.
7. Bloom DA, Seeley WW, Ritchey ML, McGuire EJ. Toilet habits and continence in children: an opportunity sampling in search of normal parameters. J Urol. 1993;149(5):1087–90.
8. Hoebeke P, Bower W, Combs A, de Jong T, Yang S. Diagnostic evaluation of children with daytime incontinence. J Urol. 2010;183(2):699–703.
9. Association AP. Fifth edition of the diagnostic and statistical manual of mental disorders (DSM-5). Arlington: American Psychiatric Pub; 2013.
10. World Health Organization. Multiaxial classification of child and adolescent psychiatric disorders: the ICD-10 classification of mental and behavioural disorders in children and adolescents. Cambridge: New York Cambridge University Press; 2008. p. 302.
11. Von Gontard A, Baeyens D, van Hoecke E, Warzak WJ, Bachmann C. Psychological and psychiatric issues in urinary and fecal incontinence. J Urol. 2011;185(4):1432–6.
12. Heaton KW, Radvan J, Cripps H, Mountford RA, Braddon FE, Hughes AO. Defecation frequency and timing, and stool form in the general population: a prospective study. Gut. 1992;33(6):818–24.
13. Chang SJ, Hsieh CH, Yang SS. Constipation is associated with incomplete bladder emptying in healthy children. Neurourol Urodyn. 2012;31(1):105–8.
14. Burgers RE, Mugie SM, Chase J, et al. Management of functional constipation in children with lower urinary tract symptoms: report from the standardization Committee of the International Children's continence society. J Urol. 2013;190(1):29–36.
15. Akbal C, Genc Y, Burgu B, Ozden E, Tekgul S. Dysfunctional voiding and incontinence scoring system: quantitative evaluation of incontinence symptoms in pediatric population. J Urol. 2005;173(3):969–73.
16. Farhat W, Bägli DJ, Capolicchio G, et al. The dysfunctional voiding scoring system: quantitative standardization of dysfunctional voiding symptoms in children. J Urol. 2000;164(3 Pt 2):1011–5.
17. Mayoglu L, Dulabon L, Martin-Alguacil N, Pfaff D, Schober J. Success of treatment modalities for labial fusion: a retrospective evaluation of topical and surgical treatments. J Pediatrc Adolesc Gynecol. 2009;22(4):247–50.
18. Aj K, Bochove-Overgaauw D, Winkler-Seinstra PL, Dik P, de Jong TP. Urethral meatus deformities in girls as a factor in dysfunctional voiding. Neurourol Urodyn. 2012;31(7):1161–4.
19. Hoebeke P, Van Laecke E, Raes A, Van Gool JD, Vandewalle J. Anomalies of the external urethral meatus in girls with non-neurogenic bladder sphincter dysfunction. BJU Int. 1999;83(3):294–8.
20. Parekh DJ, Pope JC IV, Adams MC, et al. The role of hypercalciuria in a subgroup of dysfunctional voiding syndromes of childhood. J Urol. 2000;164(3 Pt 2):1008–10.
21. Klijn AJ, Asselman M, Vijverberg MA, et al. The diameter of the rectum on ultrasonography as a diagnostic tool for constipation in children with dysfunctional voiding. J Urol. 2004;172(5 Pt 1):1986–8.
22. Yeung CK, Sreedhar B, Leung VT, Sit KY. Correlation between ultrasonographic bladder measurements and urodynamic findings in children with recurrent urinary tract infection. BJU Int. 2007;99(3):651–5.

23. Vincent SA. Postural control of urinary incontinence. The curtsy sign. Lancet. 1966;2(7464): 631–2.
24. De Jong TP, Klijn AJ, Vijverberg MA. Lower urinary tract dysfunction in children. Eur Urol Supplements. 2012;11:10–5.
25. Feldman AS, Bauer SB. Diagnosis and management of dysfunctional voiding. Curr Opin Pediatr. 2006;18(2):139–47.
26. Hinman F, Baumann FW. Vesical and ureteral damage from voiding dysfunction in boys without neurologic or obstructive disease. J Urol. 1973;109(4):727–32.
27. Hinman F Jr. Nonneurogenic neurogenic bladder (the Hinman syndrome)—15 years later. J Urol. 1986;136(4):769–77.
28. Allen TD. The non-neurogenic neurogenic bladder. J Urol. 1977;117(2):232–8.
29. Jayanthi VR, Khouri AE, Mc Lorie GA, Agarwal SK. The nonneurogenic neurogenic bladder of early infancy. J Urol. 1997;158(3 Pt 2):1281–5. Review.
30. Al Mosawi AJ. Identification of nonneurogenic neurogenic bladder in infants. Urology. 2007;70(2):355–6.
31. Bernasconi M, Borsari A, Garzoni L, et al. Vaginal voiding: a common cause of daytime urinary leakage in girls. J Pediatr Adolesc Gynecol. 2009;22(6):347–50.
32. Sher PK, Reinberg Y. Successful treatment of giggle incontinence with methylphenidate. J Urol. 1996;156(2 Pt 2):656–8.
33. Berry AK, Zderic S, Carr M. Methylphenidate for giggle incontinence. J Urol. 2009;182(4 Suppl):2062–32.
34. Chandra M, Saharia R, Shi Q, Hill V. Giggle incontinence in children: a manifestation of detrusor instability. J Urol. 2002;168(5):2184–7.
35. Richardson I, Palmer LS. Successful treatment for giggle incontinence with biofeedback. J Urol. 2009;182(4 Suppl):2062–6.
36. De Gennaro M, Capitanucci ML, Silveri M, Morini FA, Mosiello G. Detrusor hypocontractility evolution in boys with posterior urethral valves detected by pressure flow analysis. J Urol. 2001;165(6 Pt 2):2248–52.
37. Holmdahl G, Sillén U. Boys with posterior urethral valves: outcome concerning renal function, bladder function and paternity rates at ages 31 to 44 years. J Urol. 2005;174(3):1031–4.
38. Peters CA, Bolkier M, Bauer SB, Hendren WH, Colodny AH, Mandell J, Retik AB. The urodynamic consequences of posterior urethral valves. J Urol. 1990;144(1):122–6.
39. Parkhouse HF, Barratt TM, Dillon MJ, Duffy PG, Fay J, Ransley PG, Woodhouse CR, Williams DI. Long-term outcome of boys with posterior urethral valves. Br J Urol. 1988;62(1):59–62.
40. Nguyen MT, Paylock CL, Zderic SA, Carr MC, Canning DA. Overnight catheter drainage in children with poorly compliant bladders improves post-obstructive diuresis and urinary incontinence. J Urol. 2005;174(4 Pt 2):1633–6.
41. Koff SA. Estimating bladder capacity in children. Urology. 1983;21:248–50.
42. Grafstein NH, Combs AJ, Glassberg KI. Primary bladder neck dysfunction: an overlooked entity in children. Curr Urol Rep. 2005;6(2):133–9.
43. Donohoe JM, Combs J, Glassberg KI. Primary bladder neck dysfunction in children and adolescents II: results of treatment with alpha-adrenergic antagonists. J Urol. 2005;173(1):212–6.
44. Van Batavia JP, Combs AJ, Horowitz M, Glassberg KI. Primary bladder neck dysfunction in children and adolescents III: results of long-term alpha-blocker therapy. J Urol. 2010;183(2):724–30.

Congenital and Iatrogenic Incontinence: Ectopic Ureter, Ureterocele, and Urogenital Sinus

21

Keara N. DeCotiis, Liza M. Aguiar, and Anthony A. Caldamone

21.1 Ectopic Ureter

21.1.1 Embryology

During fetal development, the ureters and the collecting system of the kidneys differentiate from the ureteric bud. At about 28 days of gestation, the ureteric bud develops from the caudal end of the mesonephric duct in response to signals from the metanephric mesenchyme. Bifurcation of the ureteric bud occurs after the developing bud penetrates the metanephric mesenchyme and begins proliferating into the primitive collecting system. Direction of development of the ureteric bud has been demonstrated by manipulation of Gdnf and the Ret receptor, Foxc1/2, Bmp4, Eya1, and Hox11 and expression of other molecules implicating their involvement in appropriate maturation and location. Failure of the interactions between the ureteric bud and nephrogenic and stromal mesenchyme can cause renal agenesis. Early bifurcation of a single ureteric bud causes a bifid ureter which joins into one ureter distally before entering the bladder.

Should the mesonephric duct have two distinct ureteric buds develop, complete duplication occurs as each bud independently penetrates the metanephric mesenchyme. The upper pole of the kidney is induced by the cranial bud, and the lower pole is induced by the caudal bud. As development continues, the common excretory duct enters the posterior wall of the urogenital sinus. The caudal ureteric bud is incorporated first, and earlier incorporation allows for more migration laterally within the bladder. The cranial bud is incorporated at a later stage and has less time for migration. As a result, this ureteral orifice is located more medially and caudally

K.N. DeCotiis, M.D. • L.M. Aguiar, M.D. • A.A. Caldamone, M.D. (✉)
Division of Pediatric Urology, Hasbro Children's Hospital,
Warren Alpert School of Medicine, Brown University, Providence, RI, USA
e-mail: acaldamone@lifespan.org

© Springer International Publishing AG, part of Springer Nature 2018
G. Mosiello et al. (eds.), *Clinical Urodynamics in Childhood and Adolescence*, Urodynamics, Neurourology and Pelvic Floor Dysfunctions,
https://doi.org/10.1007/978-3-319-42193-3_21

within the bladder or sometimes ectopically located into any structure that derives from the caudal mesonephric duct. This relationship between the two ureteral orifices is constant and called the Weigert-Meyer rule. Abnormal insertion sites of ureters into the urogenital sinus may be asymptomatic or be associated with vesicoureteral reflux, incontinence, obstruction, or recurrent infections.

In males, ectopic ureters insert above the external sphincter muscle; therefore, incontinence does not occur. Common sites of insertion of an ectopic ureter are the bladder neck, prostatic urethra, ejaculatory duct, vas deferens, and seminal vesicle. For females an ectopic ureter may insert into the bladder neck, vestibule, vagina, or uterus as these are the differentiated organs of the caudal mesenteric duct. Because some of these insertion sites are distal to the external sphincter mechanism, incontinence may occur. If both right and left ureters in single system kidneys fail to incorporate into the posterior bladder wall, then the trigone and bladder neck do not develop properly. In this scenario, an incompetent bladder outlet leads to poor bladder capacity and incontinence. Although incontinence from a unilateral ectopic ureter occurs only in females, it should be noted that males may be incontinent if bilateral single system ureters fail to enter the bladder properly.

While the majority of ectopic ureters are associated with duplicated systems, ectopy can occur with single systems. During development, a single ureteric bud that is located in a more cranial position, and is carried with the mesonephric duct, will migrate ectopically. Single system ectopic ureters are more commonly seen in males and are associated with a higher incidence of associated anomalies. When an ectopic ureter from a single system is unilateral, then the bladder neck is likely intact, and incontinence relates to the insertion of the ectopic ureter. In the situation where bilateral ectopic ureters are associated with a single system, the bladder neck is compromised, and severe incontinence is seen.

21.1.2 Clinical Presentation

Ectopic ureters occur more often in females and can be associated with draining a single kidney or more commonly with draining a duplex kidney, which occurs 80% of the time [1, 2]. When the ureteral orifice is above the external sphincter in the bladder neck, incontinence is less likely. Obstruction of the ureter, however, can occur due to increased surrounding musculature of the bladder neck, which is contracted most of the time. More than half of girls present with persistent urinary leakage even though they have been appropriately toilet trained without feeling urgency or incomplete emptying [3]. The incontinence may only occur when standing if the ureter is able to accommodate urine while the child is supine. For those not presenting with incontinence, an ectopic ureter may be discovered in evaluation of hydronephrosis, frequent urinary tract infections, cysts within the vestibule, foul odors, or purulent discharge from the perineum. Infections may occur with low-grade fevers with periodic spikes [4]. In females, continuous leakage is the symptom that most often prompts investigation of a possible ectopic ureter.

Since males do not experience urine leakage due to an ectopic ureter, presentation can vary. Complaints include recurrent epididymitis, frequency of urination due to persistent urine in the posterior urethra, recurrent UTI, prostatitis, and calculi. For those children with the rare condition of bilateral ectopic ureters draining single systems, presentation consists of other genital, renal, anal anomalies and incontinence [5]. The incontinence is this scenario is generally more continuous and severe than that occurring with an ectopic ureter draining a duplex system.

21.1.3 Diagnosis

Diagnosis of an ectopic ureter may prove to be difficult due to the presence of nonspecific symptoms or the absence of symptoms. Because the ectopic ureter does not drain into the bladder, the urine culture may be negative in the presence of infection [6]. Imaging usually starts with an ultrasound, but VCUG can also be helpful. Ultrasound is useful for diagnosis of ectopic ureter by visualizing a dilated ureter, and occasionally one can identify the insertion at the bladder neck or more distally (Fig. 21.1). Hydroureter associated with an upper pole moiety of a duplicated renal unit in the absence of a ureterocele is most commonly caused by an ectopic ureter. Because ectopic ureters have a high association with a nonfunctional moiety in males [7], ultrasound may show a dilated ureter to this unit. VCUG may be suggestive of an ectopic ureter which inserts into the bladder neck or urethra showing reflux only upon voiding. Isolated reflux into the upper pole of a completely duplicated system is diagnostic of an ectopic ureter (Fig. 21.2).

The identification of unilateral and bilateral single ectopic ureters may require supplemental tests or invasive procedures. If ultrasound and VCUG are not conclusive, alternative imaging studies such as MRI, CT, vaginogram, vasogram, or IVP may be useful. Cystoscopy or vaginoscopy with an exam under anesthesia may be needed. In the rare instance of bilateral single ectopic system ureters, a VCUG would show an open bladder neck and a small bladder. The ureters may or may not reflux. Cystoscopy in these patients will show a small capacity bladder and funnel-shaped bladder neck [4].

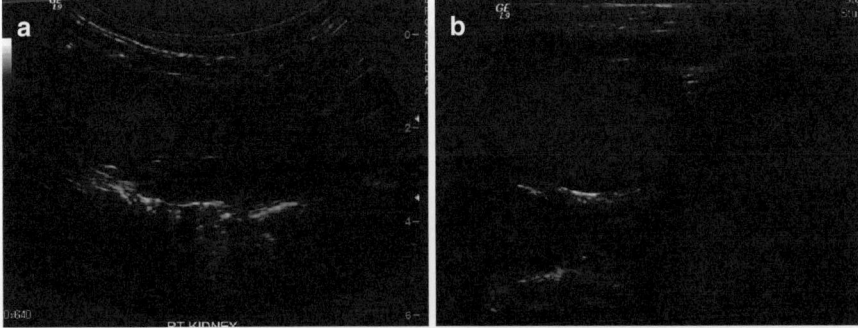

Fig. 21.1 Ultrasound of an ectopic ureter associated with a duplicated system. (**a**) Shows hydronephrosis of an upper pole moiety; (**b**) demonstrates a large dilated ureter located behind the bladder

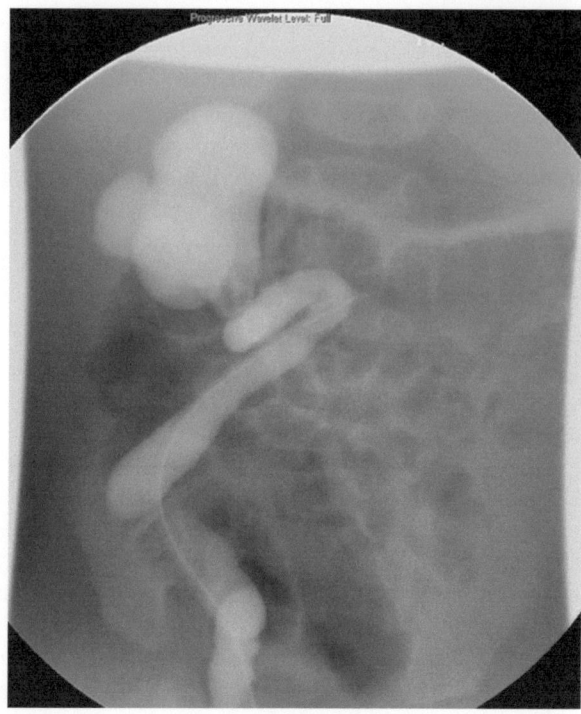

Fig. 21.2 VCUG of a patient with an ectopic ureter. Due to the ureteral opening at the bladder neck, the catheter was inserted directly up the ureter

21.1.4 Intervention

It is important to note that surgical treatment of an ectopic ureter should be individualized, as patients have variations of complex anatomy and function. When planning surgery, one must consider the function of the associated renal unit. For those single system ectopic ureters associated with a poorly functioning renal unit, nephroureterectomy is appropriate with attempt to remove as much of the ectopic ureter as possible [8]. This may be more effectively accomplished with a laparoscopic or robotic approach. Patients with functional renal units associated with single system ectopic ureters are candidates for reimplantation into the bladder. Functional status must also be assessed in a duplex kidney associated with ectopic ureter. For those without adequate function, partial nephrectomy is performed [9]. The goal with a functional renal unit is diversion of urine from the upper pole into the lower pole system via ureteropyelostomy or ureteroureterostomy. Surgical intervention for unilateral ectopic ureters provides a high rate of dryness following the procedure [4]. The use of dextranomer/hyaluronic acid subureterically for vesicoureteral reflux for ectopic ureters with entrance at the bladder neck is not recommended, as studies have shown low success rates in this scenario [10]. Bilateral single ectopic ureters with incompetent bladder necks and incontinence are intricate cases. Depending on the degree of bladder outlet incompetence and bladder capacity, surgical correction can range from ureteral reimplantation to bladder neck reconstruction with or without augmentation to urinary diversion to achieve continence.

21.2 Ureterocele

21.2.1 Embryology

A ureterocele is a cystic dilation of the intravesical portion of the ureter. In 1927, Chwalle postulated the embryologic origin of a ureterocele was the persistence or incomplete dissolution of a distal membrane that separates the ureteral bud from the urogenital sinus, known as the Chwalle's membrane, leading to the formation of a ureterocele. More recent investigations have brought forth the idea that the Chwalle's membrane may be a derivative of luminal cells in the ureter undergoing apoptosis at a late stage [4]. Delayed development of a lumen in the ureteral bud with the mesonephric duct may cause expansion of the ureter into the bladder [11]. Although both models provide partial explanation of ureteroceles, neither accounts for all anatomical variations seen. Ureteroceles may be associated with a single system or a duplex system.

21.2.2 Clinical Presentation

The incidence of ureteroceles is approximately 0.02%, with 80% occurring in females [4]. The majority of ureteroceles are associated with the upper pole of a duplicated system, and about 60–80% of ureteroceles are ectopic in that they extend beyond the bladder neck [12]. They are frequently associated with obstruction of the system which they subtend. Prenatal diagnosis of hydronephrosis is the most common presentation. Postnatally, ureteroceles most often present with urinary tract infections, hematuria, or a palpable bladder mass. The most worrisome presentation is acute outlet obstruction caused by the ureterocele prolapsing into the bladder neck. When this occurs, it may be possible to see a purple red or necrotic mass protruding from between the labia [5]. A large ureterocele may distort the bladder neck and manifest with incontinence, although this is a more rare presenting scenario [13].

21.2.3 Diagnosis

Ureteroceles are most often diagnosed on prenatal ultrasound. Investigation of a possible ureterocele relies heavily on imaging, which may include ultrasound, VCUG, renal scan, IVP, CT, and possibly MRI. Ultrasound is normally utilized first to assess the kidneys and bladder. It is important to note that ultrasounds should be done with a full bladder so that the lining of a large ureterocele within the bladder is not misinterpreted as bladder mucosa. On ultrasound, a ureterocele appears as a round lucent structure sitting within the bladder (see Fig. 21.3). The next step in

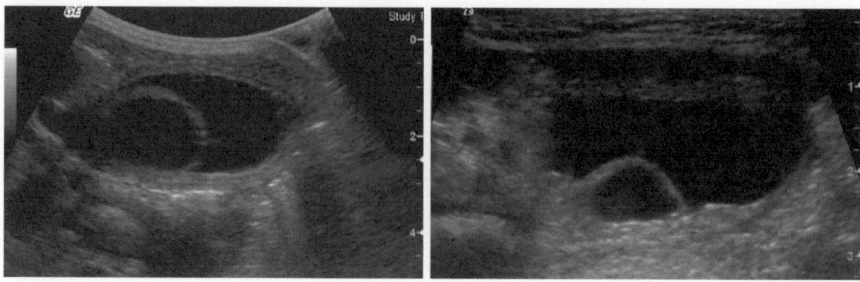

Fig. 21.3 Two ultrasound images showing intravesical ureteroceles; it is important to note that the bladders in both patients are distended which allows differentiation between normal bladder mucosa and ureterocele

Fig. 21.4 A VCUG during the voiding phase showing a space occupying lesion of the posterior bladder, representing the ureterocele

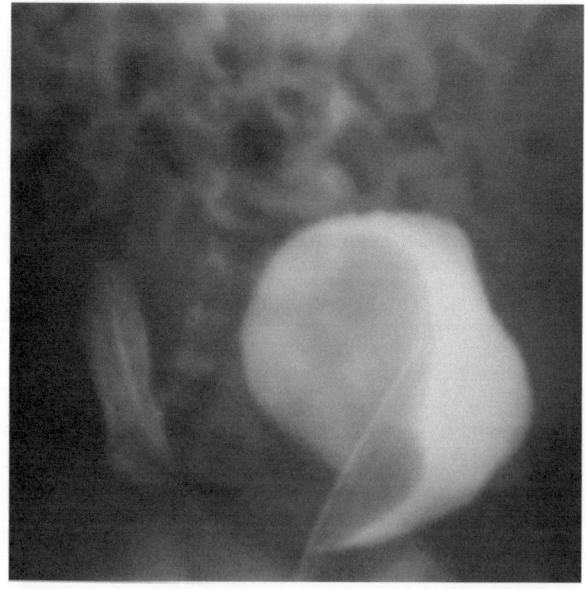

diagnosis is a VCUG which may show a ureterocele as a rim enhancing shadow within the bladder (see Fig. 21.4). Because ureteroceles are mostly associated with duplicated systems, VCUG may also serve to demonstrate vesicoureteral reflux to the lower pole of the kidney or into the contralateral system. On the voiding phase, one should note if prolapse of the ureterocele into the bladder neck is causing outlet obstruction. Nuclear scans are most often used to assess the function of the associated renal unit. Diuretic renograms may be used to diagnose or rule out obstruction. Direct visualization of ureteroceles using cystoscopy may be misleading. The size of the ureterocele may make it difficult to assess laterality, identify the ureterocele, or distinguish it from the bladder diverticulum or trigonal cysts. If further anatomical detail is necessary, magnetic resonance urography can be considered.

21.2.4 Intervention

The principal reasons for surgically intervening on a ureterocele are preservation of renal function, elimination of infection, obstruction, and maintaining urinary continence. Ureteroceles which present with moderate to severe hydronephrosis prenatally are managed initially with antibiotics to reduce the risk of infections. In order to preserve renal function, one must correct the obstruction and prevent reflux. Acute decompression and resolution of the obstruction may be required in those patients with sepsis or those with bladder outlet obstruction by performing a transurethral incision of the ureterocele. Transurethral incision of a ureterocele may be definitive treatment for 77–93% of cases depending on the anatomy, as there are lower rates of secondary procedures for the intravesical ureterocele [6, 14]. Nonemergent treatment options include transurethral incision, ureterocele excision, common sheath ureteral reimplantation, ureteroureterostomy, partial nephrectomy for nonfunctioning upper poles, and observation. Some studies have shown observation in patients with a nonfunctioning, minimally hydronephrotic, or cystic dysplastic upper tract segment associated with a ureterocele managed nonoperatively may have a benign clinical course [15].

Although the majority of ureteroceles do not present with incontinence, as stated previously, large ureteroceles may distort the bladder neck causing urinary leakage. Incontinence may be iatrogenic, or initial incontinence may fail to improve after surgical correction or excision, due to an incompetent bladder neck. These surgical procedures may also cause bladder dysfunction due to bladder hypertrophy and hyperactivity, subsequently leading to incontinence. Urinary leakage may be seen with ectopic ureteroceles, as their insertion sites may be distal to the external sphincter. Ureteroceles may also be associated with inherent bladder dysfunction such as detrusor instability, which may be associated with incontinence.

21.3 Urogenital Sinus

21.3.1 Embryology

The urogenital sinus is a normal structure during embryonic development. A portion of the developing hindgut expands into the cloaca, lined with endoderm, by the second week of gestation. Between the fourth and sixth weeks of fetal life, the cloaca is separated by the urorectal septum into the anorectal canal dorsally and the urogenital sinus ventrally. It is theorized that the fusion of yolk sac extra embryonic mesoderm and allantois membrane is what comprises the urorectal septum [16]. The urorectal septum grows down toward the cloacal membrane but before the two merge the cloacal membrane ruptures, allowing the urogenital sinus and the anorectal canal to reach the exterior at the level of the primitive perineum. The urogenital sinus will eventually become the bladder and two separate segments. The superior segment gives rise to the proximal urethra, and the inferior will differentiate into the penile urethra in males and the vestibule of the vagina in females.

In females, the urogenital sinus interacts with the uterovaginal primorium, forming the Müllerian tubercle which induces the formation of the sinovaginal bulbs. These bulbs become the vaginal plate, which will canalize in a caudal to cranial direction to form the proximal two thirds of the vagina. The inferior aspect of the urogenital sinus becomes the vestibule of the vagina, so the urethra and vagina develop separate external openings. The disruption or cessation of vaginal differentiation can cause persistence of the urogenital sinus. Interruption at an early stage of development may lead to a long urogenital sinus with a short vagina. Comparatively, females may have a short urogenital sinus with a near normal vaginal vestibule, if the disruption occurs later in development [9].

21.3.2 Clinical Presentation

The persistence of the urogenital sinus is often diagnosed prenatally on ultrasound. It is crucial, however, to note that urogenital sinus abnormalities are most often seen with disorders of sexual differentiation, most commonly with congenital adrenal hyperplasia (CAH). CAH is a group of rare inherited autosomal recessive disorders characterized by abnormalities of adrenal steroid biosynthetic enzymes. Given that CAH may be life-threatening, the presence of ambiguous genitalia warrants a thorough newborn physical exam, maternal history, karyotype, measurement of serum electrolytes, and evaluation of hormone levels.

In addition to urogenital sinus seen with ambiguous genitalia, there is a pure form of persistent urogenital sinus, urogenital sinus associated with cloacal abnormalities, and urogenital sinus associated with female exstrophy. Palpation for abdominal masses may reveal a distended bladder or hydrometrocolpos, which can be the first sign of urogenital sinus abnormality. Due to the association of spinal cord and urogenital sinus abnormalities, it is important to inspect the back and spine. Genital examination should include evaluation of the clitoris or phallus and the status of the erectile bodies, presence of gonads, status of the labioscrotal folds, placement of the sinus opening, and examination of the rectum (see Fig. 21.5a).

21.3.3 Diagnosis

Although the diagnosis of persistent urogenital sinus can be confirmed by physical exam, it is important to have a thorough understanding of a patient's anatomy before attempting surgical intervention. Key pieces to each individual's puzzle include length of the common urogenital sinus or conversely the distance between the bladder neck and the confluence of the urinary and genital cords, urethral and bladder anatomy, and the relationship between the urethra, bladder, and vagina. The location of the vagina in reference to the bladder neck may be essential to guiding surgical reconstruction. Ultrasound is the first step to assess the status of the kidneys, adrenals, ovaries, bladder, and ureters. Retrograde genitogram (see Fig. 21.5b) or MRI

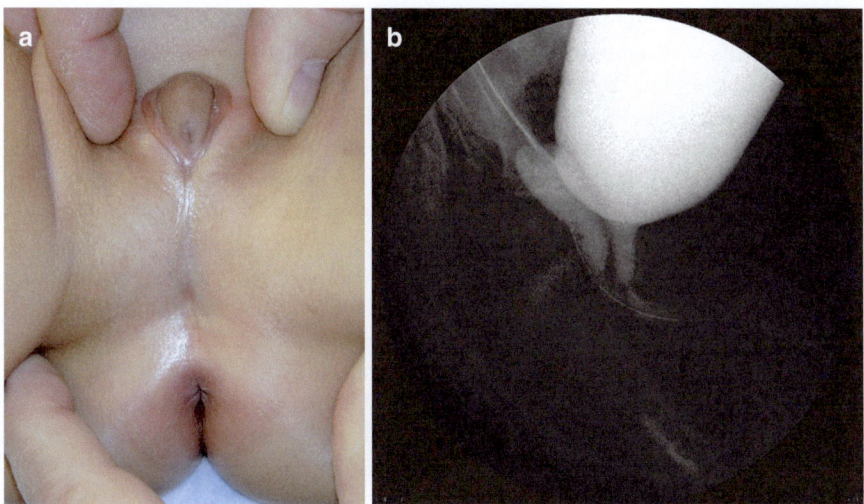

Fig. 21.5 Persistent urogenital sinus (**a**) on physical exam; there is one common orifice with clitoral hypertrophy and abnormal labial folds. Associated genitogram (**b**) shows a moderately high confluence with a clear separation of the bladder and vagina

will help outline anatomy and identify the length and extent of abnormality, define spinal abnormalities, and investigate sphincteric muscle development of the anus should there be concordant disruption. Cystoscopy and vaginoscopy should also be performed in all patients to evaluate the vaginal confluence under direct vision and to observe the number and structure of the vaginal canal.

21.3.4 Treatment

Persistent urogenital sinus is a complex malformation with a wide anatomic spectrum. The goal of surgical reconstruction is separation of the urinary and genital tracts while trying to preserve all sphincteric mechanisms for urinary and anal continence. Often, females born with urogenital sinus and ambiguous genitalia require some combination or variation of clitoroplasty, labiaplasty, and vaginoplasty. The spectrum of abnormality can vary greatly, so the extent of surgery is individualized and timing of surgical reconstruction is debatable. Vaginoplasty techniques involve four main types of repair: the cutback, the flap, the pull-through, and the complete vaginal replacement. During mobilization of the urogenital sinus, injury may occur to neural fibers or sphincter mechanisms. Interruption of pelvic floor anatomy may also lead to stress incontinence after toilet training. It is important to note that patients undergoing vaginoplasty prepubertally may require a secondary procedure postpubertally due to vaginal introital stenosis. Other complications such as incontinence, poor sexual function, and poor cosmetic outcomes can result. Extensive counseling and discussions with parents should take place preoperatively.

Persistent urogenital sinus is typically identified before toilet training age and rarely presents with incontinence. A high vaginal confluence can be associated with a hypospadiac urethra causing urinary leakage. The major concern for incontinence, however, is iatrogenic during surgical repair. Postoperative incontinence may be seen with a myriad of pelvic surgeries but notably can occur in both total urogenital mobilization (TUM), described by Peña, and partial urogenital mobilization (PUM), described by Rink [17]. Using TUM, the urogenital sinus is mobilized and brought to the perineum en bloc, so that vaginal separation using a pull-through vaginoplasty is no longer required. Similarly, PUM avoids the need for vaginoplasty but differs in that dissection does not extend beyond the pubourethral ligament and external sphincter, preserving delicate innervation. While pediatric urologists have shifted more toward PUM, recent literature has suggested that the outcomes between the two procedures may be comparable [17]. What is indisputable with persistent urogenital sinus is that iatrogenic urinary incontinence is an important complication to consider when choosing a surgical approach.

References

1. Keating MA. Ureteral duplication anomalies: ectopic ureters and ureteroceles. In: Clinical pediatric urology. London: Informa Healthcare; 2007. p. 593–648.
2. Ellerker AG. The extravesical ectopic ureter. Br J Surg. 1958;45(192):344.
3. Kim S. Observations on ureteral ectopy in children: R. S. Malek, P. P. Kelalis, G. B. Stickler, and E. C. Burke. J. Urol. 107: 308–313 (February), 1972. J Pediatr Surg. 1973;8(3):457.
4. Peters CA, Mendelsohn C. Ectopic ureter, ureterocele, and ureteral anomalies. In: Wein AJ, et al., editors. Campbell-Walsh urology. 11th ed. Philadelphia, PA: Elsevier Saunders; 2012. p. 3075–101.
5. Kesavan P. Ectopia in unduplicated ureters in children. Br J Urol. 1977;49(6):481.
6. Renzo DD, Ellsworth PI, Caldamone AA, Chiesa PL. Transurethral puncture for ureterocele—which factors dictate outcomes? J Urol. 2010;184(4, Supplement):1620–4.
7. Boston V. Ureteral duplication and ureterocele. Philadelphia: Mosby Elsevier; 2006. p. 1758–70.
8. Li J, Hu T, Wang M, Jiang X, Chen S, Huang L. Single ureteral ectopia with congenital renal dysplasia. J Urol. 2003;170(2, Part 1):558–9.
9. Subramaniam R. Ureteral duplication and ureteroceles. In: Coran AG, Scott Adzick N, editors. Pediatric surgery. 7th ed. Philadelphia, PA: Elsevier Mosby; 2012. p. 1441–51.
10. Perez-Brayfield M, Kirsch AJ, Hensle TW, Koyle MA, Furness P, Scherz HC. Endoscopic treatment with dextranomer/hyaluronic acid for complex cases of vesicoureteral reflux. J Urol. 2004;172(4, Supplement):1614–6.
11. Tanagho EA. Embryologic basis for lower ureteral anomalies: a hypothesis. Urology. 1976;7(5):451–64.
12. Holcomb G Jr. Ureteroceles in infants and children: J. Mandell, A. H. Colodny, R. Lebowitz, et al. J Urol 123:921–926, (June), 1980. J Pediatr Surg. 1981;16(2):216.
13. Husmann DA, Ewalt DH, Glenski WJ, Bernier PA. Ureterocele associated with ureteral duplication and a nonfunctioning upper pole segment: management by partial nephroureterectomy alone. J Urol. 1995;154(2):723–6.
14. Shokeir AA. Ureterocele: an ongoing challenge in infancy and childhood ureteroceles in infancy and childhood. BJU Int. 2002;90(8):777.
15. Coplen DE, Austin PF. Outcome analysis of prenatally detected ureteroceles associated with multicystic dysplasia. J Urol. 2004;172(4, Supplement):1637–9.

16. Schoenwolf GC, Bleyl SB, Brauer PR, Francis-West PH. Development of the urinary system. In: Schoenwolf GC, Bleyl SB, Brauer PR, Francis-West PH, editors. Larsen's human embryology. 5th ed. Philadelphia, PA: Churchill Livingstone/Elsevier; 2014. p. 375–93.
17. Palmer BW, Trojan B, Griffin K, Reiner W, Wisniewski A, Frimberger D, et al. Total and partial urogenital mobilization: focus on urinary continence. J Urol. 2012;187(4):1422–6.

Suggested Reading

Nepple KG, Cooper CS, Snyder HM. Ureteral duplication, ectopy, and ureteroceles. In: Gearhart JP, Rink RC, Mouriquand PDE, editors. Pediatric urology. 2nd ed. Philadelphia, PA: Saunders/Elsevier; 2010. p. 337–52.

Peters CA, Mendelsohn C. Ectopic ureter, ureterocele, and ureteral anomalies. In: Wein AJ, et al., editors. Campbell–Walsh urology. 11th ed. Philadelphia, PA: Elsevier Saunders; 2012. p. 3075–101.

Subramaniam R. Ureteral duplication and ureteroceles. In: Coran AG, Scott Adzick N, editors. Pediatric surgery. 7th ed. Philadelphia, PA: Elsevier Mosby; 2012. p. 1441–51.

Bladder Exstrophy

22

Alan Dickson

22.1 Introduction

Bladder exstrophy is a congenital abnormality of the urinary tract and is the most common of the conditions within the bladder exstrophy-epispadias complex (BEEC), the other two being epispadias and cloacal exstrophy. It is a rare but very serious anomaly which causes significant urological, sexual and psychological problems.

The embryology of bladder exstrophy remains unclear and various theories have been suggested. The evidence is that it starts developing early in embryonic life. Marshall and Muecke [1] have postulated an overdevelopment of the lower part of the cloacal membrane, which obstructs the medial migration of mesenchymal tissue, thereby preventing normal growth of the lower abdominal wall. More recently, Manner et al [2] developed this theory more, demonstrating in chick embryos a mechanical obstruction of the medial migration of the lateral layers of the abdominal wall.

Whilst most births with exstrophy are sporadic, there are multiple reports [3] of familial cases, clearly showing that there is a genetic basis to the condition. The incidence of bladder exstrophy is about 1 in 40,000 live births [4] and is three times more common in males than girls.

22.2 Anatomy of Bladder Exstrophy

The features of classic bladder exstrophy are shown and listed in Figs. 22.1 and 22.2. There is a lower anterior abdominal wall defect through which the open bladder herniates. In the male, the epispadias aspect of the abnormality includes the

---

A. Dickson, BSc, MBChB, FRCS(Ed), FRCS(Eng)
Consultant Paediatric Urologist, Royal Manchester Childrens Hospital,
Stony Littleton, Bath, UK
e-mail: alan.dicksonmedleg@btinternet.com

© Springer International Publishing AG, part of Springer Nature 2018
G. Mosiello et al. (eds.), *Clinical Urodynamics in Childhood and Adolescence*,
Urodynamics, Neurourology and Pelvic Floor Dysfunctions,
https://doi.org/10.1007/978-3-319-42193-3_22

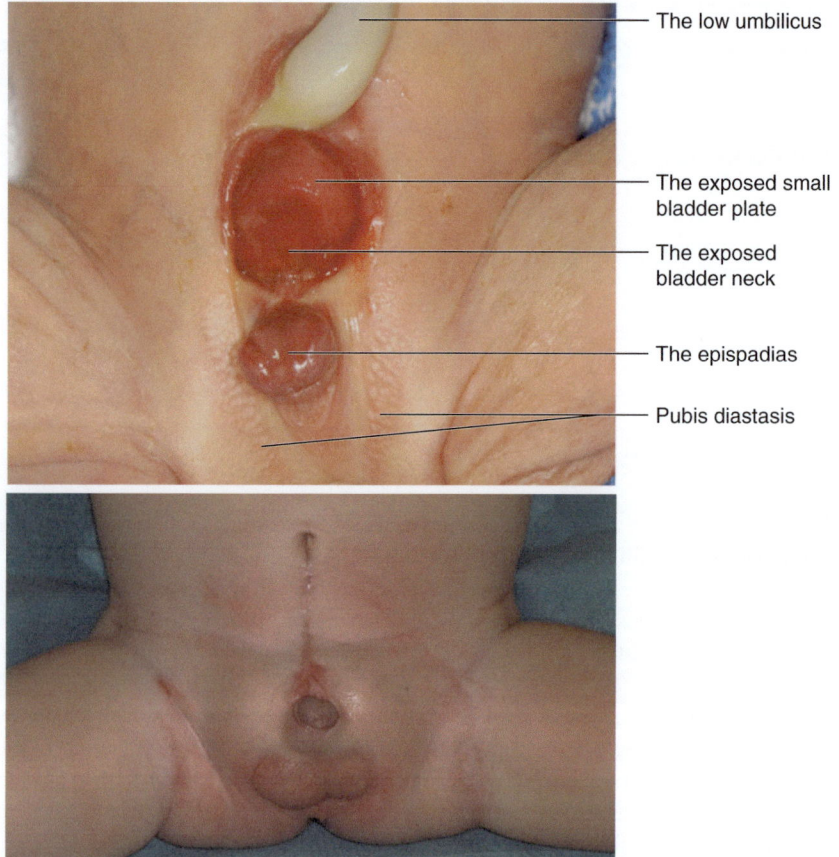

Fig. 22.1 Male bladder exstrophy (*Top*). Male exstrophy, 6 weeks after primary repair (*Bottom*)

open dorsal penis and the open bladder neck. In the female, the bladder, bladder neck and urethra are similarly open and the clitoris is bifid.

Associated congenital anomalies are uncommon but include renal anomalies, cardiovascular anomalies, spinal anomalies, anorectal malformations and undescended testes.

22.3 Presentation of Bladder Exstrophy

The features of bladder exstrophy on antenatal scanning are well-defined and some babies are therefore diagnosed antenatally. These features include, in particular, inability to visualise urine in the foetal bladder but also a low-set umbilical cord, a pubic diastasis, a short wide penis and a bulging bladder plate [5]. Indeed, the features are so well-defined that it is surprising that only 25% are detected on maternal ultrasound [5].

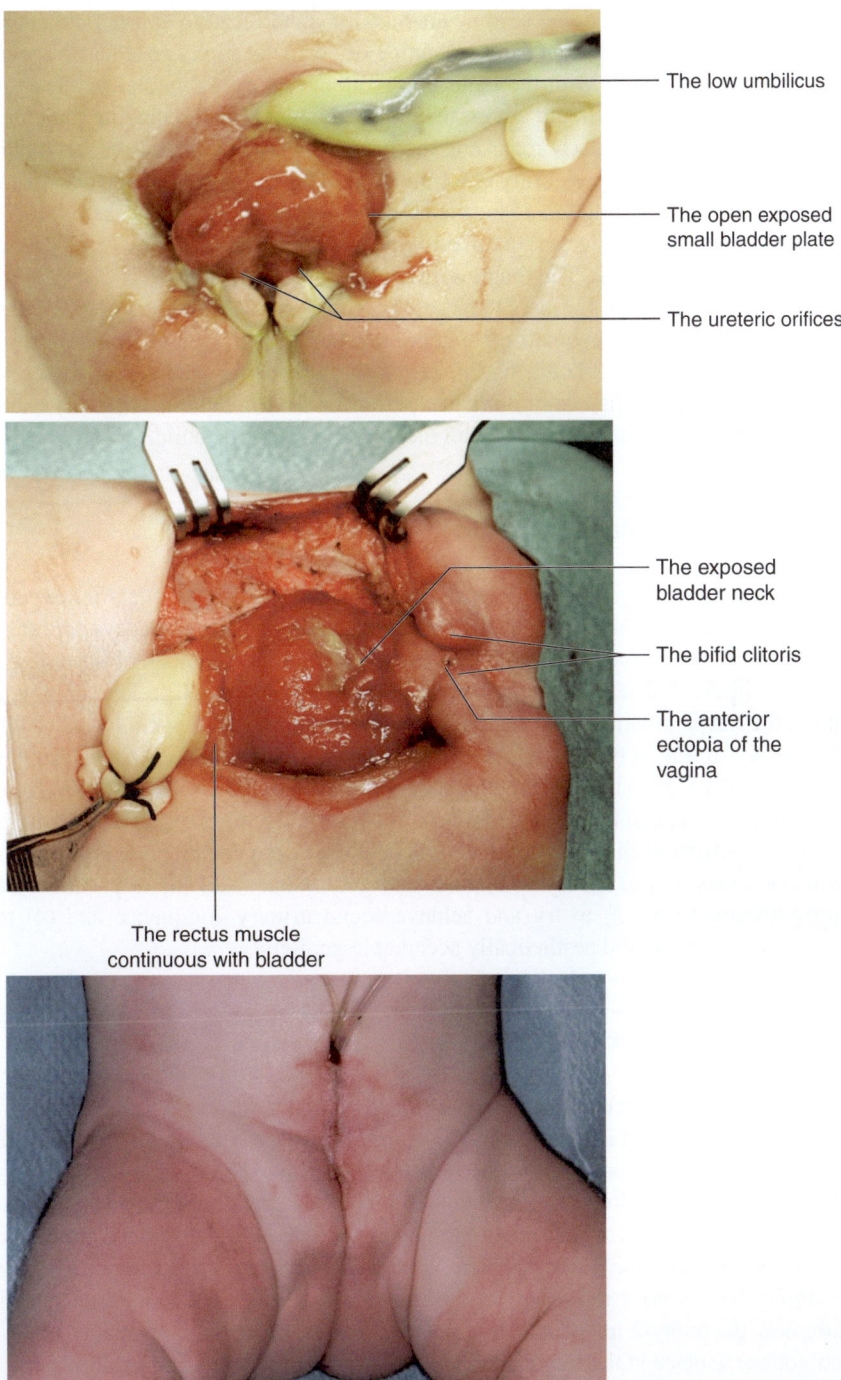

Fig. 22.2 Female bladder exstrophy (*Top*). The rectus muscle continuous with the bladder (*Middle*). Primary closure of female exstrophy, 4 weeks after operation (*Bottom*)

The detection of bladder exstrophy antenatally should lead to appropriate counselling for parents and, if applicable, planning of postnatal care. A paediatric urologist should be involved with the counselling, along with nursing and psychology professionals, and they should advise the parents about the nature and implications of the condition, particularly regarding the prognosis and the impact of the condition on family life. The possibility of termination of pregnancy should be discussed, but the decision regarding this is for the parents and not the professionals.

As implied above, however, the majority of babies with bladder exstrophy present unexpectedly at birth. The diagnosis should usually be fairly clear, but in practice, it is not uncommon for there to be some confusion. The diagnosis of a disorder of sexual development is sometimes entertained, but the visible bladder plate below a low-set umbilical cord confirms the diagnosis. Sometimes, the sex of the child may be unclear to the first examining inexperienced doctor, but this is usually clarified when a doctor who is familiar with the condition sees the child.

22.4 Surgical Management

Because of the small number of affected children and the many difficulties experienced in the care of bladder exstrophy children, many countries nowadays are rationalising the management of bladder exstrophy to a small number of specialised centres with multidisciplinary teams and psychology support [6]. This approach allows the development of experience and expertise amongst a few clinicians, along with the possibility of better clinical and laboratory research, and the hope is that this will eventually lead to improved outcomes for the children. The early evidence, from such initiatives, is that better outcomes can be achieved in more experienced hands.

The objectives of the management of bladder exstrophy are directed to the long-term outcomes: (1) to close the bladder and abdominal wall, (2) to preserve the upper urinary tract, (3) to try and achieve social urinary continence and (4) to construct functional and aesthetically acceptable genitalia.

22.5 Surgical Techniques

Immediately after birth until the bladder is closed, whether this is performed immediately in the days after birth or on a more delayed basis (see below), the bladder plate should be covered and protected with a non-adherent film of plastic wrap such as cling film or a hydrated gel dressing. The baby should be checked for associated congenital abnormalities, some of which might require urgent attention. Ultrasound should be performed to check the kidneys. There is no indication to prescribe antibiotics for exstrophy babies prior to closure as the urine drains freely, and urine infection is extremely uncommon in this situation. Indeed, inappropriate antibiotics may lead to antibiotic resistance in the future and facilitate the development of fungal infection.

The most serious risk for children with bladder exstrophy is damage to the upper renal tracts. It is imperative that clinicians are aware that major reconstructions of the lower urinary tract carry significant risks for the kidneys. Clinicians have a responsibility to monitor the upper tracts of children with exstrophy and particularly so in the first 12 months after any major lower tract reconstruction.

Most surgeons attempt to reconstruct bladder exstrophy with a view to providing the patient with the possibility (and hope) of volitional continent urethral micturition. There is presently however no universally agreed surgical approach and several have been described. It is not even agreed now that the bladder should be closed in the newborn period, with some clinicians reporting better primary closure outcomes at age 3–6 months, without any loss of bladder capacity or other complications [6].

In summary, however, there are two general approaches. The first is to approach the problem in a staged way, thereby dividing the reconstruction into two or three operations. Examples of this approach include the most popular approach, the so-called modern staged repair of bladder exstrophy (MSRE) [7, 8] and also the radical soft tissue mobilisation (RSTM), commonly known as the Kelly operation [9, 10]. The alternative approach is to perform a complete primary repair of bladder exstrophy (CPRE) in the newborn period as popularised by Mitchell [11, 12] in the 1990s and now practised in several major units.

22.6 Staged Approaches

The first stage in these operations is the primary closure of the bladder. In general, the bladder is closed in the neonatal period, but this can be delayed for either clinical reasons to do with the baby's health or the size of the bladder plate or the preference of the surgeon. Most specialist units now first perform pelvic osteotomy to facilitate pelvic bone reconstruction and include epidural anaesthesia for intraoperative and postoperative pain relief as routine. Prophylactic broad-spectrum antibiotics should be administered, and the ureters are protected with stents of the surgeon's choice. Sometimes the bladder mucosa is covered with hamartomatous polyps that hinder closure and reduce the eventual capacity of the bladder, and they should be removed and the mucosa then meticulously repaired.

An incision is made around the margins of the bladder plate. The bladder plate is then dissected off the skin and then sharply off the rectus muscles on either side in the properitoneal plane. In the male, the dissection is carried down to the level of the verumontanum on either side of the proximal urethral plate but making sure not to leave the urethral plate too narrow for eventual reconstruction. In the female, the dissection stops just above the vaginal opening, again making absolutely sure not to leave the urethral plate too narrow for eventual reconstruction. The final step in mobilization is to dissect deeply on either side of the bladder neck, dividing the thick fibromuscular attachments to the pubic symphysis on either side. This final step releases the bladder from the pubic bones, thereby enabling the bladder and proximal urethra eventually to be closed without tension. The bladder and proximal urethra are then reconstructed over ureteric and bladder drainage, followed by apposition of the pubic symphysis and closure of the abdominal wall.

The low-set umbilicus can be a source of infection postoperatively and should be removed during the mobilization. At the end of the operation, an umbilicoplasty should be fashioned in the correct position.

Recently, some centres have reported delaying the primary closure until age 3–6 months and perform bilateral ureteric reimplantation at the same time in order to improve the primary outcomes [6].

(Surgeons who are planning to pursue the RSTM as the second stage do not perform osteotomies and may not appose the pubic bones during this first stage.)

22.6.1 Modern Staged Repair of Bladder Exstrophy (MSRE)

In the girl, the primary bladder closure is essentially a complete repair, including the urethra, but without any formal bladder neck functional reconstruction. In the boy, however, the primary bladder neck closure leaves the epispadias unrepaired. Therefore, at age 1 year, the epispadias and full urethral reconstruction is completed using the modified Cantwell-Ransley method (see below).

In the third stage (or second stage in the female), bladder neck reconstruction (BNR) is performed only if the bladder develops a satisfactory capacity of at least 100 mL. This operation generally includes two key parts: first, bilateral cephalad ureteric reimplantation to correct/prevent vesicoureteric reflux (if not previously performed), and second, the bladder neck reconstruction itself which is constructed by tubularisation of the mucosal and muscle layers of the trigone, cephalad to the internal urethral meatus. Although some surgeons regard it as only creating a partial obstruction, the BNR is an attempt to create a form of sphincter function, and the author has seen volitional controlled micturition achieved in patients who were completely incontinent prior to the reconstruction. There is not a fixed point when the third stage should be performed. It is dependent on the child and the parents, and nurse specialists should be available to prepare the families and also to advise them about the possibility of prolonged clean intermittent catheterisation (CIC). Although the aim of MSRE is for the child to have gained continence by school age, in reality, it is often later. Although MSRE is probably the safest surgical approach to bladder exstrophy, perhaps its most negative feature is that the child often remains incontinent of urine when he starts school.

22.6.2 Radical Soft Tissue Mobilisation (RSTM)

The RSTM repair aims at achieving a more definite form of physiological sphincteric function. The exstrophy is closed in the neonatal period as described above. The RSTM itself is ideally performed around age of 9–12 months. The operation includes two key parts: (1) a dissection of the pelvic floor is performed, releasing the muscles, the pudendal pedicles and the corpora cavernosa off the pubic rami, thereby allowing (2) a tension-free reconstruction of the pelvic floor around the posterior urethra. The release of the urethral plate from the corpora in the male leaves a significant hypospadiac external urethral meatus which later requires a further two major operations to reconstruct, using the Bracka method. The protagonists for this approach offer potential external lengthening of the penis by the release of the short corpora from the pubic rami, as a significant benefit. However, there is also a major risk of iatrogenic penis damage secondary to the radical mobilisation of the pudendal pedicles.

22.6.3 Complete Primary Repair of Bladder Exstrophy (CPRE)

This technique, like the RSTM, aims to provide a more normal physiological sphincter function. It is based on the principle that bladder exstrophy represents a hernia of the open bladder through the defect in the anterior abdominal wall, and therefore, repair should be based on repositioning the bladder posteriorly into the pelvis, thereby allowing the relocation of anterior pelvic floor structures anterior to the posterior urethra. The operation does not include bladder neck reconstruction. The bladder, bladder neck and urethra are mobilised as a single unit off the two corpus cavernosum bodies. The intersymphyseal ligaments are then seen and incised and the bladder and urethra are placed posteriorly into the pelvis, and the anterior perineal muscular complex may be reconstructed around the posterior urethra. The mobilization of the urethra with the bladder off the corpora leads to a similar hypospadiac situation as occurs in the RSTM, and the majority of boys later require further two major operations to reconstruct, using the Bracka method.

22.6.3.1 Urodynamics and Outcomes

The application of urodynamic assessment in bladder exstrophy patients is relatively recent. Historically, static volume assessment of the bladder under general anaesthetic was the standard, allowing objective measurement of the bladder capacity at 20 cm pressure H_2O under image intensifier control. This has been, and still is in some centres, the assessment tool used to determine if BNR can be undertaken in children following the MSRE protocol. The majority of children do however achieve sufficient capacity to proceed with BNR.

The continence outcomes of MSRE after BNR are difficult to assess from the literature. This is partly because there are few papers which assess that issue directly and also because researchers are not always assessing the same issues. The best results are from Johns Hopkins, where MRSE has been developed over the years [9, 10].They report 70% of patients with minimum 5 years follow-up achieving dryness, day and night, following neonatal closure, Cantwell-Ransley and BNR, without need for augmentation or clean intermittent catheterisation (CIC), with a further (10%) being dry by day but damp at night. The Manchester group [6] in the UK recently reported a group of 26 patients following MRSE of which 16/26 (62%) are continent and able to micturate per urethra but 6 of which also need to perform urethral CIC.

Most other reports include patients who have had bladder augmentations following MRSE and are dependent on CIC for bladder drainage. Continence is therefore not volitional urethral continence but rather dryness. Most groups report only 20–25% of patients passing urine per urethra and being continent.

The RSTM and the CPRE both attempt to achieve the exciting possibility of a more normally functioning pelvic floor and sphincter in bladder exstrophy patients. Investigators have reported evidence of physiological synergic bladder function based on formal urodynamic assessment, following both of these operations. Long-term outcomes of the CPRE however seem to be disappointing. Although undoubtedly some children do achieve normal urethral voiding with continence, several reports suggest little improvement in outcomes compared to MRSE, and indeed some are worse. Many patients require further bladder neck procedures as well as bladder augmentation and catheterisation regimes. Several groups have also found that there is an increased risk of upper tract complications, secondary to bladder outlet and urethral issues. There are also reports that the extensive penile dissection can sometimes result in significant permanent penile damage.

The Great Ormond Street Hospital group have also reported normal urodynamic synchronised bladder function following their RSTM operation. They have also reported much better results than previously reported RSTM series with approximately 75% of their children becoming completely normally dry by day and 40% completely continent by night at 10 years follow-up [10]. A further noteworthy finding is that bladder function seems to improve as the child grows. As with the CPRE, interested observers are worried as to possible penile damage occurring secondary to the radical pudendal dissection required during the RSTM.

There is no easy solution to bladder exstrophy. At this point in time, the units with best-reported continence outcomes are the Johns Hopkins performing the MRSE and Great Ormond Street performing the RSTM. As long-term follow-up develops, and hopefully will be reported, it will be extremely important to define what happens to these patient groups after puberty and as they progress into adult life. Formal urodynamic assessment of some intact exstrophy bladders shows variable significant detrusor dysfunctions including low compliance, detrusor overactivity and, in some, even detrusor failure. Time will tell if exstrophy children who achieve voiding continence in childhood will continue to have good enough bladder function as they grow up, to allow them the normality of urethral micturition to be their life's experience.

The fallback operation for all children with bladder exstrophy, if normal continence cannot be achieved, is bladder augmentation, bladder neck repair/closure and a Mitrofanoff catheterisable continent stoma. The development of this operation in the 1990s provided a significantly improved outcome for exstrophy children than was available before [13] and can still offer a good quality of life if normal voiding cannot be achieved.

22.7 Epispadias

22.7.1 Male Epispadias

Epispadias is part of classic male bladder exstrophy but also occurs as an isolated lesion (Fig. 22.3). It is a very rare anomaly occurring in 1:120,000 live births [4].

In classical epispadias, the urethra is open on the dorsum of the penis, the foreskin is hooded on the ventral aspect and is significantly deficient on the dorsal aspect (Fig. 22.3) and the diagnosis is clear at birth. The urethra opens distally on the glans in the least severe variety; in the least common variety, it opens on the penile shaft; or in the most severe variety, it opens at the junction of the penis with the abdominal wall (complete or penopubic), and in this situation, the open urethra extends into the bladder neck. In this severe form, the verumontanum is often displaced proximally onto the bladder neck or even sometimes into the bladder. Sometimes there may be

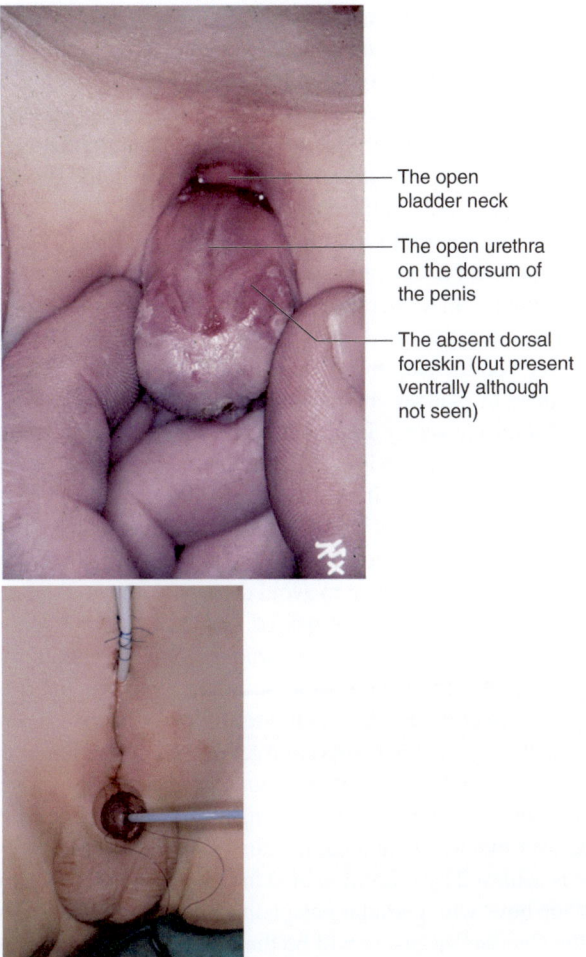

Fig. 22.3 Male epispadias (*Top*). Post Cantwell-Ransley Repair of Primary Epispadias (*Bottom*)

- The open bladder neck
- The open urethra on the dorsum of the penis
- The absent dorsal foreskin (but present ventrally although not seen)

a degree of pubic diastasis. Although the likelihood of incontinence is obvious in penopubic epispadias, in all forms, there may be degrees of incompetence of the bladder neck and sphincter function, and parents should be informed at diagnosis that the risk of incontinence exists, even in the less severe forms.

The penis is short with dorsal curvature of the corpora cavernosa (known as chordee) in all varieties of epispadias. Occasionally in glanular or penile epispadias, the foreskin may be intact and covers and conceals the deficient dorsal urethra, so that the diagnosis is missed. Because the penis is naturally short, the appearance may be similar to that of a buried penis or even a mega-prepuce. Doctors should be aware of the possibility of underlying epispadias when they are contemplating these two other diagnoses.

22.7.1.1 Surgery for Male Epispadias

Male epispadias is usually operated around the age of 1 year. The surgical objective is to repair the penis and achieve optimal lengthening, straightening and appearance of the penis. Eventually in many, there is requirement, as in exstrophy, to achieve urinary continence without compromising the upper urinary tracts.

The CPRE and RSTM approaches as described above in relation to exstrophy are also applicable to epispadias. Indeed the CPRE was first described for epispadias [11] and then extended later into full bladder exstrophy repair. The benefit again of these two operations, as primary approaches, is that they offer an attempt at achieving continence from the first operation, particularly for the more severe degrees. In practice, however, outcomes for CPRE and RSTM in epispadias have sometimes not led to urinary continence, and children have subsequently undergone formal bladder neck repairs or bladder augmentations and Mitrofanoff.

The *Cantwell-Ransley repair* is probably the most preferred primary operation used for epispadias. The first step is careful smooth incision along the lateral edges of the urethral plate extending proximally to around the margin of epispadiac external urethral meatus. The critical steps is meticulous sharp dissection of the urethral plate off the corporeal bodies up to the level of the glans distally and to the prostatic urethra proximally. It is extremely important to avoid damage to the urethral plate during this mobilisation in order to minimise the risk of fistula or stricture complications. The urethral plate is then tubularised, and the corporeal bodies are then rotated medially and over the urethra, thereby ventralising the urethra, burying the suture line of the urethroplasty and correcting the dorsal chordee. A caverno-cavernostomy should be performed to maintain the medial corporal rotation and correction of the chordee. At all times, it is important to be aware of the neurovascular bundles and to know exactly where they are, in order to avoid damage during the extensive dissections. Finally, the glans is closed over the urethra and the meatus is ventralised into a normal position. Skin coverage is achieved by utilisation of skin flaps, created from the foreskin.

In some of the boys with glanular epispadias, the child will develop normal continence, and the Cantwell-Ransley will be the only operation that is required. Most however require ongoing assessment and eventual bladder neck repair or bladder augmentation with Mitrofanoff.

22.7.2 Female Epispadias

In female epispadias (Fig. 22.4), the urethra is open on its dorsal surface, and the clitoris is split and is bifid, each side being attached to its labium minorum. Externally, the mons pubis appears flat and there may be some pubic diastasis. Internally, the bladder neck is deficient and open, and the bladder capacity is usually small and the children do not achieve continence. Sometimes the bladder wall is extremely thin and deficient in detrusor fibres, and its detrusor contractions are weak.

The diagnosis should really be clear at birth, but it is often missed. As a result, the diagnosis is not made until the child presents with dribbling incontinence. All girls presenting with a history suggestive of dribbling incontinence should undergo careful examination of the vulva in order to exclude or diagnose epispadias. In older

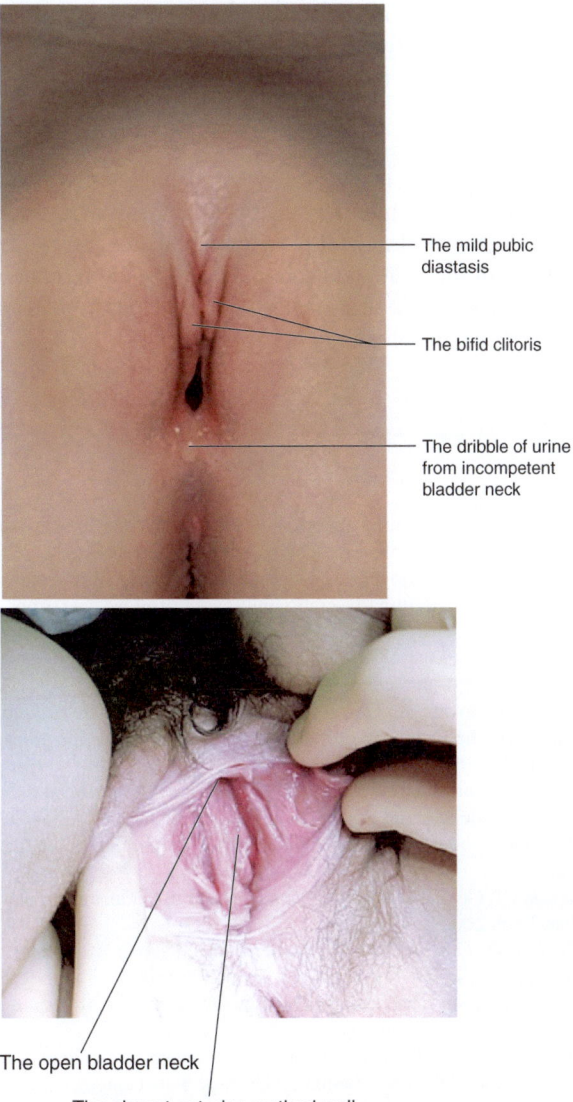

Fig. 22.4 Female Epispadias at birth and after being diagnosed in puberty

girls, this may necessitate examination under general anaesthetic. The author has the experience of seeing girls presenting in puberty with undiagnosed epispadias.

The standard surgical approach to female epispadias is primary anatomical repair in the first year of life. As in male epispadias, the children are followed up and can undergo bladder neck repair later.

The CPRE and RSTM principles have been applied to female epispadias in the same way as they are applied to female exstrophy so that the girls have an attempted all-in-one repair in the first year.

Occasionally bladder neck repair achieves its aim of volitional urethral continence in a girl, but for most, dryness is achieved by a bladder augmentation, bladder neck tightening or closure and then CIC through a Mitrofanoff.

Conclusions

Bladder exstrophy and epispadias are serious anomalies, which cause multiple problems. It is important to monitor the upper tracts following lower urinary tract reconstruction. Many children will require several surgeries to achieve dryness. The management of these and related conditions should be concentrated in specialist units with multidisciplinary teams in order to allow them to develop experience and expertise and hopefully improve outcomes.

References

1. Marshall VF, Muecke E. Congenital abnormalities of the bladder. In: Handbuch der Urologie. New York: Springer; 1968. p. 165.
2. Manner J, Kluth D. The morphogenesis of the exstrophy-epispadias complex: a new concept based on observations made in early embryonic cases of cloacal exstrophy. Anat Embryol (Berl). 2005;210:51–7.
3. Reutter H, et al. Seven new cases of familial isolated bladder exstrophy and epispadias complex (BEEC) and review of the literature. Am J Med Genet A. 2003;120(2):215–21.
4. Cervellione RM, Mantovani A, Gearhart J, Bogaert G, Gobet R, Caione P, Dickson AP. Prospective study on the incidence of bladder/cloacal exstrophy and epispadias in Europe. J Pediatr Urol. 2015;11(6):337.e1–6.
5. Goyal A, Fishwick J, Hurrell R, Cervellione RM, Dickson AP. Antenatal diagnosis of bladder/cloacal exstrophy: challenges and possible solutions. J Pediatr Urol. 2012;8(2):140–4.
6. Dickson AP. Bladder exstrophy: the Manchester experience. J Pediatr Surg. 2014;49(2):244–50.
7. Baird AD, Nelson CP, Gearhart JP. Modern staged repair of bladder exstrophy: a contemporary series. J Pediatr Urol. 2007;3:311–5.
8. Purves JT, Baird AD, Gearhart JP. The modern staged repair of bladder exstrophy in the female: a contemporary series. J Pediatr Urol. 2008;4(2):150–3.
9. Kelly J. Vesical exstrophy: repair using radical mobilisation of soft tissues. Pediatr Surg Int. 1995;10(5):298–30.
10. Cuckow P, Featherstone N, Ryan K, Desai D. Attainment of volitional voiding—15 years of the Kelly operation. Abstract: Paediatric Urology Fall Congress. Society of Paediatric Urology; 2014.
11. Mitchell MI, Bägli DJ. Complete penile disassembly for epispadias repair: the Mitchell technique. J Urol. 1996;155:300–4.
12. Grady RW, Mitchell ME. Complete primary repair of exstrophy. J Urol. 1999;162(4):1415–20.
13. Cervellione RM, Bianchi A, Fishwick J, Gaskell SL, Dickson AP. Salvage procedures to achieve continence after failed bladder exstrophy repair. J Urol. 2008;179(1):304–6. Epub 2007 Nov 19

Posterior Urethral Valves

23

Mario De Gennaro, Maria Luisa Capitanucci, Giovanni Mosiello, and Antonio Zaccara

23.1 Introduction

Posterior urethral valve (PUV) is a congenital condition which very often deals with bladder problems, not only due to neonatal bladder outlet obstruction but also because of a number of consequences on bladder function during infancy and childhood, often persisting through adolescence and long life. For the above reasons, PUV should be considered one of the main issues of clinical urodynamic in children. The condition is early detected prenatally by obstetric ultrasound but can be diagnosed later on.

Despite early relief of bladder outlet obstruction, remaining pathological changes in the bladder can cause significant bladder dysfunction resulting in incontinence and impaired upper tract drainage. A considerable quote of children (about 20%) suffer from urinary incontinence, and urodynamic bladder dysfunction was seen in many patients (55%, 0–72%) after primary treatment.

While a certain degree of bladder recovery will occur in most patients, some have long-term issues severe enough to result in compromise of the upper urinary tracts and renal function. The progressive slow deterioration that some of these patients present over years in renal function has been showed as a result of bladder dysfunction. Bladder function is often compromised since infancy as low compliant or overactive, with possible consequent delayed toilet training. Later in life the bladder tends to become oversized and empties poorly. Polyuria which is associated with renal failure as well as secondary changes in the bladder neck also has an effect on bladder function and emptying.

M. De Gennaro (✉) • M.L. Capitanucci • A. Zaccara
Division of Urology, Surgery for Continence and Urodynamics,
Bambino Gesù Children Hospital, Rome, Italy
e-mail: mario.degennaro@opbg.net

G. Mosiello
Pediatric NeuroUrology Research and Clinic, Bambino Gesù Children Hospital, Rome, Italy

23.2 Posterior Urethral Valves in Neonate

Demography. Posterior urethral valves (PUV) are the commonest etiology of urinary tract obstruction in the neonate. It is the commonest cause of chronic kidney disease secondary to urinary obstruction in children. A population-based study found the incidence to be 2.48 (2.14–2.81) per 10,000 live births [1].

Antenatal diagnosis. Prenatal ultrasound scanning has increased detection rate of PUV: in a population-based study, prenatal diagnosis rate was 46.9% [1]. Sonographic features of PUV include thick-walled bladder, bilateral hydronephrosis, scanty liquor, dilated bladder and posterior urethra, and echo-bright kidneys (Fig. 23.1a, b).

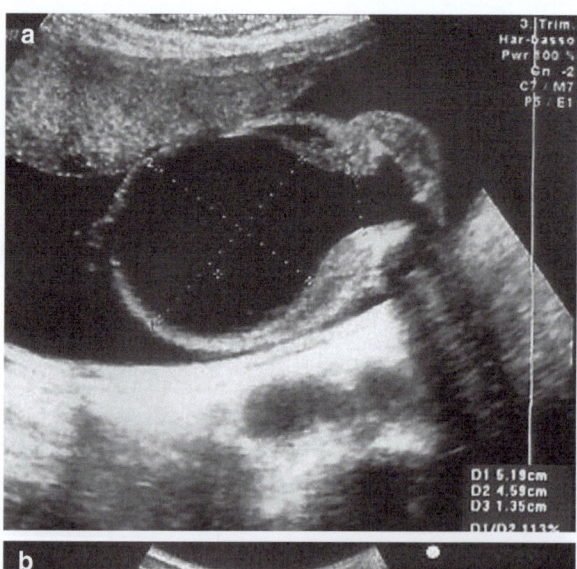

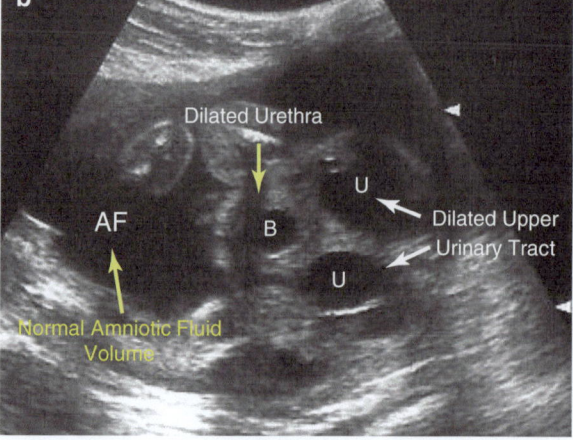

Fig. 23.1 Ultrasound antenatal diagnosis. (**a**) Antenatal US of a male fetus at 20 weeks of gestational age, showing an enormously dilated bladder and dilated posterior urethra with normal amniotic fluid volume. (**b**) Antenatal US (21 weeks g.a.) shows a dilated upper urinary tract and dilated posterior urethra (arrow), under a not severely dilated bladder (B) but dilated ureters (U), with normal amniotic fluid volume (yellow arrow)

Prenatal interventions. Interventions on the fetuses, like vesico-amniotic shunt/ vesicocentesis, have been done for many years. The rationale was that early drainage of obstructed system would allow improvement in renal function and survival with prevention of lung damage [2], but among survivors, prenatal drainage did not alter renal function status. An extensive randomized trial (PLUTO) did not answer questions on benefit of prenatal intervention in bladder outflow obstruction [3]. Nowadays, oligohydramnios should be considered the main prognostic factor in terms of kidney function and survival, but prenatal diagnosis has not globally improved long-term outcomes.

23.2.1 Neonatal Management

After delivery, bladder is catheterized, and it is no longer a surgical emergency. By this way, babies with urosepsis, dehydration, and acidosis can be managed. Rarely, it may not be possible to catheterize the urethra, and some newborns require suprapubic catheter. If kidneys fail to drain despite adequate bladder drainage, upper tract drainage can be required, especially if the kidney is infected.

Diagnosis. The first imaging needed is *ultrasound* scan, which may demonstrate enlarged/thick-walled bladder, dilated urethra, dilated kidneys and ureters, and bladder diverticula. Urinary ascites and/or urinoma may also be seen on US, presumably due to high-pressure systems with rupture of the upper urinary tract. *Voiding cystourethrogram* (VCUG) is the mainstay of diagnosis for PUV: it shows dilated/small bladder, reflux, trabeculations of bladder, dilatation of posterior urethra, and bladder neck hypertrophy (Fig. 23.2a–c). At this stage, *isotope scans* are not necessary.

23.2.2 Endoscopic Interventions in Neonate

Endoscopic valve ablation remains the definitive intervention in PUV. Earlier, cutting loops were used, while these days, bugbee electrode is preferred, and some surgeons prefer to use cold knife. Valves are incised at 5 o'clock and 7 o'clock position (Fig. 23.3). The role of bladder neck incision is controversial (see paragraph): even if it is supposed to represent a further aid to remove obstruction, little information are available regarding subsequent late retrograde ejaculation in adolescence/adulthood.

Complications with valve ablation/fulguration can occur with significant morbidity in the neonate: strong current, excessive destruction of tissue can lead to stricture formation. Other complications, as urinary extravasation and bladder injury, are rare. Urethral stricture occurring in a long term can be successfully treated endoscopically [4].

Minimal invasive laser ablation. To prevent complications, an alternative approach is to ablate the obstructive tissue by laser energy, with minimal invasive procedure. Few series are published, the largest on 40 children aged average 2 years [5] and a more recent one on 17 neonates [6]. Both used the holmium:YAG laser,

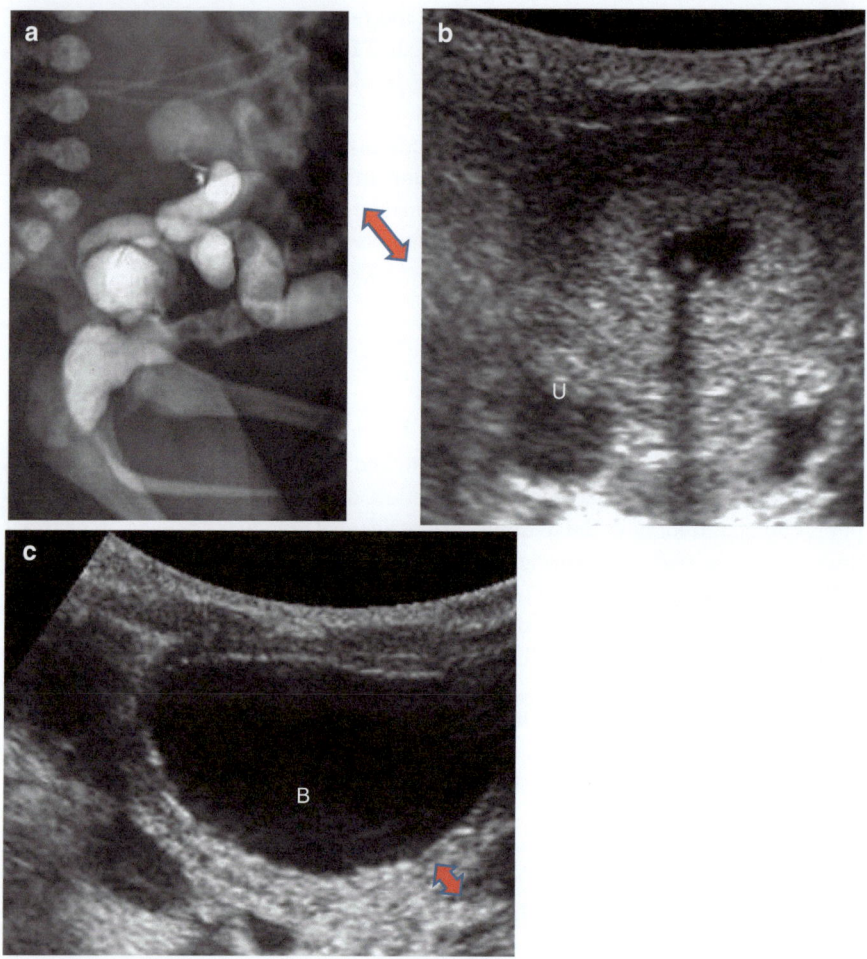

Fig. 23.2 Newborn with PUV: voiding cystourethrography and ultrasound. (**a**) VCUG of a newborn (2 days) with severe PUV, diagnosed prenatally. Evidence of posterior urethra dilatation and narrowing under the sphincteric area; severe bilateral redundant ureteral reflux. (**b**) US at 2 days: very small bladder, with severe thickened bladder walls and widely dilated ureters (U). (**c**) US at 15 days, after endoscopic valve section: the bladder is wide (B) and dilated, bladder wall is thickened (red arrow), but much less than prior to valves resection and only one ureter is still dilated

which is recommended for soft tissues. We currently use this technique, with apparent good immediate results on voiding after removal of catheter and no hematuria. We are confident that minimal invasive ablation is a preventive tool also in terms of late bladder dysfunction.

Fig. 23.3 Endoscopy for posterior urethral valves ablation by classical fulguration

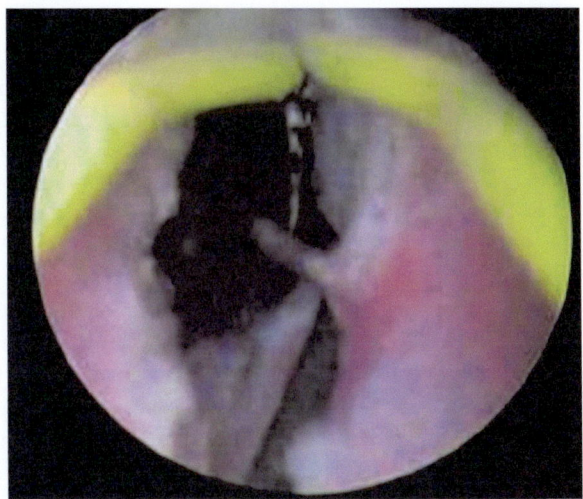

23.2.3 Early Diversion in PUV?

In preterm babies, small neonates may not be suitable for endoscopic valve ablation. These babies can be managed with indwelling bladder catheter till they are able to undergo cystoscopic ablation. Failing this, supravesical diversion (i.e., cutaneous vesicostomy) provides for adequate low-pressure bladder drainage, and patients can undergo valve ablation and diversion closure at a later date. Vesicostomy can be closed whenever conditions are favorable. It is a procedure of choice in developing countries, and mini-vesicostomy facilitates clean intermittent catheterization (CIC) and overnight bladder drainage [7]. Some patients with enormously dilated ureters and poor drainage may benefit by ureterostomy: a high ureterostomy provides better drainage of kidney, but low "loop ureterostomy" provides kidney drainage while some urine drains into the bladder allowing cycling, which is good for late bladder function.

Nephrostomy is an alternative in very small/sick children, but it is associated with chronic infection and difficult subsequent reconstruction.

Long-term outcome of early diversion. Supravesical drainage has not been conclusively shown to improve outcomes and is at best a temporizing measure in those babies with fragile kidneys. In a prospective study over 6 years, vesicostomy and fulguration were compared in 45 neonates with PUV: patients did not have significant difference of renal function and somatic growth [8]. In summary, very few cases of valve bladder actually have obstructed ureters, dictating that upper tract diversions are rarely necessary. On the contrary, studies showed that, compared to valve ablation alone, temporary vesicostomy or supravesical diversion led to less bladder instability and better compliance and capacity on urodynamics, later on [9].

23.2.4 Postneonatal Follow-Up

All patients are followed for improvement of renal function. *Urodynamic* evaluation is performed when the child is older, while a check *VCUG* or *cystoscopy* may be required 3–6 months following initial cystoscopy.

23.3 Bladder Dysfunction

Despite early relief of bladder outlet obstruction, remaining pathological changes in the bladder can cause significant bladder dysfunction resulting in incontinence and impaired upper tract drainage. While a certain degree of bladder recovery will occur in most patients, some have long-term issues severe enough to result in compromise of the upper tracts. Different studies have indicated that the progressive slow deterioration that some of these patients present over years in RF is a result of bladder dysfunction [10, 11]. Over time, one or a combination of three abnormal urodynamic patterns of myogenic failure, detrusor hyperreflexia, and decreased compliance/small capacity may develop [12]. In addition, bladder function has been shown to change with time from poor compliance in newborns to instability from hypercontractility in older children to myogenic failure in postpubertal patients. Myogenic failure, in conjunction with increasing capacity and poor emptying, is primarily a later phenomenon and is most likely to be secondary to increased urine production and decreased frequency of voiding with advancing age [13].

Despite early and correct valve ablation, a large proportion of boys treated for PUV have gradual detrusor 'decompensation' and/or secondary bladder neck outlet obstruction leading to obstructive voiding and finally underactive detrusor [14].

The bladder neck was once recognized as the major cause of bladder outlet obstruction in patients with PUV. It may be evident since newborn age, at postoperative bladder ablation cystogram (Fig. 23.4), and/or may occur later on, at videourodynamic studies carried out because of persistence urinary incontinence and signs of outlet obstruction, where it isn't easy to differentiate between bladder neck and residual urethral obstructions. The concept was largely disputed by Glassberg [15], and many pediatric urologists suspect that ongoing bladder neck dysfunction is responsible of obstruction subsequent to valves ablation. Various treatments have been directed at the bladder neck, including alpha blockers, bladder neck incision (BNI), and clean intermittent catheterization (CIC) which is difficult to establish in boys with PUVs. In 2007, Kajbafzadeh evaluated the effects of simultaneous BNI and valve ablation on urodynamic abnormalities in 46 patients with posterior urethral valves: he concluded that simultaneous valve ablation and BNI effectively reduces bladder hypercontractility and prevents development of myogenic failure [16]. The concept is attractive, thinking in terms of late outcome of possible bladder decompensation due to residual obstruction. But, in the absence of clear long-term data on continence and regular ejaculation, this procedure should be avoided or reserved to peculiar patients with persisting poor bladder compliance or high residuals demonstrating anatomical obstruction or nonobstructive retention. In fact, several patients ameliorate spontaneously, thus conservative management should be preferred or a temporary measure as Botox injection can be considered.

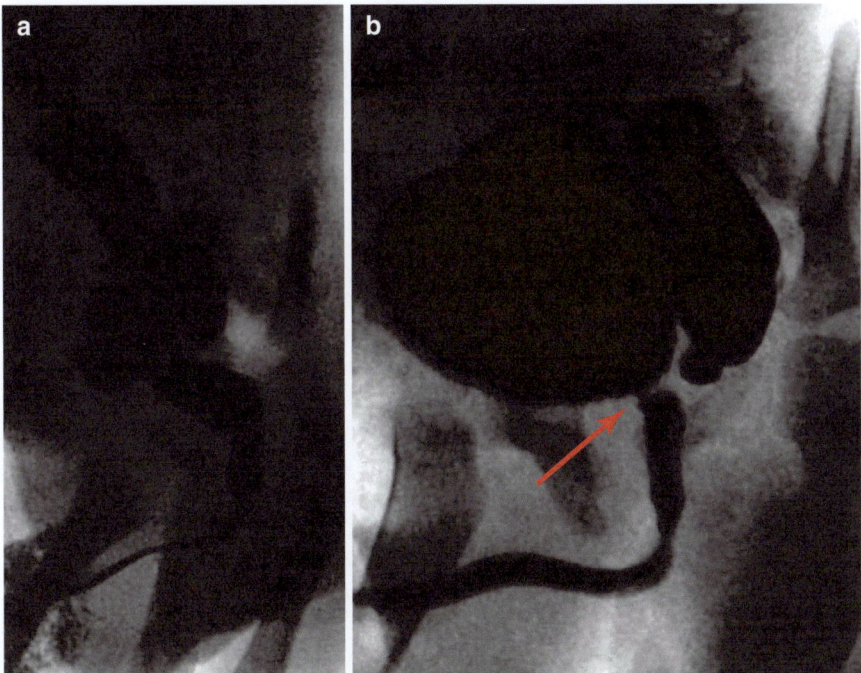

Fig. 23.4 (**a**) Cystogram of a newborn with severe valves: dilated posterior urethra, small bladder and regularly opening bladder neck, and gross reflux. (**b**) The same boy 1 year following successful endoscopic valves ablation. The VCUG shows a very narrow bladder neck (red arrow) at voiding, and the urethra shows a nice caliber with resolution of valves obstruction, with persistence of gross reflux

23.3.1 Bladder Dysfunction and Renal Failure

Several studies have shown the predictability of the development of renal failure based on specific detrusor patterns seen on urodynamic evaluation. Persistent poor compliance, high detrusor pressures, bladder outlet obstruction (BOO), and or chronic failure of the detrusor to adequately contract during voiding with increased post-voiding residual (PVR) are the most likely causes of deterioration [12]. Consequently, bladder dysfunction will be a determinant of the development of long-term renal dysfunction in some patients with treated PUV.

23.3.2 Urodynamics in PUV

Since lower urinary tract dysfunction is long established and possibly related to deterioration of upper urinary tract function, long-term urodynamic follow-up is widely recommended in boys with PUV. The clinical challenge is to identify those individuals at risk for long-term bladder dysfunction and its deleterious side effects [17]. Timing of urodynamic follow-up, however, are still undefined. Some literature argues that the use of a urethral catheter in urodynamics falsely increases voiding pressure. But there are findings which support voiding pressure as a valid independent urodynamic parameter in this population that can be objectively measured before and after therapeutic intervention [18]. All children with PUV are different and do not necessarily follow any schedule in terms of deteriorating bladder function, but it is clear that different patterns of bladder pathology are seen specifically in children with PUV.

Noninvasive urodynamic. Due to catheterization of a sensate urethra, boys with PUV usually experience strong discomfort during urodynamic study so that many decline further invasive studies. Noninvasive urodynamic evaluation is considered effective in detecting non-neurogenic LUTD. Noninvasive urodynamic evaluation, which is widely recommended as a first-line assessment, avoids some of the pitfalls of invasive urodynamics, including the complex methodology and the lack of cooperation of children undergoing a painful examination [19]. Additionally, it was recently reported that invasive urodynamics did not correlate better than noninvasive techniques in terms of clinical diagnosis and outcome in children with OAB and dysfunctional voiding [20]. Findings in a longitudinal series of 28 children, half monitored conservatively by noninvasive urodynamics, support the safety and effectiveness of this strategy in detecting LUTD and preventing late-onset renal failure in boys with PUVs. Moreover, noninvasive studies promote the reassessment and involvement of patients in diagnostic evaluation and treatment; regular contacts with patients promote also awareness of lower and upper urinary tract, encouraging repeated evaluations and appropriate rehabilitative and pharmacological treatments. Based on these findings, it may be possible to limit invasive urodynamic testing to cases of progressively deteriorating LUTD or worsening upper urinary tract function [21].

23.3.3 Pharmacotherapy

Oxybutynin. The beneficial effects of anticholinergics on bladder wall compliance in patients with PUVs have been documented [22]. Theoretically if one acts early to improve the bladder dynamics associated with hypertrophic muscle in the bladder wall, then more rapid remodeling of bladder muscle will occur. A study demonstrates that the early use of anticholinergic therapy in infants with high voiding pressures and/or small bladder capacity after primary PUV ablation has beneficial effects on bladder and compliance [23].

Alpha-blockers. Accumulating data have shown the efficacy of alpha-blockers in improving voiding dysfunction and upper tract dilatation in patients with PUV, presumably through decreasing intravesical pressure and outlet resistance [24]. Terazosin has recently proved to be safe and results in significant improvement in bladder emptying in patients with posterior urethral valves [25].

Botox. The use of Botox to treat bladder neck obstruction would be effective and present an alternative to other more aggressive bladder neck procedures. An interesting study on children with VUPs and persistent BOO looked at this difficult group of patients and randomized 20 patients to receive a bladder neck injection of 100 units of Botox at the time of their check cystoscopy and followed them for a further 6 months: both the Botox and control groups improved during the follow-up period, but there was no additional benefit demonstrated by the Botox injection [26].

23.4 Reflux in PUV Boys

Vesicoureteral reflux (VUR) secondary to PUV is known to affect the ultimate outcome of treatment and renal function status after correction of PUV [27] and is present in up to 72% of cases. The relationship between PUV and VUR should be considered taking into account the urodynamic phenomena which occur into the lower and upper urinary tracts. It seems that bladder function is a key determinant of renal outcome in children with VUR secondary to PUV [28]. Increased storage and/or voiding pressures caused by lower urinary tract symptoms may lead to a spectrum of intravesical anatomic disorders possibly predisposing the patient to VUR. Contrary to the results in primary VUR cases, no difference in the resolution of VUR was observed among different grades of secondary reflux, and moreover, even high-grade secondary VURs can resolve with conservative therapy in some cases [29]. Accordingly, attempts should be focused on correction of bladder function rather than performing invasive procedures for the correction of the radiologic findings regarding VUR.

Overall, conservative therapy can be regarded as the mainstay of reflux treatment after successful valve correction as it is associated with a 66% success rate [30].

The best option is an observation with management of bladder/bowel dysfunction (BBD), in addition to treatment of urinary tract infections (UTI), as they occur [31]. In children with PUVs, bladder surgery should be in general avoided, to prevent deterioration of bladder function, which may lead with the necessity of bladder augmentation.

23.5 Urinary Continence

The natural evolution of urinary continence in boys following posterior urethral valves ablation is difficult to investigate, due to the various conditions present in the single patient. Due to early treatment of valves and bladder dysfunction, nowadays children with have better outcome in terms of continence achievement. No doubt that recent groups of patients, who receive an accurate toilet training program and strict follow-up, achieve continence earlier compared with older series of boys who are now adults and didn't receive that treatment.

Anyway, continence achievement is delayed in PUV children, compared to normal population, especially in those who have chronic renal failure (high creatinine level at 5 years). There are no data regarding significant difference in boys with/without initial reflux or who underwent temporary ureteral diversion.

The impression is that a conservative management after valve ablation, limiting surgery on the bladder, is a big help to avoid urinary incontinence. Boys with PUVs can achieve regular voiding and continence, if early but conservatively treated, if they don't have initial renal impairment with consequent polyuria, and if receiving adequate toilet training and subsequent close follow-up with urotherapy and noninvasive urodynamic assessment.

23.6 Bladder and Renal Function Relationship

Posterior urethral valves (PUV) account for almost 17% of children with end-stage renal failure [32]. A pathophysiological relationship has been suggested between lower urinary tract dysfunction and late-onset renal failure. Furthermore, the polyuria occurring for CRF determines high volumes into the (dysfunctional) bladder, not only leading with urinary incontinence but also deteriorating the upper tract itself.

23.6.1 Polyuria and Bladder Volume-Dependent Obstruction

The urinary concentrating capacity is impaired in about 75% of PUV children, and tubular damage worsens with age, despite early relief of obstruction in many patients [33]. An increased daily urine volume can exacerbate bladder dysfunction, increasing the hydrostatic pressure transmitted to the kidneys in the presence of the decreased bladder capacity and compliance, and lead to progressive renal injury. For patients with salvageable RF, it is essential to control bladder pressure. Overnight catheter drainage in patients with persistent hydronephrosis and polyuria will allow bladder and UUT decompression for at least a third of each day and relieve a possible negative effect on renal function [34, 35].

23.6.2 Renal Transplant

It is unclear whether the initial valve intervention in children with PUVs has an effect on the development renal graft failure. One hypothesis is that primary valve ablation alone would lead to higher graft success, perhaps by resulting in less bladder dysfunction compared to that in patients with a non-functionalized bladder due to diversion. The impact on transplant kidney survival of valve treatment approaches and the impact of bladder dysfunction and its treatments have been studied. Graft survival at 5 years was 50% in those children with PUVs, while a control group with ESRD due to non-genitourinary causes had 75% graft survival, and it would be argued that the effect of the valve bladder may explain these findings [36]. Children with PUVs who received transplants have a significantly increased incidence of ureteral obstruction. Furthermore, pyelonephritis graft loss seems to be more frequent in PUV patients who underwent augmentation cystoplasty. Thus, provided that adequate surveillance of BD and high PVR is obtained, avoiding augmentation may be protective. Preemptive augmentation is not a first option, and it should be constructed only if there is great risk associated with increased bladder pressures, higher than the risk associated with augmentation. Moreover, since a considerable number of PUV patients with high-pressure bladders eventually develop myogenic failure, it seems logical to postpone surgical options. On the contrary, an adequate management of BD is essential to improve bladder function and to minimize UTIs [37].

23.7 Transitional Care

23.7.1 Hyperfiltration Injury

Another factor that can contribute to the late onset of renal failure in PUV patients is the hyperfiltration injury due to the increased metabolic demands of puberty. Over the long term, and with time, hyperfiltration would produce proteinuria and focal segmentary glomerulosclerosis and result in renal failure. Proteinuria has been demonstrated to be a good indicator of the hyperfiltration. Early use of angiotensin-converting enzyme inhibitors or antagonists in patients who present proteinuria during follow-up may attenuate these hemodynamic alterations and delay or even avoid CRF [38].

23.7.2 Sexual Function and Fertility

Nowadays, more PUV boys reach adolescence and adulthood, and their sexual function and fertility have become relevant. However, information on these issues is still scant. In adolescents with treated PUV, the posterior urethra can remain widely dilated and the bladder neck open, despite adequate valve ablation, which will result in ejaculatory dysfunction. Furthermore, reflux into the vasa deferentia may be present, affecting testicular or prostatic components of semen. In a series of 21 men (mean age 24.6 years), 48% complained of slow or dry ejaculation, even if erections and orgasm were normal [39]. In another series of 16 patients (mean age 24 years), all experienced erections and orgasm, but 2 ones (1 on dialysis) had mild and 2 patients medium erectile dysfunction. Ejaculation was normal in all patients, except in the patient on dialysis [40]. The analysis of semen may show abnormally viscous semen, high pH, and increased liquefaction time, as possible reduction in prostatic or seminal vesicle fluid. Sexual function and fertility remain a matter of speculation owing to the scarcity of studies and the discrepancies in results. However, it would seem that these patients have normal sexual function (some with slow ejaculation).The ability to father children appears to be more dependent on RF than on PUV dysfunction.

References

1. Malin G, Tonks AM, Morris RK, et al. Congenital lower urinary tract obstruction: a population-based epidemiological study. BJOG. 2012;119:1455–64.
2. Clark TJ, Martin WL, Divakaran TG, et al. Prenatal bladder drainage in the management of fetal lower urinary tract obstruction: a systematic review and meta-analysis. Obstet Gynecol. 2003;102:367–82.

3. Pluto Collaborative Study Group, Kilby M, Khan K, Morris K, et al. PLUTO trial protocol: percutaneous shunting for lower urinary tract obstruction randomised controlled trial. BJOG. 2007;114:904–5.
4. Sarhan O, El-Ghoneimi A, Hafez A. Surgical complications of posterior urethral valve ablation: 20 years experience. J Pediatr Surg. 2010;45:2222–6.
5. Mandal S, Goel A, Kumar M, et al. Use of holmium YAG laser in posterior urethral valves: another method of fulguration. J Pediatr Urol. 2013;9:1093–7.
6. Pagano MJ, van Batavia JP, Casale C. Ablation in the management of obstructive uropathy in neonates. J Endourol. 2015;29(5):611–4.
7. Nanda M, Bawa M, Narasimhan KL. Mini-vesicostomy in the management of PUV after valve ablation. J Pediatr Urol. 2012;8:51–4.
8. Narasimhan KL, Kaur B, Chowdhary SK, et al. Does mode of treatment affect the outcome of neonatal posterior urethral valves? J Urol. 2004;171:2423–6.
9. Kim YH, Horowitz M, Combs A, et al. Comparative urodynamic findings after primary valve ablation, vesicostomy or proximal diversion. J Urol. 1996;156:673.
10. Parkhouse HF, Barrat TM, Dillon MJ, et al. Long-term outcome of boys with posterior urethral valves. BJU Int. 1988;62:59.
11. Ghanen MSA, Wolffenbuttel KP, Vylder A, et al. Long-term bladder dysfunction and renal function in boys with posterior urethral valves based on urodynamic findings. J Urol. 2004;171:2409–12.
12. Ansari MS, Gulia A, Srivastava A, et al. Risk factors for progression to end-stage renal disease in children with posterior urethral valves. J Pediatr Urol. 2010;6:261–4.
13. De Gennaro M, Capitanucci ML, Mosiello G, et al. The changing urodynamic pattern from infancy to adolescence in boys with posterior urethral valves. BJU Int. 2000;85:1104.
14. Androulakakis PA, Karamanolakis DK, Tsahouridis G, et al. Myogenic bladder decompensation in boys with a history of posterior urethral valves is caused by secondary bladder neck obstruction? BJU Int. 2005;96(1):140–3.
15. Glassberg KI. The severe bladder dysfunction: 20 years later. J Urol. 2001;166:1406–10.
16. Kajbafzadeh A, Payabvash S, Karimian G, et al. The effects of bladder neck incision on urodynamic abnormalities of children with posterior urethral valves. J Urol. 2007;178:2142–9.
17. De Gennaro M, Mosiello G, Capitanucci ML, et al. Early detection of bladder dysfunction following posterior urethral valve ablation. Eur J Pediatr Surg. 1996;6:163.
18. De Gennaro M, Capitanucci ML, Capozza N, et al. Detrusor hypocontractility in children with posterior urethral valves arises before puberty. Br J Urol. 1998;81:81.
19. Nevéus T, von Gontard A, Hoebeke P, et al. The standardization of terminology of lower urinary tract function in children and adolescents: report from the Standardisation Committee of the International Children's Continence Society. J Urol. 2006;176:314.
20. Bael A, Lax H, De Jong TP, et al. The relevance of urodynamic studies for urge syndrome and dysfunctional voiding: a multicenter controlled trial in children. J Urol. 2008;180:1486.
21. Capitanucci ML, Marciano A, Zaccara A, et al. Long-term bladder function followup in boys with posterior urethral valves: comparison of noninvasive vs invasive urodynamic studies. J Urol. 2012;188:953–7.
22. Kim YH, Horowitz M, Combs AJ, et al. Management of posterior urethral valves on the basis of urodynamic findings. J Urol. 1997;158:1011.
23. Jessica TC, Jennifer AH, Max M, et al. Early administration of oxybutynin improves bladder function and clinical outcomes in newborns with posterior urethral valves. J Urol. 2012;188:1516–20.
24. Misseri R, Combs AJ, Horowitz M, et al. Myogenic failure in posterior urethral valve disease: real or imagined? J Urol. 2002;168:1844–7.
25. Abraham MK, Nasir AR, Sudarsanan B, et al. Role of alpha adrenergic blocker in the management of posterior urethral valves. Pediatr Surg Int. 2009;25:1113–5.
26. Mokhless I, Zahran AR, Saad A, et al. Effect of Botox injection at the bladder neck in boys with bladder dysfunction after valve ablation. J Pediatr Urol. 2014;10:899–905.

27. Sarhan OM, El-Ghoneimi AA, Helmy TE, et al. Posterior urethral valves: multivariate analysis of factors affecting the final renal outcome. J Urol. 2011;185:2491–5.
28. Ghanem MA, Wolffenbuttel KP, De Vylder A, et al. Long-term bladder dysfunction and renal function in boys with posterior urethral valves based on urodynamic findings. J Urol. 2004;171:2409–12.
29. Fast AM, Nees SN, Van Batavia JP, et al. Outcomes of vesicoureteral reflux in children with non-neurogenic lower urinary tract dysfunction with targeted treatment at their specific LUT condition. J Urol. 2013;190:1028–33.
30. Tourchi A, Kajbafzadeh AM, Aryan Z, et al. The management of vesicoureteral reflux in the setting of posterior urethral valve with emphasis on bladder function and renal outcome: a single center cohort study. Urology. 2014;83(1):199–205.
31. Hunziker M, Mohanan N, D'Asta F, et al. Incidence of febrile urinary tract infections in children after successful endoscopic treatment of vesicoureteral reflux: a long-term follow-up. J Pediatr. 2012;160:1015–20.
32. Yohannes P, Hanna M. Current trends in the management of posterior urethral valves in the pediatric population. Urology. 2002;60(6):947e53.
33. Dinneen MD, Duffy PG, Barrat TM, et al. Persistent polyuria after posterior urethral valves. BJU Int. 1995;75:236–40.
34. Koff SA, Mutabagani K, Jayanthi VR. The valve bladder syndrome: pathophysiology and treatment with nocturnal bladder emptying. J Urol. 2002;167:291–7.
35. Hale JM, Wood DN, Hoh IM, et al. Stabilization of renal deterioration caused by bladder volume dependent obstruction. J Urol. 2009;182:1973–7.
36. Reinberg Y, Gonzalez R, Fryd D, et al. The outcome of renal transplantation in children with posterior urethral valves. J Urol. 1988;140:1491.
37. Pippi Salle JL, Jesus LE. Pre-transplant management of valve bladder: a critical literature review. J Pediatr Urol. 2015;11:5–11.
38. Wühl E, Schaefer F. Therapeutic strategies to slow chronic kidney disease progression. Pediatr Nephrol. 2008;22:705–16.
39. Woodhouse CR, Reilly JM, Bahadur G. Sexual function and fertility in patients treated for posterior urethral valves. J Urol. 1989;142:586–8.
40. Lopez Pereira P, Miguel M, Martinez Urrutia MJ, et al. Long-term bladder function, fertility and sexual function in patients with posterior urethral valves treated in infancy. J Pediatr Urol. 2013;9:38–41.

Hypospadia and Urethral Stricture

24

Carlos Arturo Levi D'Ancona, Juliano Cesar Moro, and Caio Cesar Citatini de Campos

24.1 Introduction

Hypospadias is the second most common malformation in male genitalia. It is defined as an abnormal ventral opening of the urethral meatus between the distal glans and perineum, caused by an abnormal development of urethral spongiosum and ventral prepuce associated to an arrest on the physiological correction of the ventral curvature [1, 2].

A congenital defect involving the fusion of urethral plates causes the abnormality, although its origin still remains uncertain. The critical process of hypospadias happens between the 8th and 12th week of gestation [1]. The prevalence varies among different regions, from 4 cases per 10,000 births in Japan up to 74 cases per 10,000 births in the United States, with an average of 40 cases per 10,000 births worldwide [3–5].

The etiology is unclear, but some evidence can suggest that low birth weight, maternal hypertension, preeclampsia, and placental insufficiency as important factors [6, 7].

Hypospadias diagnosis is based on clinical examination, which is first suspected by the lack of ventral prepuce and confirmed by the proximal meatus (Fig. 24.1). Other anomalies can also be found, such as ventral curvature (chordee), downward glans tilt, and deviation of the median penile raphe [1, 8].

Duckett's classification is the most used in clinical practice. Urethral defects are divided in anterior (50%), middle (30%), and posterior (20%), according to the following example (Fig. 24.2).

C.A.L. D'Ancona (✉) • J.C. Moro • C.C.C. de Campos
Division of Urology, Universidade Estadual de Campinas—UNICAMP, Campinas, São Paulo, Brazil

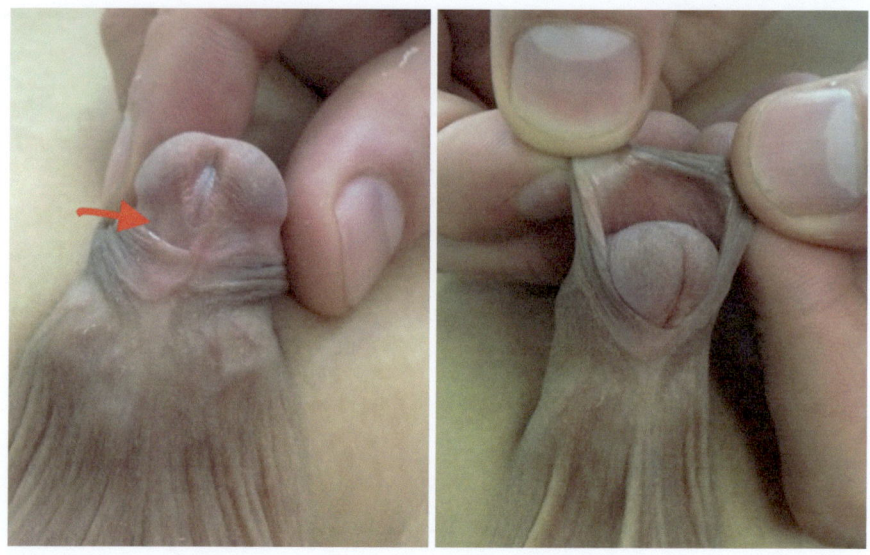

Fig. 24.1 Hypospadias with proximal meatus (arrow) and lack of ventral prepuce

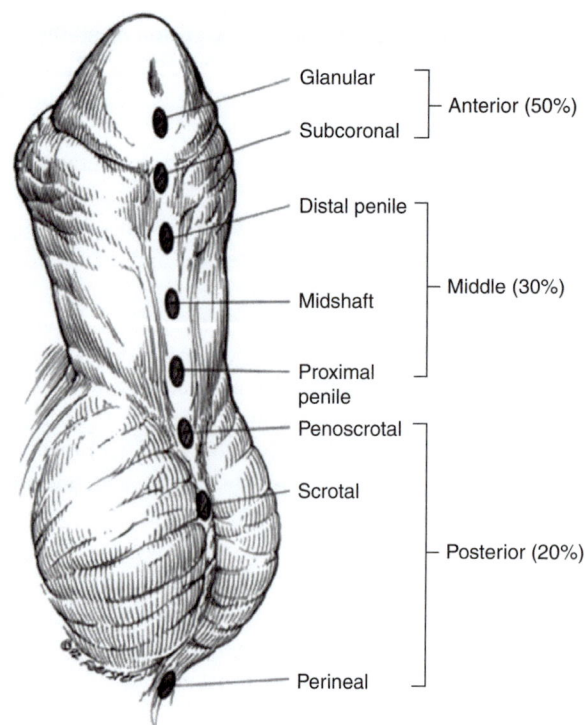

Fig. 24.2 Hypospadias Duckett's classification based on meatus position

Despite surgical success in childhood, some patients develop problems related to self-image, sexual and lower urinary tract function, and stenosis of urethra, discussed below.

24.2 Self-Image, Psychosocial Features, and Psychosexual Development Related to Hypospadias

The cosmetic results are of fundamental importance in the treatment of hypospadias, considering that surgery leads to major changes in the aesthetic appearance of the penis. The impact of these changes in self-image and sexual function in patients has been the subject of research of several authors. So many are investigating in very different ways to answer these questions.

A systematic review analyzed 13 studies, and it was noted that none of them made analyzes related to health-related quality of life (HRQoL) [9]. Moreover, the results of the psychosocial and psychosexual data were inconsistent, although many have demonstrated negative impact on sexual development by evidence that patients have a very negative impression on the genitalia and suffer from sexual inhibitions.

The questionnaires used to evaluate psychosocial adjustment in these studies were many, the Children's Depression Inventory (CDI), State-Trait Anxiety Inventory for Children (STAIC), Minnesota Multiphasic Personality Inventory (MMPI), Junior Dutch Personality Questionnaire (PDS-J), Social Anxiety Scale for Children (SAS-C), and other scales and countless questionnaires developed by different authors.

The great lesson of this study, however, is in finding the lack of standardization in research of psychosocial and psychosexual risk factors in order to correlate them properly with the results obtained in hypospadias surgery.

Another revision analyzing 20 studies that sexual function was satisfactory in 81% of the total hypospadias group but in control group, the satisfaction rate was 93% [10]. Erectile dysfunction was significantly higher in the hypospadias group. Moreover, patients with severe hypospadias often had less intimate relationships compared to the control group.

Contrary data to the negative impact on sexual development have also been published by others authors [10–12], which show that hypospadias does not influence the age of sexual initiation nor on the sexual behavior of patients.

The problem with evaluating sexual development begins with the patient's own penile perception. The instrument most commonly used for this purpose is the Pediatric Penile Perception Score (PPPS). This, for example, has shown that its results can vary among children, parents, and surgeons [9]. In this study, the perception of children is better than that of the parents and surgeons.

Data on sexual development are heterogeneous [13], showing greater satisfaction in sexual life of treated patients, despite the negative perception of the penis' appearance. Another unexplored aspect is the ejaculatory function, which has shown to be different in some studies [11, 12, 14–16]. The most frequently were weakness of the ejaculation or the need to milk semen out of the urethra.

The purpose of presenting these data, as heterogeneous and divergent, does not exhaust the subject, but attention must be paid to the importance of consideration to these aspects (self-image and sexual function) in clinical practice and stress the need to establish standardized methods for the evaluation of these data in order to generate more consistent future results.

Urethral meatus position is considered a major concern to men but is not of great importance to women. In a recent study developed by Ruppen-Greef NK [17], 105 women questioned through a standardized questionnaire, 10 standard photos of penis with hypospadias repaired and 10 photos of circumcised penis. The results obtained by this interesting methodology demonstrated that women consider the position of the meatus and shape of the gland as of low importance. This information seems to be decisive in starting the treatment of minor forms of hypospadias and on patients' counseling after surgery.

24.3 Role of Urodynamics in Patients with Hypospadias

Historically, urinary symptoms are not part of the preoperative medical history of patients with hypospadias. The vast majority who have their correction in childhood and patients at this age do not know how to explain their symptoms. The anomalous position of the meatus is the main reason for medical appointments, and the main goal of treatment at this time is the functional and cosmetic result. However, several studies state that the incidence of urinary symptoms is significantly higher in patients undergoing hypospadias correction, and this fact cannot be neglected, especially when considering long-term results.

In a retrospective survey of 167 patients with hypospadias compared to 169 controls, at least one urinary symptom was observed in approximately 33% of patients treated for hypospadias, compared to 15% of patients in the control group. Furthermore, it was observed that in treated groups, maximum flow rate (Q_{max}) was 18.8 mL/s, compared to 26.2 mL/s in the control group. This data reveals that urinary function can be abnormal in both subjective and objective aspects [18].

Despite several articles on urine flow in hypospadias patients, this method provides important information for the diagnosis and posttreatment; however, the isolated interpretation of the data must be carefully interpreted. Study showed that only 32% of the urinary flow curves were normal and 46% of them demonstrated uncoordinated voiding, at least until the end of the first year of life [19]. Children's urine flow standard at this age remains uncertain. Other similar studies support this data. We need to remark that only articles based on urinary flow of similar age comparison groups should be emphasized.

The way to measure the urinary flow in boys up to 1 year is based on ultrasound probe positioned on the base of the penis. Twenty-one boys with distal hypospadias and 19 normal were analyzed. Maximum urinary flow was significantly lower in those with hypospadias (2.4 vs. 4.4 mL/s, $p < 0.01$). A surprisingly higher number of uncoordinated flow curves in the control group (64% vs. 36%, $P < 0.01$) were also found. An old hypothesis that meatal size should correlate to Q_{max} became unreal [20]. From these data, the authors speculated that the decrease of both urethral and corpus spongiosum complacency could reduce the maximum urinary flow. They could also act as a voiding uncoordinated agent [20].

Urinary flow is barely reported on patients' follow-up. Regular flowmetry values in young teenagers are not established yet [21]. Uroflowmetry was performed in 17 young boys, age range from 13 to 15. The average flow rate of the control group was 29.19 mL/s (range from 14 to 54), while urine flow of 60 patients who underwent correction of hypospadias as children and evaluated at the same age was 22 mL/s (range from 2 to 64). Eighty-eight percent of the patients with hypospadias were 1 standard deviation (SD) below the control group, and 14% were 2 SD below. The location of the urethral meatus before surgery probably does not influence the flow rates, but the presence of chordee, moderate and severe, perhaps does.

In conclusion, the flowmetry is a useful tool for the long-term evaluation of urethral function after correction of hypospadias [21], and its practice should be encouraged.

Just a few articles exist using urodynamics in preoperative evaluation of hypospadias. In a prospective survey of 65 children with hypospadias, 60 underwent urodynamic evaluation, while the other 5 did not, due to the small diameter of the urethral meatus. Detrusor overactivity was the most frequent abnormality, observed in 48% (28 patients) of the children; 39% (11 patients) also had stenosis of the urethral meatus. Authors point out that this might be the cause of bladder dysfunction [22]. However, significant differences between the position of meatus and detrusor overactivity were not observed in other studies. On the other hand, the authors also found detrusor overactivity in 57% of children with obstruction compared to 33% without it. 60.8% of patients had the abnormality previously mentioned (detrusor overactivity) [23].

Based on these results, urodynamics should be performed in special situations. In hypospadias with no other anatomical or functional abnormalities, it does not affect the prognosis or treatment.

24.4 Neourethral Stricture

Late dysfunction of the neourethra has become a significant issue according to many publications, showing that the development of the genital tubercle is an essential parameter in long-term hypospadias reconstruction evaluation [24]. Symptoms like dysuria, poor urine stream, weak stream, spraying stream, long micturition time, dysuria, and urine infection must be considered and investigated, as they are probably related to stricture of the urethra [24].

The fundamental characteristic of hypospadias surgery in children is that it is made in growing tissues. Studies have demonstrated that genital tubercle grows between the age of 1 and 10. The growth of the genital tubercle is almost double in length and width [25]. This fact should be considered when selecting the

Fig. 24.3 Mictional cystography demonstrates meatus stenosis

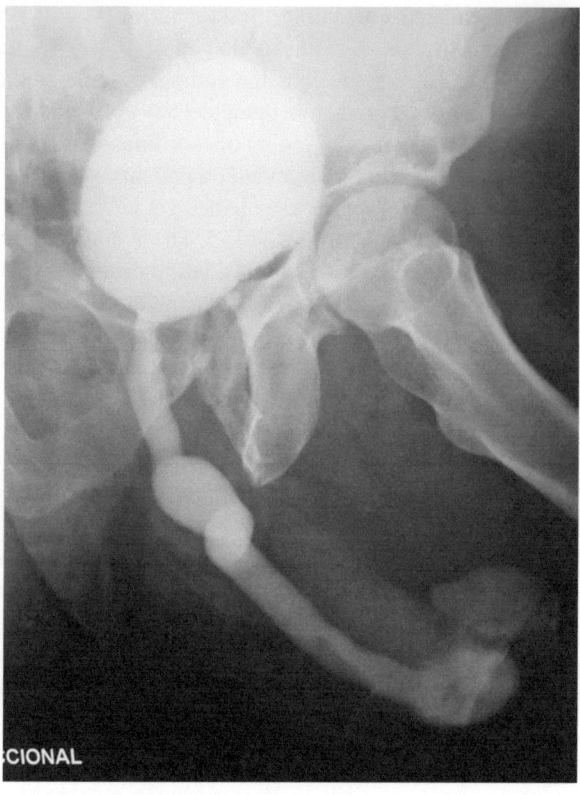

reconstruction technique. The whole development of the tissue used must be considered. One explanation is that the proximal tissue responds well to androgen stimulation, whereas the tissue beyond the corpus spongiosum division responds poorly to androgenic stimulation [24].

Early complications (less than 1 year) are related to urethral fistula and suture dehiscence. Later complications (more than 1 year) are linked to stenosis of the urethra (Fig. 24.3) and penile curvature [24]. In a retrospective study, 578 urethroplasties by Duplay technique performed in a single institution with a mean follow-up of 25.6 months (ranging from 6 months to 17 years) reported 8.5% stenosis for distal hypospadias, 19.1% for penile, and 45% for proximal hypospadias, a total of 10.2% of stenosis [24].

Another series of 57 adults treated for hypospadias with a mean of 37 years follow-up (range 18–74) represent a heterogeneous group. More than half of adults with complications related to hypospadias had several operations, one of the toughest challenges for reconstructive surgery (Fig. 24.4). About 30% of patients with an initially successful repair in childhood have recurring problems in adulthood, suggesting that the reconstruction results may not be as durable as estimated by short-term follow-up series [26].

Fig. 24.4 Multiples scars due to many surgeries

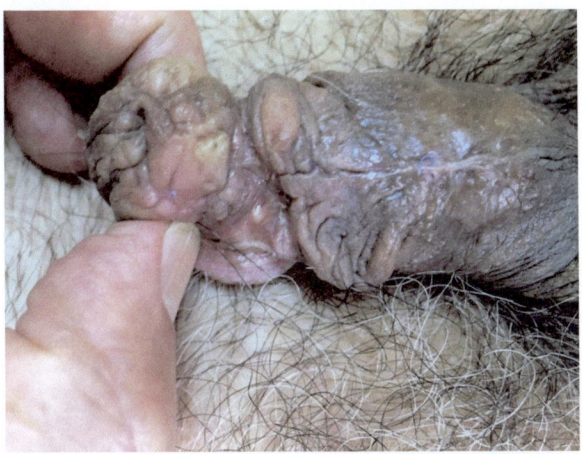

It is also important to state that all patients with urethral stricture should be carefully evaluated to identify lichen scleroses (balanitis xerotica obliterans) before treatment. They correspond to 4–15% of the postoperative strictures. In such cases, the urethroplasty with buccal mucosa is recommended [27]. Lichen sclerosus is more prevalent in patients treated for hypospadias compared to the control group, 42.9% compared with 8.7% [26].

Conclusion

Patient medical care must go beyond the repositioning of the urethral meatus. Several more evident functional aspects such as penis size and aspect of the glands can cause psychological damage related to self-image, leading to sexual disorders. In addition, unusual functional aspects of the lower urinary tract, less explored in clinical practice, should be considered. Urine flow, detrusor activity, and urethral stricture should also be evaluated for their potential to cause urinary symptoms in these patients.

References

1. McDougal SW, Wein AJ, Kavoussi LR, Novick AC, Partin AW, Peters CA, Ramchandani P. Campbell-Walsh urology. 10th ed. Philadelphia: Saunders Elsevier; 2012.
2. dos Reis RB, Zequi SC, Filho MZ. Urologia moderna. 1a ed. São Paulo: Lemar; 2013.
3. Kurahashi N, Murakumo M, Kakizaki H, et al. The estimated prevalence of hypospadias in Hokkaido, Japan. J Epidemiol. 2004;14:73–7.
4. Canon S, Mosley B, Chipollini J, et al. Epidemiological assessment of hypospadias by degree of severity. J Urol. 2012;188:2362–6.
5. Kalfa N, Sultan C, Baskin LS. Hypospadias: etiology and current research. Urol Clin North Am. 2010;37(2):159–66.
6. Macedo A Jr, Rondon A, Ortiz A. Hypospadias. Curr Opin Urol. 2012;22(6):447–52.

7. Baskin LS. Hipospadias. In: Antono Macedo Jr., Salvador Vilar Correia Lima, Descio Streit, Ubirajara Barroso Jr., editors. Urologia Pediátrica. 1a ed. São Paulo: Roca; 2004. p. 193–194.
8. Baskin LS, Ebbers MB. Hypospadias: anatomy, etiology, and technique. J Pediatr Surg. 2006;41:463–72.
9. Weber DM, Schonbucher VB, Landolt MA, Gobet R. The pediatric penile perception score. An instrument for patient self-assessment and surgeon evaluation after hypospadias repair. J Urol. 2008;180:1080–4.
10. Rynja SP, De Jong TPVM, Bosch JLHR, De Kort LMO. Functional, cosmetic and psychosexual results in adult men who underwent hypospadias correction in childhood. J Pediatr Urol. 2011;7:504–15.
11. Kumar MV, Harris DL. A long term review of hypospadias repaired by split preputial flap technique. Br J Plast Surg. 1994;47:236–40.
12. Aho MO, Tammela OK, Somppi EM, Tammela TL. Sexual and social life of men operated in childhood for hypospadias and phimosis. A comparative study. Eur Urol. 2000;37(1):95–100.
13. Kiss A, Sulya B, Szasz AM, Romics I, Kelemen Z, Tóth J, et al. Long-term psychological and sexual outcomes of severe penile hypospadias repair. J Sex Med. 2011;8:1529–39.
14. Aulagne MB, Harper L, de Napoli-Cocci S, Bondonny JM, Dobremez E. Long-term outcome of severe hypospadias. J Pediatr Urol. 2010;6(5):469–72.
15. Hoag CC, Gotto GT, Morrison KB, Coleman GU, Macneily AE. Long-term functional outcome and satisfaction of patients with hypospadias repaired in childhood. Can Urol Assoc J. 2012;2(1):23–31.
16. Lam PN, Greenfield SP, Williot P. 2-stage repair in infancy for severe hypospadias with chordee: long-term results after puberty. J Urol. 2005;174(4 Pt 2):1567–72.
17. Ruppen-Greeff NK, Weber DM, Gobet R, Landolt MA. What is a good looking penis? How women rate the penile appearance of men with surgically corrected hypospadias. J Sex Med. 2015;12(8):1737–45.
18. Örtqvist L, Fossum M, Andersson M, Nordenström A, Frisén L, Holmdahl G, Nordenskjöld A. Long-term follow up of men born with hypospadias: urological and cosmetic results. J Urol. 2015;193(3):975–81.
19. Olsen LH, Grothe I, Rawashdeh YF, Jørgensen TM. Urinary flow patterns in first year of life. J Urol. 2010;183(2):694–8.
20. Olsen LH, Grothe I, Rawashdeh YF, Jørgensen TM. Urinary flow patterns in infants with distal hypospadias. J Pediatr Urol. 2011;7(4):428–32.
21. Perera M, Jones B, O'Brien M, Hutson JM. Long-term urethral function measured by uroflowmetry after hypospadias surgery: comparison with an age matched control. J Urol. 2012; 188(4 Suppl):1457–62.
22. Gupta L, Sharma S, Gupta DK. Is there a need to do routine sonological, urodynamic study and cystourethroscopic evaluation of patients with simple hypospadias? Pediatr Surg Int. 2010;26(10):971–6.
23. Ozkurkcugil C, Guvenc BH, Dillioglugil O. First report of overactive detrusor in association with hypospadias detected by urodynamic screening. Neurourol Urodyn. 2005;24(1):77–80.
24. Grosos C, Bensaid R, Gorduza DB, Mouriquand P. Is it safe to solely use ventral penile tissues in hypospadias repair? Long-term outcomes of 578 Duplay urethroplasties performed in a single institution over a period of 14 years. J Pediatr Urol. 2014;10:1232–7.
25. Damon V, Berlier P, Durozier B, Francois R. Study of the dimensions of the penis from birth to adult age and as a function of testicular volume. Pediatrie. 1990;45(7–8):519–22.
26. Ching CB, Wood HM, Ross JH, Gao T, Angermeier KW. The Cleveland Clinic experience with adult hypospadias patients undergoing repair: their presentation and a new classification system. BJU Int. 2011;107(7):1142–6.
27. Cimador M, Vallasciani S, Manzoni G, Rigamonti W, De Grazia E, Castagnetti M. Failed hypospadias in paediatric patients. Nat Rev Urol. 2013;10:657–66.

Part III

Therapies

Cognitive Behavioral Therapy on the Basis of Urotherapy

25

Anka J. Nieuwhof-Leppink and M.A.W. Vijverberg

25.1 Introduction

The loss of urine during the day in children is a complex process. Children who wet themselves during the day have in almost every case a functional problem in the lower urinary tracts. Accurately mapping out and understanding the issues are essential to arriving at a correct diagnosis, which is critical to formulate an adequate treatment plan. The basic strategy for children with incontinence is urotherapy, that is a therapeutic treatment method. In addition to medical treatment, in the last decade, it has found itself in an important position in the range of treatment options for children with lower urinary tract dysfunctions. It is a treatment that uses techniques from cognitive behavioral therapy. Urotherapy appears to make a successful contribution to the improvement or disappearance of symptoms.

25.2 What Is Cognitive Behavioral Therapy?

25.2.1 Cognitive Therapy

Cognitive therapy is mainly based on the premise that what we think affects our emotions and what we choose to do or avoid. The therapy focuses on irrational, dysfunctional thoughts and beliefs. The aim of the therapy is to find alternative thoughts or beliefs that are more functional than the dysfunctional ones. At the same time one strives to have a good understanding of the experience someone is facing [1]. The therapy involves a series of techniques, such as "self-monitoring" (observation and

A.J. Nieuwhof-Leppink (✉) • M.A.W. Vijverberg
Pediatric Psychology and Social Work, Wilhelmina's Children Hospital,
University Medical Center Utrecht, Utrecht, The Netherlands
e-mail: a.nieuwhof-leppink@umcutrecht.nl

recording), "activity planning" (organization of activities), and "labeling" (with the help of positive suggestive statements) and homework arrangements.

25.2.2 Behavioral Therapy

In behavioral therapy, the focus is on the behavior of the person. How a person acts determines to a large extent how a person feels. The therapy concentrates on observable behavior and the circumstances in which the behavior occurs. It focuses on changing observable behavior through various techniques, such as "classical conditioning" and "operant conditioning", which basically mean learning through success, and can be achieved by using positive or negative reinforcement strategies. Baselining and monitoring are also effective techniques used in cognitive behavioral therapy. Merely observing and recording actually have a therapeutic effect and reduce many symptoms just as they are observed [2].

Next, the therapist helps the patient react with more suitable behavior patterns in those circumstances. Various exercises and homework assignments are used to both identify the problematic behavior and invent and practice a new, more appropriate behavior to substitute instead.

25.2.2.1 A Good Combination
Cognitive therapy combined with behavioral therapy can influence a person's mindset, interpretations, and/or actions. Sometimes the emphasis is on thinking, sometimes more on behavior or avoiding behaviors. In other cases, one works simultaneously with both aspects. Cognitive therapy techniques are used in the treatment of children with urinary problems. The goal of urotherapy is to regulate the patterns of bladder management and prevent all aspects of psychological and physical damage. Therefore, basic training always starts with explanation of bladder function and possible dysfunction. Therefore, basic training always starts with explanation of bladder functions and dysfunctions. Insight into the problem helps with further motivation for treatment. Urotherapy takes the overall process of potty training into account, from filling to emptying the bladder [3].

Urotherapy is described as a therapy that is designed for children with lower urinary tract syndrome (LUTS) and is aimed at improving bladder dysfunction [4]. In the standardization of terminology of lower urinary tracts in children, the International Children's Continence Society (ICCS) defines urotherapy as a non-pharmacological, nonsurgical treatment of dysfunctions of lower urinary tracts.

The program is divided into standard therapy and specific interventions such as pelvic floor training, behavioral training, and biofeedback training [5, 6].

25.3 Assessment

Assessment is a very wide ranging term which will be common to a broad variety of different practitioners each having their own understanding, professional codes and practices and spectrum of investigations. Caregivers that offer urotherapy must have knowledge of the anatomy, physiology, and pathophysiology of the entire urogenital system, including the lower and upper urinary tracts [7]. Additionally, they must understand all forms of functional incontinence and have insight into the psychological and behavioral influences of incontinence on children.

It is the task of the urotherapist to seek out the child's problem and to decide. Whether the whole spectrum or only part of urotherapy is needed for the individual bladder problem. The following elements should be identified before starting treatment:

1. Identify the subtype of incontinence, come to a diagnosis.
2. Is bladder training suitable for this problem?
3. Is the development of the child suitable to endure treatment.

It will be useful to look at each of the elements separately but it is important to note that these elements are interrelated.

1. Identify the Subtype of Incontinence
   Voiding and defecation diary: Before treatment it is essential to look at defecation frequency for 1 week at home. Voiding diary with fluid intake, voiding frequency and voided volumes needs to be done for 2 days.

   Voiding history: Through the voiding and defecation diary, micturition history and repeated uroflowmetry followed by ultrasound to measure residual urine, a complete picture is obtained of the urinary problem. After this, one should be able to come to a diagnosis. This urinary incontinence is a heterogeneous disease with different subtypes (defined by the ICCS). A proper diagnosis is important in order to start an adequate treatment. In addition, a distinction should be made between the different sub-types of incontinence. Possible diagnoses are overactive bladder (OAB) dysfunctional voiding (DV), voiding postponement (VP) and underactive bladder (UAB). An child with overactive bladder (OAB) requires a different focus of treatment than one with dysfunctional voiding.

2. Is Bladder Training Suitable for the Problem?
   In the majority of incontinent children, no obvious reason for this incontinence can be found, and there is a considerable overlap between the different lower urinary tract conditions presenting with daytime incontinence. Non-pharmacological treatment options and the pharmacological therapy as well as the combined therapy are recommended. The majority of the children will require a combination of these treatment options to achieve continence during the day. A bladder training is a form of specific urotherapy, it is a combination of behavioral training, and biofeedback training.

   A bladder training is being applied by a less invasive and a child-friendly approach.

   Before starting a bladder training, anatomical and neurological causes of incontinence should be excluded.

   Constipation and/or urinary tract infections must be identified and treated before a child is eligible for bladder training. It is advisable to analyze defecation issues according to the Bristol score list and the Rome IV criteria.

3. Is the development of the child suitable to endure treatment?
   Assessing psychosocial history is important to judge that the child has the sufficient psychological ability and motivation to sustain the training before it begins.

Important events such as moving or the arrival of a little brother or sister may be reasons to postpone the start of treatment. Interactive problems within the family can also have a negative impact on treatment results. Additionally, psychological and psychiatric aspects play an important role in caring for children and adolescents with either nocturnal enuresis or urinary incontinence. Correct assessment is essential both from the point of view of the diagnosis and the point of view of treatment of interest. Behavioral and emotional disorders are seen more often in children with incontinence than anatomical or neurological causes and this comorbidity. Research shows that 20–30% of children with bed-wetting, 20–40% with urinary incontinence, and 30–50% with fecal incontinence meet the criteria of psychiatric disorders as classified in the ICD-10 and DSM-IV [8] Because of the high prevalence of comorbidity, each child should be screened as a part of routine assessment. Questionnaires are effective screening tools for gathering information even though they offer no diagnosis. A broad and validated questionnaire is the Child Behavior Checklist (CBCL) [8–10].

25.4 Treatment

25.4.1 Standard Treatment

Standard treatment can be given to children over 6 years old. When the child is younger than 6 years, the clinician would give parents advice about sitting on the toilet, medications, urinary frequency, fluid intake, and constipation.

In addition to instruction on relaxation of the pelvic floor, urinary frequency, and drinking patterns, there must also be a change in behavior in which the child learns to consciously react to urges and wet incidents. Repetition and reinforcements are part of the therapy.

1. Constipation
   When kids have constipation problems in addition to issues wetting the bed, it is advisable to treat this at the start of treatment. Constipation can cause voiding dysfunction or worse. The child receives advice to go to the toilet two to three times daily after meals to try to defecate. The child also gets an explanation about good pushing techniques during defecation [5]. The results are recorded, so that the Bristol score list can be a helpful tool for the child and parents. Simultaneously, eating and drinking patterns can be modified, and sometimes medication must be added for extended periods of time [11].

2. Urinary Tract Infections
   Urinary tract infections must be treated, and eventually prophylaxis is administered to prevent recurrence of infection.

3. Psycho-Education
   Educate the child about his or her disorder, and help to understand normal and abnormal functions of the bladder (Fig. 25.1). When parents and the child

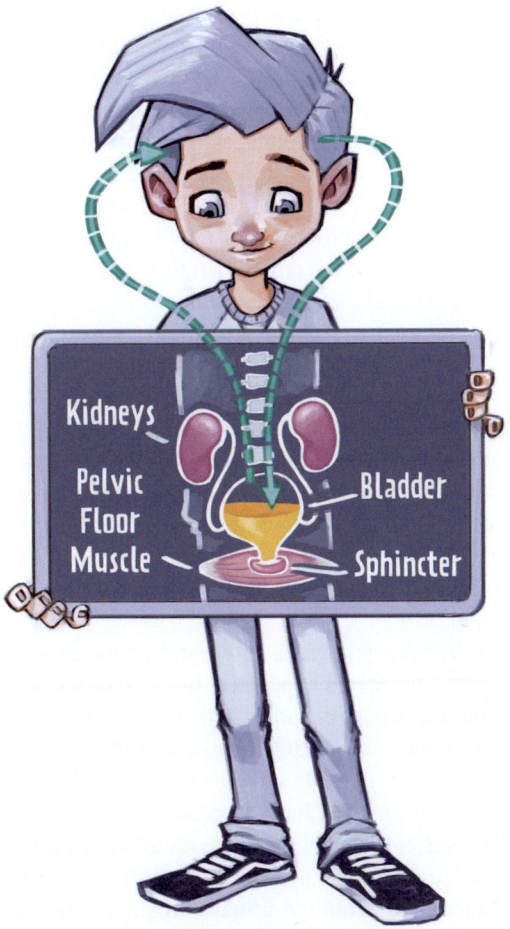

Fig. 25.1 The pee factory

understand why symptoms arise, they will exhibit a higher commitment and adherence to training. The following are the main components to be covered in explaining urotherapy to the child and parents [12–18]:
- Explain normal and abnormal function.
- Discuss survival strategies.
- Fluid intake.
- When and how often to urinate.
- Toilet position.
  - *Explain the normal and abnormal function* of the bladder by using age-appropriate drawings or videos. A clear and child-oriented explanation will increase the child's motivation to carry out the training instructions.
  - *Discuss the survival strategies used by the child.* Many children have given up the courage to go to the toilet in time. They tend to pretend that wet pants do not bother them. Others have found a way to cope with unexpected

urges. For example, when a child "wobbles" or "squats" upon urges ("holding it" techniques), parents see this and want to send the child to the bathroom, but the child does not want to go because they unconsciously know they will be wet. When the feelings of urges are gone, the child does not go to the toilet. Children and parents learn to understand why the child cannot walk to the toilet on time of imperative urgency. Sometimes the bladder may also not be totally filled, and the child feels he or she can wait to go pee. If parents understand the abnormal functions of the bladder and know that it is not the fault of the child, then they will be able to respond appropriately and effectively apply the training rules.

- *Drink regularly with a recommended* fluid intake of approximately 1.5 L per day. (About 1200–1500 mL depending on child's age).

  Children with an overactive bladder have an instinctive, unconscious habit of not drinking a lot. They are most likely thinking, "If I don't drink too much, I won't have to pee as often and will be less wet." As a result this creates a vicious circle, because the lack of fluid intake prevents the bladder from getting the chance to build volume. Additionally, highly concentrated urine has a stimulating effect and can cause irritation.

- *Teach when and how often one should urinate.*

  When to Void

  The urinary frequency is often different, because children have symptoms of an overactive bladder, a hypoactive bladder, or abnormal urination. They either are not sensitive to the urges of their bladder or go pee every time they feel the need, for fear of wetting their pants. Other children pay no attention to whether or not they should urinate (avoidance behavior). From a kind of survival mechanism, they have learned to ignore the sense of urgency, because they suffer too much from the issue. They need to learn to let go of this survival strategy and instead become aware again of this sense of urgency. Since many children urinate irregularly and do not know which bladder signals to react too, setting times to go pee is a good method to add to the other instructions.

  How Often

  On average the child should go to the toilet six to seven times, in accordance with regular daily routines such as school, breaks, eating, and sleeping times. The child will try to urinate with or without urge. If it doesn't work to pee, that is alright. If the child has to pee at another time (not scheduled), naturally they should go then too. "Time voiding" leads to positive results because the child does not wet their pants as often. If it is difficult for the child to adhere to these set times, it is helpful to have them wear a special watch with a vibrating alarm to remind them to go to the toilet. These watches can be set at random times. By keeping a voiding diary as homework, the child gets insight into the frequency of urination and allows for normal urinary frequency to be learned.

- *Instructions of a relaxed toilet position.* Relaxation of the pelvic floor muscles and sphincter during urination is necessary to properly empty the bladder. Children are instructed to sit on the toilet in a relaxed manner by

supporting the feet on the floor or on a stool so that the thighs are horizontal with the lower legs and form an angle of 90° (see Fig. 25.2). Accidents are also recorded in the voiding diary to assess improvement after standard advice and to make children and parents aware of the frequency of these accidents.
– Tacking can also provide insight as to what times there is leakage, which can lead to discussions of specific interventions.

The basis of the training consists of three learning elements (Table 25.1), each with its own feedback mechanisms. It is essential that all three learning elements are

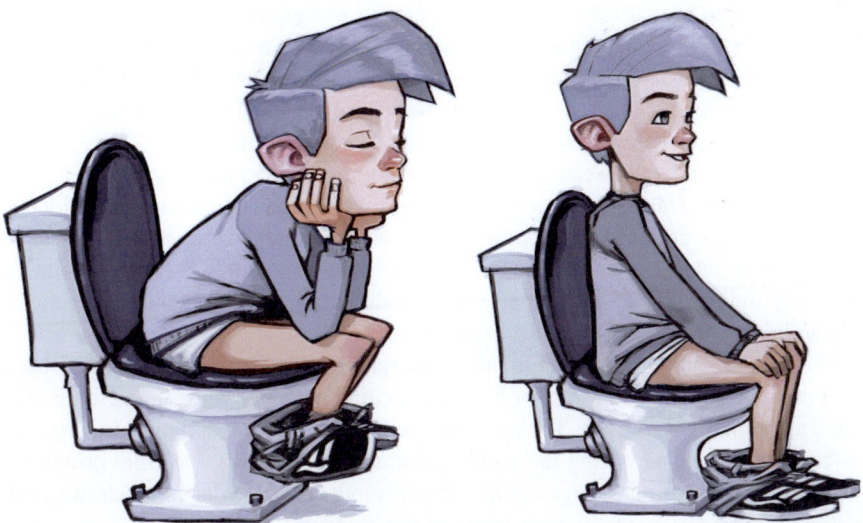

Fig. 25.2 Correct and wrong voiding posture

Table 25.1 Learning elements

Learning element	Goal	Tools	Child action
1. When do you pee	Adequate reactions to signals from bladder	– Voiding diary – Detection of underwear/pants control	– Record every urination accident
2. How should you pee	Relaxed peeing, empty the bladder	– Flowmeter – Specific physiotherapy,	– No straining – Relaxed stomach – Listen to the urine stream – Feet on a stool and thighs horizontal
3. How often do you pee	Learning about regular urination frequency	– Voiding diary – Timed voiding/peeing watch	– Record every urination

carried out simultaneously; otherwise optimum results will not be expected. Depending on the diagnosis, one or more of these elements will be emphasized. It is important that the children themselves can explain what they will be learning during training.

25.4.2 The First Learning Element: When Do You Urinate

Children learn to recognize the signal to urinate with a reaction of going to the toilet. The concentration and awareness of the bladder need to be relearned. This relearning process can be disrupted by infections, an overactive bladder, and thickened bladder walls or through abstaining urination in response to detector pants, which is a kind of bed-wetting alarm that can be worn during the day and responds immediately with a beeping sound when the child loses a drop of urine. In an outpatient setting, wearing a bed-wetting alarm is not recommended, because it is socially unacceptable if the child goes to school during the day. It is therefore advised to use the detector underwear only in a hospital setting.

A detector underwear can be replaced at home by underwear inspections (after every pee turn). This is also a good way to receive feedback on urination accidents. Wet underwear or pants are recorded in the voiding diary list as a small cloud or "W" for wet, and a dry part of the day deserves a small sun or "D" for dry. Notating the diary in this manner helps analyze the gradual process. For example, one could see an improvement from grade 3 to grade 1.

Keeping a voiding diary is more than just recording information. It is a feedback tool that makes the child aware of his or her peeing behavior while at the same time adds a competitive element. The facilitator will act as a coach and must incorporate a "race-type" feeling during the child's treatment. In this way the child brings the avoiding and ignoring of urge signals to consciousness in order to reach the goal, which is good management and control of the bladder.

25.4.3 The Second Learning Element: How Should You Pee

The child will receive instructions on proper toilet, because good posture can best relax the pelvic region during urination (Fig. 25.2). Let the child listen to their stream of pee and explain to them that they can't strain during urination and to keep the stomach relaxed. The child is instructed to let the urine fall or come out on its own.

Biofeedback of the Urination Pattern

In children with dysfunctional voiding and urge symptoms, the pelvic floor muscles are usually overactive. Biofeedback of the urination pattern is an essential learning element. Children learn to urinate with a relaxed pelvic floor. It certainly makes sense to explain toilet posture instructions repeatedly during training to achieve optimal relaxation of the pelvic muscles and prevent straining. Using a balloon as an example, it is possible to visualize the functions, straining and emptying of the bladder [13–15].

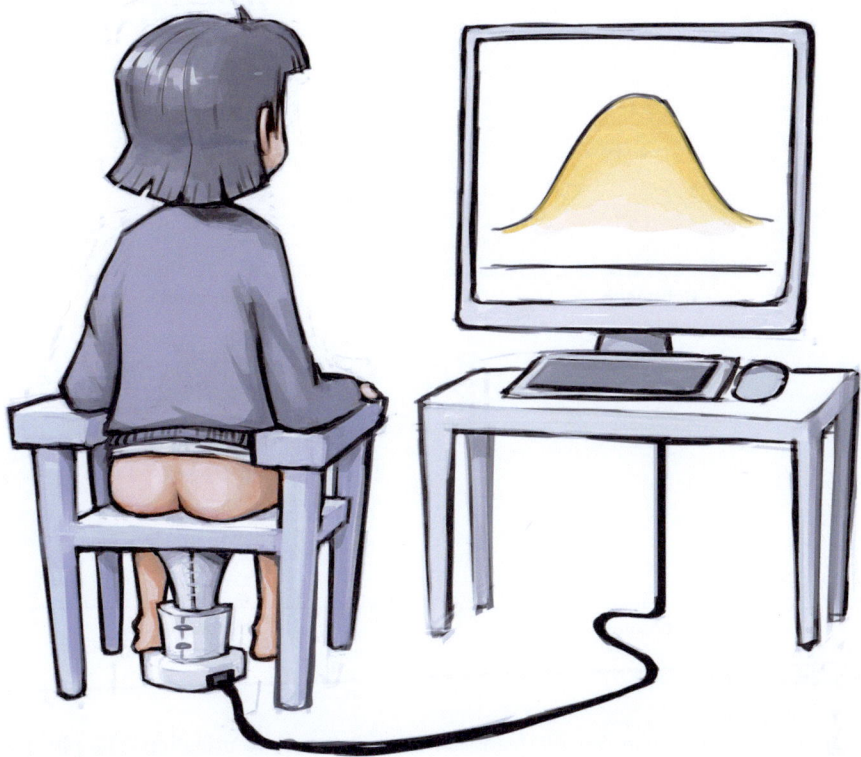

Fig. 25.3 Realtime uroflowmetry = biofeedback

The feedback from good urination can be given in two ways:

1. Flowmeter
   The flowmeter (pee computer) (Fig. 25.3) measures the stream, speed, and volume during urination and can be used with or without the EMG (electromyogram). The flow curve can be used for diagnosis, and during training the curve is used as biofeedback. The child learns to recognize when they urinate incorrectly and will keep on trying (through a relaxed posture and possibly softly blowing or whistling) until they achieve a nice, continuous, bell-shaped curve (Fig. 25.4). Eventually the child learns to urinate with a relaxed pelvic floor and normal urine volume, and the straining and sloppy peeing is deliberately forgotten. Ultrasound can be used to check if the bladder is empty after urination. Using the EMG provides additional information on the use of the pelvic floor during urination. It should be noted that some EMGs give an unreliable picture, and analyzing of this biofeedback requires some experience [5].

2. Physiotherapy
   When giving instructions about toilet posture and feedback through flowmetry yields insufficient results (or when a flow meter is not available), physiothera-

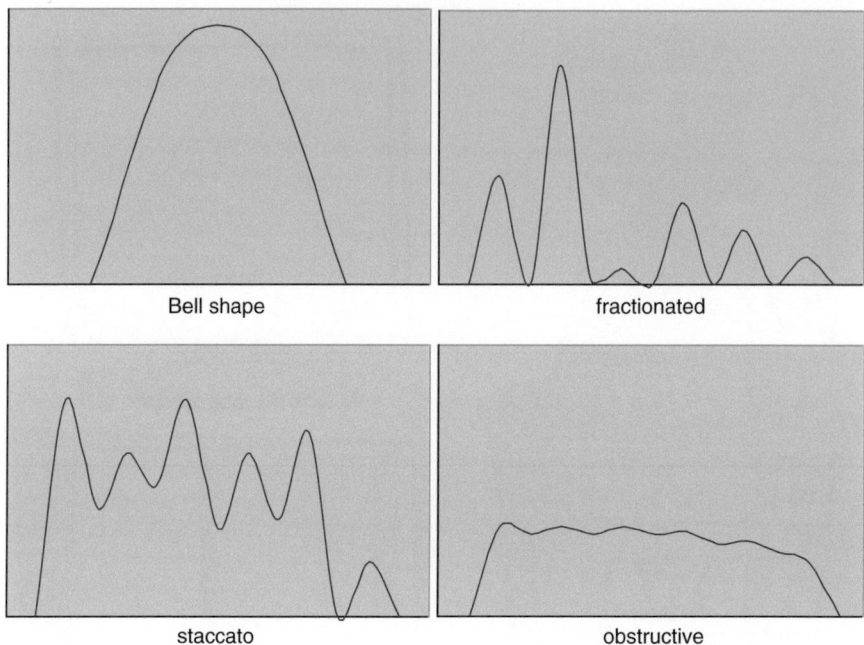

Fig. 25.4 Flowpatterns

peutic guidance can provide feedback on the manner of urination. The physiotherapist analyzes the movement patterns during micturition and looks at whether the child is physically capable of learning a new, correct motor program, that is, micturition with the pelvic floor relaxed and without abdominal straining. Experience shows that nearly all children over 6 years can learn how to use their pelvic floor muscles through exercise therapy. With older children, additional biofeedback can be attained using an anal pressure probe. The children receive low-frequency physiotherapy (one time per week/per 2 weeks) and have clear homework assignments, which they complete daily under the guidance of their parents [15, 16].

25.4.4 The Third Learning Element: How Often Should You Urinate

This third element is very essential to the training process. Children often have to learn a new micturition frequency. The frequency of urinations is made visible by having children keep voiding lists of every urination on the toilet and every time they wet their pants so that they become aware of the urinary frequency and wet accidents. Achieving good results gives the child motivation to continue. Depending on the form of functional incontinence, the child must learn to urinate more or less often. A normal urination frequency at a fluid intake of 1.5 L per day should be on average six to seven times. The micturition diary should serve not only as a recording tool but also as immediate feedback for the child to see the results they have achieved so far. After about 3 weeks, results should show that a regular urination pattern is forming. The list can then be gradually reduced until the child can go to the bathroom six to seven times a day without using it. If the list is not being completed or no results are being achieved, training no longer makes sense, and the child should follow further consideration.

25.4.5 Timed Voiding

If children have the tendency to hold their pee endlessly, like with children who have hypoactive bladders or dysfunctional voiding, then an initially fixed time frame for urination is an important tool. These children need to learn to urinate when it's time to do so and not when they sense urgency. In this way, the child will not wait until the bladder is too full but will attempt to pee with a more relaxed pelvic floor. Toilet instructions should also be given so that the child won't strain just to produce urine. A watch can help to remind the child to go to the toilet. Some children don't get the feeling of urgency back and will need to urinate at set times for an extended period of time.

25.4.6 Small Bladder Volume

Children with extremely small bladder volume will have trouble holding their pee endlessly. They urinate very often high voiding frequency but it can be helpfull to become dry for a period. When the child is confident that he or she can be dry, they then begin the second stage, which is training to increase bladder volume. The child is instructed to hold their pee as long as they can once a day and once a week after holding it for the maximum possible time, to measure bladder volume by capturing the urine. By making the result visible (recording the measurement and converting it into graphics), the child is motivated to keep practicing. With bladder volume build-up training, it is imperative to drink enough. The experience teaches children with overactive bladders that 1.5 L of fluid intake per day is an enormous quantity (they have usually become accustomed to not drinking a lot). In this case it can be chosen to increase the number of drinking cups (e.g., one additional cup every week). Many children will also be treated with anticholinergics in order to achieve the maximum effect of urotherapy.

25.5 Intensive Therapy: Group Training

Group training is for children who have the most persistent form of urinary incontinence and for whom outpatient training and drug treatments had no effect. The learning process includes the same three learning elements but is more intensive, and observation and feedback are given several times a day so that a change in behavioral response to pressure, urinary frequency, and method of urination is taught. This should ultimately lead to continence. Because of the intensive approach and commitment, there is a greater chance of success [12–14, 19, 20]. It's important that the children are screened early to determine whether or not they can handle the learning process. Usually two till four children are being trained at the same time because of the solidarity-enhancing effect. In the beginning the children are helped and instructed by the therapist a lot. In the course of time, they have to try to do it by themselves more and more, so that when they are at home they can handle training instructions independently. In the clinical treatment course, a follow-up period of regular telephone contact is maintained between the child and the permanent trainer. The follow-up period is as important as the treatment period. During this period the child and parents are still being guided, while training is reduced slowly.

25.6 Rewards and Support

Finally, children do not need to be rewarded with gifts for performing the required tasks. Instead the reward lies in the confirmation that they have done well or not done well, to which they have the chance to do it better. It is necessary that the doctor and parents fully support the child. Through encouragement and positive assessment of the results, the child remains motivated to persevere. It's just like practicing sports, where you also need a coach to motivate you to keep going. It is important for parents to make clear that results can decline during exciting times like in a movie, new school, or birthdays. When parents and children know what to do in these situations, like tightening up training rules or taking a "training vacation" for a few days, it prevents a negative spiral in the sense of "see, it's not working."

25.7 Ending the Therapy

Urotherapy can be tried for an episode of 3 months. During this period, the child needs to be controlled regularly by the urotherapist. Weekly follow-up could be done by telephone, chat, or email. Counseling is a part of this follow-up, results should be evaluated, and instructions are repeated. Finally feedback takes place on the outpatient clinic. At these visits, uroflowmetry with ultrasound residual urine assessment is done. Training results can be assessed on the basis of the following ICCS criteria:

- No improvement (0–49% reduction of symptoms)
- Partial response (50-99% reduction of symptoms)
- Good response (100% improvement or first symptom occurs less than 1 time per month)

The success of treatment is not only dependent on the above criteria. Treatment success is determined especially by the extent that the child and parents are satisfied with the result. Treatment and cure are not synonymous. When urotherapy fails, it is important for the therapist to identify the cause or consult with the referring physician. It may be that the child is still too immature to complete the training.

Sometimes, there needs to be more psychological support. It is also possible that an underlying medical issue is the cause of the inability to maintain instructions [21].

25.8 The Role of the Therapist

The first step in any diagnostic and therapeutic process is to create a good relationship between the child and his or her parents. One should enquire and openly discuss all relevant facts, signs, and symptoms as well as subjective meanings and connotations. Next, the provision of information is essential. Parents as well as children need to understand what may be responsible for the bed-wetting. This should be provided in words and concepts that a child can absorb and in a format that is attractive. Increasing motivation and alleviation of stress and guilty feelings are all part of the dissemination of knowledge process. Counseling is already part of the treatment process, which has been defined as the provision of assistance and guidance in resolving personal, social, or psychological difficulties. Sometimes, it can be helpful to enhance the verbal counseling by other techniques, such as "demonstration" and "coaching." Other techniques might include "modeling" and "role-playing." The learning effect is much greater in these interactive forms of teaching than in solely verbal counseling.

25.9 The Role of the Parents

The success of the training and the proper execution of the instructions are partly dependent on the coach-like role of the urotherapist and the parents. The parents need to be explained what is incorporated in the coaching role. For parents of children with long-standing incontinence, this is not always easy. Parents generally have tried many options before they report to a pediatrician or specialist. Often they will do anything to get the child to stay dry. Some parents have dealt with this topic for years with their child. During the training the goal is for children to begin to sense themselves when they need to go, and with a little help from their surroundings, take the initiative to go to the toilet. The urotherapist can play a supporting role by providing parents explanations on how they should react to the urinary behavior and training efforts of the child. In this training the child is instructed to have the same type of commitment as when winning a contest. The contest "to keep the pants dry" is the ultimate end goal. The parents, just like with regular sports, must take on the role of the supporter by giving encouragement and feedback to the child every day. Children will be more committed and keep training for longer with a good support system.

In the training children have a degree of responsibility, but they cannot do it alone. Especially younger children, children with anxiety, and children with behavioral problems such as ADHD or ADD need support from parents [10]. Parents may need help when explained which comments work positively and which reactions stimulate performance anxiety. Parents should be warned that training takes a lot of time and effort, and it will affect daily routines. By comparing the training to a professional sport, where even participants in the Olympic Games have a coach, facilitators, and supporters to achieve the best results, the child and parents can better understand the level of commitment that is expected to be maintained during the entire training program for "the bladder to become the boss."

25.10 Results

A systematic review has shown that virtually no reliable studies exist concerning the best method of treatment of children with OAB [17]. The WHO-ICI refers to diverse studies about different forms of urotherapy [3]. These studies show that training produces very different positive outcomes. There are also many different program descriptions. Various combinations of cognitive training, biofeedback, central inhibition training, physical therapy, and fixed urination times are not supported by pharmacotherapy. Scientific evidence about the effectiveness of biofeedback in comparison with pharmacotherapy or placebo treatment is lacking almost entirely. The only randomized study found no difference in results between monotherapy with oxybutynin and biofeedback [14].

There are few controlled studies in the area of dysfunctional voiding (DV). A randomized prospective study shows that cognitive outpatient training for DV in 144 children has a success rate of 55%. Awareness of the problem is an important part of success [13]. Combined cognitive and biofeedback training in the clinical setting (in a retrospective study) saw this percentage rise to 68%, and in which children over 8 years old did significantly better [14]. Another prospective study examined the effect of both outpatient and inpatient bladder training in 60 children with urge incontinence and DV. The study revealed the same results. Sixty-four percent showed better or good results due to outpatient or inpatient urotherapy. Older children had better results than children under 8 years old [22]. A recent study to the effect of an inpatient cognitive and biofeedback training program for children with overactive bladder (OAB) after failed earlier treatment found a higher age during clinical training as a predictor for good training outcome [20].

There are a number of published, uncontrolled studies which report success rates of over 90% [19, 23]. The gold standard approach (according to WHO-ICI) is a combination of instruction, biofeedback, and physical therapy combined with pharmacological treatment of constipation and infections.

25.11 Drawbacks

It is the main task of the therapist to make a clear distinction between the different types of functional incontinence. An overactive bladder (OAB) requires a different focus in urotherapy than a child with dysfunctional voiding. A child with the DV generally recognizes urges but is used to continuously tightening the pelvic floor muscles and is not able to relax sufficiently during micturition. In this urotherapy the emphasis will be on timely visits to the toilet to prevent over-contraction of the pelvic floor and makes relaxation more feasible. Moreover, this child will need to unlearn straining during urination with help from good toilet posture and biofeedback, while children with OAB must learn to suppress urges and assess when they need to go to the toilet before they lose urine.

The most difficult is the combination of a functional problem with toilet avoidance behavior. Even though the child appears cooperative, avoidance behavior can hinder the commitment needed to achieve good results.

Children who are gifted generally understand the instructions but are not accustomed to putting in much effort. Other skills are easy for them, and in order to learn this new skill, they must put in more than normal effort. Children who alongside incontinence issues also have behavioral problems such as ADHD or PDD-NOS will also have a lot of trouble putting in the necessary commitment. They find it difficult to keep up with all the instructions and particularly the concentration required to learn a new skill. If the symptoms do not improve through urotherapy, it is sometimes difficult to distinguish whether the cause of failure in treatment should be sought in the medical or behavioral problems of the child. It is important to make a clear distinction between the main problem and side issues. The correct exclusion of anatomical issues is the only fair way to say that the cause lies in behavioral aspects [10].

25.12 Intermittent Self-Catheterization

Children with an underactive bladder can have such an over-distended bladder that spontaneously urinating without straining is no longer possible. Even training cannot solve the problem of incomplete bladder emptying and incontinence overflow. The bladder needs to be emptied a few times a day with the aid of a catheter. This can be temporary, because through regularly emptying the bladder completely, the bladder is less overstretched and able to pull together again. Children of 6 years old can learn how to self-catheterize themselves well. This is recommended because self-catheterization is less painful and makes the child less dependent. Guidance in this process is very important to let the treatment integrate well into daily life. Afterwards training of urinary patterns with relaxed pelvic muscles will remain necessary [4, 5].

References

1. Beck JS. Cognitive therapy: basics and beyond. New York: Guilford Press; 1995.
2. Mahoney MJ. Constructive psychotherapy: practices, processes, and personal revolutions. New York: Guilford Press; 2003.
3. Schulman SL, Von Zuben FC, Plachter N, Kodman-Jones C. Biofeedback methodology: does it matter how we teach children how to relax the pelvic floor during voiding? J Urol. 2001;166:2423.
4. Chang S, Van Laecke E, Bauer S, von Gontard A, Bagli D, Bower W, Renson C, Kawauchi A YS. Treatment of daytime urinary incontinence: a standardization document from the international children's continence society. Neurourol Urodyn. 2017;36:43–50.

5. Austin PF, Bauer SB, et al. The standardisation of terminology of lower urinary tract function in children and adolescents: update report from the Standardisation Committee of the International Children's Continence Society. Neurourol Urodynam. 2015;9999:1–11.
6. Yang S, Chua ME, Bauer S, Wright A, Brandström P, Hoebeke P, et al. Diagnosis and management of bladder bowel dysfunction in children with urinary tract infections: a position statement from the International Children's Continence Society. Pediatr Nephrol. 2017. https://doi.org/10.1007/s00467-017-3799-9.
7. De Gennaro M, Niero M, Capitanucci ML, von Gontard A, Woodward M, Tubaro A, et al. Validity of the international consultation on incontinence questionnaire-pediatric lower urinary tract symptoms: A screening questionnaire for children. J Urol [Internet]. 2010;184(4 SUPPL.):1662–7.
8. Joinson C, Heron J, von Gontard A. Psychological problems in children with daytime wetting. Pediatrics. 2006;118(5):1985–93.
9. von Gontard A, et al. Clinical behavioral problems in day- and night-wetting children. Pediatr Nephrol. 1999;13(8):662–7.
10. von Alexander G, Dieter B, Van Eline H, William JW, Christian B. Psychological and psychiatric issues in urinary and fecal incontinence. J Urol. 2011;185(4):1432–7.
11. Klijn AJ, Asselman M, Vijverberg MA, Dik P, De Jong TP. The diameter of the rectum on ultrasonography as a diagnostic tool for constipation in children with dysfunctional voiding. J Urol. 2004;172(5 Pt 1):1986–8.
12. Van Gool JD, de Jong TPVM, Winkler-Seinstra P, Tamminen-Mobius T, Lax-Gross H, Hirche H. A comparison of standard therapy, bladder rehabilitation with biofeedback and pharmacotherapy in children with non-neurogenic bladder/sphincter dysfunction. Presented at second annual meeting of International Children's Continence Society, Denver, Colorado, August 23–26, 1999.
13. Klijn AJ, Uiterwaal CS, Vijverberg MA, Winkler PL, Dik P, de Jong TP. Home uroflowmetry biofeedback in behavioral training for dysfunctional voiding in school-age children: a randomized controlled study. J Urol. 2006;175(6):2263–8. discussion 2268
14. Vijverberg MA, Elzinga-Plomp A, Messer AP, van Gool JD, de Jong TP. Bladder rehabilitation, the effect of a cognitive training programme on urge incontinence. Eur Urol. 1997;31(1):68–72.
15. Hoebeke P, Van Laecke E, Renson C, Raes A, Dehoorne J, Vermeiren P, Vande Walle J. Pelvic floor spasms in children: an unknown condition responding well to pelvic floor therapy. Eur Urol. 2004;46(5):651–4. discussion 654
16. De Paepe H, Renson C, Hoebeke P, Raes A, Van Laecke E, Vande WJ. The role of pelvic-floor therapy in the treatment of lower urinary tract dysfunctions in children. Scand J Urol Nephrol. 2002;36(4):260–7. Review
17. Sureshkumar P, Bower W, Craig JC, Knight JF. Treatment of daytime urinary incontinence in children: a systematic review of randomized controlled trials. J Urol. 2003;170(1):196–200. discussion 200, Review
18. van der Weide M, de Jong L, Verheij P, de Gier R, Feitz W. The treatment of children with functional disorders of the lower urinary tract system according to the Nijmeegs model. A nursing method. AZN, St. Radboud; 1998.
19. Chin-Peukert L, Salle JL. A modified biofeedback program for children with detrusor-sphincter dyssynergia: 5 year experience. J Urol. 2001;166(4):1470–5.
20. Meijer EF, Nieuwhof-Leppink AJ, Dekker-Vasse E, de Joode-Smink GC, de Jong TP. Central inhibition of refractory overactive bladder complaints, results of an inpatient training program. J Pediatr Urol. 2015;11(1):21.e1–5.
21. Mulders MM, Cobussen-Boekhorst H, de Gier RP, Feitz WF, Kortmann BB. Urotherapy in children: quantitative measurements of daytime urinary incontinence. J Pediatr Urol. 2010. https://doi.org/10.1016/j.jpurol.2010.03.010.
22. Heilenkötter K, Bachmann C, Jahnsen E, Stauber T, Lax H, Petermann F, Bachmann H. Prospective evaluation of inpatient and outpatient bladder training in children with functional urinary incontinence. Urology. 2005;67(1):176–80.
23. Duel BP. Biofeedback therapy and dysfunctional voiding in children. Curr Urol Rep. 2003;4(2):142.

Pelvic Floor Rehabilitation and Biofeedback

26

Sandro Danilo Sandri

26.1 History and Background

While biofeedback (BFB) was introduced at the end of the 1970s and quickly gained favor for treatment of lower urinary tract dysfunction (LUTD), pelvic floor rehabilitation was introduced at the end of the 1980s and only slowly gained popularity.

In the 1970s the Hinman syndrome became a well-recognized functional disease, thanks to the widespread use of urodynamics. Because of the refractory response to pharmacological treatment and lack of alternatives except for surgical treatment, BFB with the aim of relaxing the urethral sphincter was proposed.

In the 1980s, Kegel exercises regained gradual success in treating adult female stress urinary incontinence and then mixed and urge urinary incontinence. It was then consequential to adopt the same therapeutic approach for urinary incontinence in the pediatric age group. But because pelvic floor hyperactivity was responsible for many dysfunctional voidings (DVs), the fear of worsening micturition delayed the use of perineal muscle training, impeding widespread use of this approach. Nevertheless, teaching how to correctly contract these muscles continued to be adopted by a few centers.

In 1998 a survey of pediatric urology centers throughout the USA found that more than half of those that responded did not offer BFB as a treatment option [1]. In the next decade, many studies favored the use of BFB, and in 2010 the importance of BFB was finally endorsed by the standardization committee of the International Children's Continence Society (ICCS) [2].

S.D. Sandri
Department of Urology and Spinal Unit, Hospital of Legnano, Legnano, Italy

Department of Urology and Spinal Unit, Hospital of Magenta, Milan, Italy
e-mail: sandro.sandri@ao-legnano.it

The main lesson derived from pediatric neurorehabilitation is that noninvasive diagnostic steps should proceed together with initial noninvasive treatment. For example, once incorrect contraction of the perineal muscles is recognized, it is time to start teaching how to use them. Furthermore when abdominal straining during voiding is observed, it is important to start at once to teach how to avoid the use of the abdominal muscles during micturition. And again, once we teach and the child learns how to avoid abdominal straining during micturition, we can better recognize the electromyographic behavior of the perineal floor.

Many studies have described combinations of treatments for different LUTDs, which makes it difficult to evaluate the results. A significant improvement in this field was achieved by the ICCS standardization of terminology in 2006 [3].

26.2 Pelvic Floor Behavior in Asymptomatic Children

Pelvic floor muscle (PFM) behavior in children without LUTD has received very poor attention in the literature. In 1997 we did research in this field with the help of a pediatrician [4]. Fifty-eight Italian children aged between 4 and 9 years examined at school or admitted to the pediatric ward for different reasons, but without urinary disorders, were asked about the position they assumed while passing urine and how they tried to resist in the event of the urge to void. They were also required to contract their perineal muscles, and we observed their ability to contract the anus or retract the perineum. Five children (two females and three males) were shy and refused to cooperate. All of the females (23) and two males passed urine in a sitting position. All of the other males (28) passed urine in a standing position. Holding maneuvers were adopted by some, such as crossing or joining the legs, especially in females, to guard against urgency. Pressing the urethral meatus with fingers or by squatting (the curtsy sign) was also frequent in females. Boys were more prone to compressing their urethra than joining or crossing their legs.

Perineal contraction was completely absent in three females and four males. In the others it was frequently weak and always associated with other muscle contractions, especially of the abdominal, gluteal and, in a few cases, adductor muscles.

Therefore the perineal muscles and their contractions are currently unknown to children (and also to many adults); nevertheless, children are usually able to control urgency by central nervous inhibition or, in the case of emergency, in different mechanical ways.

Studies with ultrasound have established that neither children [5] nor adults [6] with normal bladder control can correctly identify PFM activity or reliably recruit or relax these muscles on command. This was precisely defined by measuring the movement of a point close to the bladder neck and consequently the direction of PFM movement with transabdominal ultrasound [7]. This study demonstrated that in children apparently free of LUTD, pelvic floor displacement is highly variable, representing a difference in the capacity of children to control the PFMs. A third of 21 subjects demonstrated a posterior movement instead of an anterior movement. The use of intra-abdominal pressure and efforts to sustain a contraction of long duration increase the likelihood of downward and posterior pelvic floor movement.

26.3 Pelvic Floor Rehabilitation in Childhood

As we have just seen, even children without LUTD are not able to isolate contraction of the perineal floor. The situation is worse in those with daytime incontinence due to an overactive bladder (OAB), as was shown in a group of 49 children (27 males and 22 females aged between 4 and 16 years, mean 8 years) where only four showed normal contractions that were digitally controlled [8]. Another four showed weak contraction, and 14 were unable to contract any muscle. Nineteen used abdominal muscles and eight used adductor and/or gluteal muscles instead or simultaneously. This proportion was nevertheless not statistically different from that of the asymptomatic group of children previously described ($p = 0.085$).

In our experience, training was previously simply conducted with rectal digital or visual control without BFB instruments and contracting the perineal muscles while avoiding simultaneous contraction of other muscles. Proper contraction was judged digitally or visually, observing retraction of the perineal area. The contraction should last for 5 s followed by a pause of 10 s. At least two series of ten contractions should be performed each day. Parents were required to follow the child during home daily exercises. Seventeen children were also asked to avoid holding maneuvers to contrast urgency and to contract their perineal muscles instead. They were also trained to interrupt the stream once during each micturition. Those with recurrent urinary tract infections (UTIs) were kept on prophylactic antibiotics during the training period. Training required only 1–3 sessions lasting less than 15 min. At follow-up, which was available for 42 cases between 3 and 96 months, with a mean of 25 months, all of the children were able to properly contract the perineal muscles, nine with still a weak contraction and three with simultaneous contraction of gluteal and hip adductor muscles.

26.4 Biofeedback in Childhood

BFB is a learning process with the aim of achieving control of an involuntary or incomplete voluntary physiological function. The perception of a body function, particularly a visceral function, can be scanty or even absent, such as intestinal movements or heartbeats. Instrumentation is able to record, amplify, and visualize a body function, which helps to improve perception and then can allow achievement of control of these functions without any more need for the instrument [9]. Urodynamic or electromyographic (EMG) instrumentation allows us not only to investigate but also to give information to a child with LUTD. The relationship between the child and the therapist is crucial to achieve the best results in a shorter time. The therapist must continuously explain and encourage the child to change his voiding behavior. The child should cooperate by recording a bladder diary and understanding how to make this change.

Different types of BFB can be applied to LUTDs in the pediatric age group. PFM exercise, EMG, and BFB using patch electrodes or an anal plug can be used to increase the strength of these muscles in stress or urge urinary incontinence or to teach how to relax the same muscles in DV. Voiding BFB can be useful to eliminate abdominal straining and to learn how to relax the perineal muscles during micturition in order to achieve a bell-shaped flow curve in DV. Bladder BFB can be applied to control detrusor overactivity.

During voiding BFB the child can watch the electromyography trace (voiding EMG/BFB), the flow curve (uroflow/BFB), or both (combined voiding uroflow/EMG/BFB) on a television screen. In the first case, he/she must learn first how to contract and relax his/her PFMs and then try to relax them during voiding. When the abdominal muscles are involved during voiding, additional EMG of the abdominal muscles or monitoring of abdominal pressure through a rectal catheter can help to avoid the use of these muscles. To see only the flow curve can be useless and confusing at the beginning, because flow is the result of the teaching program. The first thing to learn is the behavior of the voluntary perineal muscles during voiding, and the flow curve should be regarded as the result obtained.

The principal disadvantage of BFB is that its success depends on patient and therapist motivation and dedication to the program. To improve adherence to the training program, the EMG unit can also be used at home [10] or connected to a computer, and the BFB program can be linked to a BioGame [11] in order to teach how to relax the muscles. This interactive modality engages children and maintains their attention by natural attraction to the game, avoiding withdrawal from the training program which, in this way, can be extended to a child as young as 4 years. But if the child is trained only in this way without observing EMG and the flow curve during micturition, improvement is seen only after a longer time [11].

26.5 Rehabilitation in Monosymptomatic Enuresis

Improvement of enuresis can happen with pelvic floor rehabilitation when enuresis is associated with daytime urinary symptoms. But many cases still remain unresolved [12–14]; therefore, pelvic floor rehabilitation is not the treatment of first choice for monosymptomatic enuresis.

26.6 Rehabilitation in Overactive Bladder (Urge Syndrome)

OAB in children can often be successfully treated with standard urotherapy and pharmacological treatment; nevertheless, approximately 20% of cases are refractory to this first approach [15]. Many published studies have shown good results by adopting different methods (pelvic floor exercises together or sequentially in difficult cases with BFB) but often without first differentiating cases with DV [16]. Children with daytime incontinence should be investigated first, starting with non-invasive functional examinations in order to rule out DV and also considering the presence of constipation and/or encopresis. The presence of these last dysfunctions (dysfunctional elimination syndrome) changes the rehabilitative treatment approach.

Uroflowmetry with ultrasound residual urine evaluation—repeated at least 2–3 times if abnormal, for confirmation—allows verification of the voiding behavior and identification of DV. This can be present even when staccato or fractionated flows are not evident, but when a low and flattened flow is associated with an unrelaxed pelvic floor during micturition [11]. If this is present, the primary target should be to remove the functional obstruction and only later address the treatment of the eventual persistent OAB. On the other hand, to perform complete urodynamic examination in all children is sometimes mistaken because of the artifacts induced by the urethral catheter, and it is useless before a rehabilitation program. It should be restricted to children with neurological disease and those refractory to a noninvasive rehabilitation program [17].

Behavioral training and bladder training (standard urotherapy) are useful tools to improve control of urgency and to increase bladder capacity in OAB, and they are usually adopted as the initial treatment.

Pelvic floor rehabilitation is the second-line treatment approach when the first has failed.

In our experience, a group of 58 children aged between 4 and 13 years, equally divided into males and females, and complaining of urge, giggle, or stress incontinence, was trained to perform proper Kegel exercises in order to be able to resist urgency [14]. Data from a mean follow-up of 25 months were available for 46 cases. Ninety-one percent showed full resolution of or a decrease in their incontinence. There was no significant difference between those who were able to perform normal perineal contraction after training and those who were not. Therefore, in our opinion, improvement did not depend only on the perineal floor behavior. Training probably helps the child to achieve better cortical control of his/her micturition centers. There was no significant improvement in enuresis and no increased rate of UTI even after suspension of antibiotic prophylaxis. As stated in another paper [18], we believe that the majority of children do not require perineal rehabilitation or even BFB to improve symptoms of daytime incontinence, thus avoiding unnecessary use of skin electrodes or invasive anal plugs, which also necessitate more numerous, time-consuming, and costly visits. These treatments should be reserved only for cases resistant to standard urotherapy.

Similar results were found in a group of 74 children, with data from a mean follow-up of 4.7 years available for 48 of them, aged from 3 to 14 years at the time of treatment, and through a self-reported questionnaire [18]. A long-term improvement in daytime urinary control was noted in 60%. Improvement in the frequency of UTI was noted in 56%. A noticeable change in symptoms occurred after a median of 3.5 weeks, but the interesting thing is that the improvement decreased over time from 74% to 60% after the first year of follow-up. This finding conflicts with the widely held belief that symptoms will spontaneously resolve with age, and suggests that the therapeutic benefit in the first year was related to the treatment and not merely the function of maturation. Unfortunately the evaluation of success was different after 1 year and later on, and there was no analytical detection of a subgroup of children (on the basis of age or stronger symptoms) in whom the results were less evident or decreased in a major proportion with time.

Girls without improvement can be treated with bladder BFB. Catheterization, especially in males, can damage the relationship between the clinician and the child.

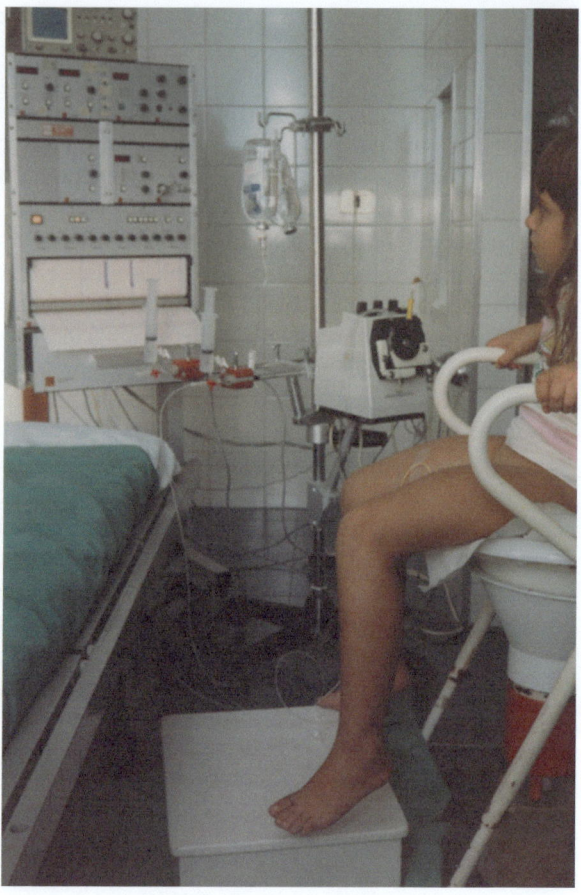

Fig. 26.1 Young girl receiving bladder biofeedback

Bladder BFB was first used in female adults by Cardozo et al. to treat detrusor instability, with good results [19].

Bladder BFB requires vesical catheterization with a dual-lumen catheter in order to fill the bladder slowly while simultaneously recording the intravesical pressure [20]. The bladder pressure recording is shown to the child, who should, in this way, recognize the onset of bladder contraction earlier and try to inhibit it by voluntary control with the eventual aid of perineal contraction (Fig. 26.1). Others teach avoidance of pelvic floor contraction at the onset of bladder contraction in order to promote cortical control of uninhibited contractions and probably for fear of inducing DV. This shift from simple OAB to increased perineal contraction during micturition has never been demonstrated except when an invasive urodynamic examination is repeated [21], but in this situation, artifacts can play a big role. This rehabilitative process requires a cooperative child. During the attempt to reduce bladder pressure, some children contract the perineal muscles, while others relax, performing deep breaths. Every session can last up to 1 h, and the bladder is usually filled two times.

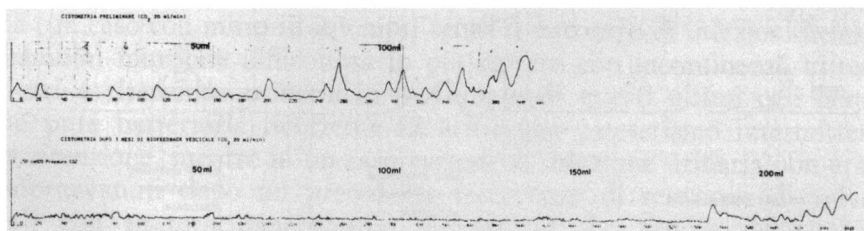

Fig. 26.2 Cystometry during the first session of bladder biofeedback and after 3 months

Then the child is told to adopt the same behavior when feeling urgency and to avoid wearing pads at home. A bladder diary recorded directly by the child can show eventual improvement, which should be emphasized by the parents, with words and rewards. Improvement can also be evident from progressive delay and reduction of bladder contractions during BFB sessions (Fig. 26.2).

Millard and Oldenburg obtained 70% resolution of daytime incontinence with bladder BFB in a mixed population of adults and children [22]. Of ten children with daytime urge incontinence and enuresis, two were cured, five were significantly improved, and three were unchanged, with persistence of enuresis.

Hellström et al. [13] used bladder BFB in children, some of them with OAB symptoms, but because of mixed symptoms and different methods, it was not possible to extrapolate the results with the different treatment modalities. They found complete success in 51% after 1 year and in 76% after 3 years, and the training program was applicable in children as young as 4 years old. They justified their good results in the younger children on the basis that the disturbed voiding pattern might not have been established as deeply as in the older children.

Our experience in five girls with daytime urge incontinence and enuresis without UTIs, one with first-degree vesicoureteral reflux (VUR), and two after correction of voiding dysfunction with micturition BFB, showed resolution of daytime symptoms after 2–4 sessions in all, but with persistence of enuresis [12].

A recent paper reviewed the results of 10 days of inpatient intensive urotherapy including BFB of the pelvic floor, which was not described further, with the aim of helping children with OAB to recognize and centrally suppress bladder overactivity, rather than using all available musculature [15]. Seventy children (mean age 9 years, range 7–13 years), of whom 69% were male, were enrolled. Eighty percent of them had undergone previous surgery, mainly endoscopic valve ablation or meatotomy. Sixty percent underwent urodynamic study demonstrating not only OAB in the majority (52%) but also obstruction (33%) and detrusor–sphincter dyssynergia (5%). Therefore the previous surgical treatment was interfering with the learning process, and some patients still had functional or mechanical obstruction. After 6 months, 43% reported a good effect of the training, and 31% were improved. After 2 years, 64% reported a good effect and 11% had improvement. Older age and motivation were found to be predictors of a good outcome.

26.7 Rehabilitation in Dysfunctional Voiding

Once uroflowmetry shows staccato or interrupted flow, if neurological signs are not present, the next step is to recognize if the child voids using also abdominal straining. Uroflow with recording of the abdominal pressure through a rectal probe easily allows identification of implication of the abdominal muscles. At this point the child should be trained to avoid the use of the abdominal muscles during voiding, using voiding BFB. To add surface pelvic floor EMG at this stage is useless because the use of the abdominal muscles interferes with the performance of the perineal muscles and can create confusion in the learning process, at least at the beginning of the rehabilitation. Once the child does not use the abdominal muscles during micturition, if the flow is still abnormal, then pelvic floor relaxation exercises or voiding BFB might be indicated either in children with only recurrent UTIs or in those with urinary retention and eventual deterioration of the upper urinary tract, unless renal failure is present and more aggressive treatment is indicated.

Contrary to what is done for daytime wetting, voiding BFB application is preceded by pelvic floor exercises and EMG/BFB with the aim of achieving muscle relaxation.

The first application of BFB to treat non-neurogenic vesical–sphincter dyssynergia was published by Maizels et al. in 1979 [23]. Three girls aged from 9 to 14 years with recurrent UTI and one with progressive hydronephrosis after bilateral ureteral reimplants because of reflux were recruited in order to observe the recording of perianal EMG and the urine flow rate during voiding. Two of the girls were able to suppress the dyssynergia and improved their urinary frequency and incontinence. In a subsequent study, Sugar and Firlit [24] applied the same technique to 10 children aged between 6 and 16 years with daytime incontinence and recurrent UTI. All but one were able to convert to synergy, eight were cured, and two were improved. A case history with good success was reported at the same time by Norgaard and Djurhuus [25]. Jerkins et al. [10] reported a 63% success rate in 35 children (including 33 girls) aged from 3 to 15 years; 17% demonstrated improvement with fewer episodes of incontinence and better control of infections. Three children relapsed within 3 months and improved again with a refresher course in which the BFB regimen was used once again for 1 month at home. After 6 months no further relapses happened.

In our first study, seven children with voiding dysfunction, six with urinary incontinence, and four with urinary retention were treated with voiding EMG/BFB [12]. Five had recurrent UTIs and two were receiving intermittent catheterization. VUR or megaureter was present in six, of whom four cases were bilateral. Two had already undergone surgical ureteral reimplantation. Antibiotic prophylaxis to prevent UTIs was adopted in three. Urodynamics showed detrusor overactivity in five and poor compliance in two. All were treated with a minimum of two and a maximum of 13 sessions of voiding EMG/BFB, and two also had bladder BFB for persistent OAB for a period of a few weeks to 6 months. With the exception of one girl aged 4 years, all of the children were able to learn to relax the perineal floor and to avoid the use of abdominal muscles during micturition. Two cases still showed fractionated flow, due to detrusor underactivity secondary to posterior urethral valve ablation in one and sacral extradural lipoma in the other. In these cases, BFB was able to reveal the real cause of the DV.

Uroflowmetry with surface perineal EMG is performed in order to observe the perineal muscle behavior and the shape of the flow curve during voiding. If these muscles are not relaxed during micturition, it is useful to perform voiding EMG/BFB, focusing the attention of the child on the perineal muscles first and explaining that the EMG trace should be flat or the loudspeakers should be silent during voiding (Fig. 26.3). Two surface electrodes are placed on the perineal skin and are better tolerated than an anal plug. The effectiveness of the perineal surface electrodes in recording PFM activity was demonstrated in a methodological study [26]. With this method the same authors were able to demonstrate the importance of leg support in the sitting position to obtain optimal relaxation of the PFMs [27]. Therefore this posture should always be adopted during the training sessions and at home. The child is trained to recognize on the instrument when the perineal muscles are contracted, observing increasing activity on the electromyographic trace. Voiding should be repeated, and the child should be invited to drink before furosemide 1 mg/kg is administered [24]. Positive verbal reinforcement is necessary throughout the training process. A little improvement can be seen after the end of the first session, especially if good rapport is established between the child and the therapist. Because of the need for the child's cooperation, this treatmenet is not suitable for children younger than 6 years. Parents should be instructed and should follow the child at home, emphasizing (gradual) progress toward short and not fractionated micturition.

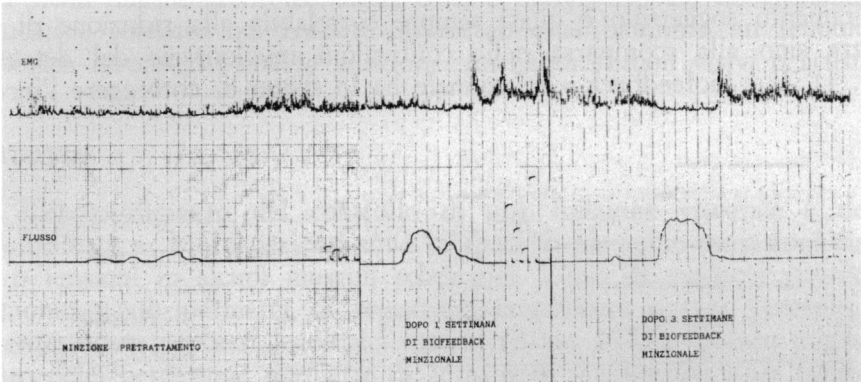

Fig. 26.3 Changes in uroflowmetry and electromyography after 1 and 3 weeks of voiding biofeedback

Kjølseth et al. [28] treated 32 children (including 28 girls) aged 5–15 years with voiding EMG/BFB and obtained a cure rate of 51.5% and pronounced improvement of symptoms in 26%, while flow was normalized in 55% and nearly normalized in 22.5%. The mean follow-up interval in 18 of the children was 4 years. Two relapses after 1.5 years and after retreatment were newly cured.

Further studies with more children treated were published starting from 1996, when Hoebeke et al. [29] treated 50 girls aged between 6 and 13 years with urodynamically proven DV. Ninety-two percent normalized their flow and bladder capacity, and their daytime incontinence disappeared with a maximum of 18 sessions in a 6-month period. After 6 months, 10% had relapsed.

In 1998, Combs et al. published their findings on the use of voiding uroflow and surface EMG/BFB in 21 children with voiding dysfunction, obtaining an excellent response in 81% in terms of both urodynamic patterns and symptoms after an average of 3.7 sessions and follow-up of 34 months [1]. Unfortunately, in 16 children, they filled the bladder through a urethral catheter in order to obtain more quickly repeated voidings.

A systematic review of randomized controlled trials treating daytime urinary incontinence in children was published in 2003 [30] and showed that only one randomized study described the use of BFB [31]. This multicenter prospective European Bladder Dysfunction Study (EBDS) published further papers in 2008 [21] and 2014 [32]. Ninety-seven children with OAB were randomly allocated to receive either standard therapy (i.e., careful explanation of the problem by a trained urotherapist, with written instructions explained by the urotherapist, emphasizing adequate intake of fluids, adherence to voiding diaries, recognition of the urge to void, proper posture during voiding, low-dose chemoprophylaxis, and/or treatment of constipation when needed, as well as personal hygiene) plus pharmacotherapy (double-blinded: oxybutynin versus placebo), or standard therapy plus bladder training (6–12 sessions with at least two voidings each), and 105 children with pelvic floor overactivity during voiding were randomly allocated to receive either standard treatment only or standard therapy plus voiding uroflow BFB. The treatment lasted for 6 months, and the follow-up period lasted for 12 months. A urodynamic study was done before treatment in all children and repeated after treatment in 69 of the first group and 82 of the second group. In the group with OAB, detrusor overactivity was present in 33% of cases and persisted in 27% after treatment, where two thirds of the cases were of new onset. In the group with DV, increased pelvic floor activity was found in 67% of children before treatment and in 56% after treatment, and in more than half, it occurred de novo. No statistically significant differences in outcome emerged between the different treatment modalities after 6- and 12-month follow-up. The conclusions of these important works were that urodynamic study is not a good witness of non-neurogenic voiding disorders in children and pharmacotherapy, and that bladder training and voiding BFB are not superior to standard therapy. Actually, urodynamic study is not useful, because many factors (anxiety, discomfort from the catheter, bowel problems, the state of hydration) can influence its results, and the outcome should be based upon clinical improvement or the cure rate instead of urodynamic changes. It is better to rely on noninvasive and repeatable tests such as uroflow and surface perineal EMG, while standard urotherapy should always be offered first to these children, with other more time-consuming or invasive treatments being reserved for refractory cases.

The first study adopting isolated pelvic floor exercises for children with DV appeared in 1991 as an abstract [33] and in 1995 as a full publication [34]. The study included only girls aged between 6 and 15 years (median 8 years), all with OAB but half [8] also with an abnormal flow pattern, shown by fractionated or slowly decaying flow curves, and 12 with EMG dyscoordination during voiding after cystometry performed in 14 cases. This difference can be due to the presence of a catheter, and once again I must underline that DV can be better assessed by simple uroflowmetry and EMG surface electrodes instead of being recognized soon after or during urethral catheterization causing obvious discomfort. These girls were treated by a physiotherapist, mostly in small groups, with the aim of increasing awareness of the PFMs and the ability to contract and relax them at will. PFM exercise, EMG, and BFB were used only at the beginning of the treatment. After 1 year, 56% of the girls were cured and the rest had improved, and after 3–4 years 75% were cured. The urinary flow pattern became normal in seven girls (88%). Symptomatic or asymptomatic bacteriuria was present in 81% of the girls before the treatment, decreasing to 69% after 1 year and to 25% after 3–4 years.

Another study published in 2000 [35] treated 20 children (including 18 girls) aged less than 5 years mainly with behavioral treatment and manual testing; eight were also treated with relaxation EMG/BFB of the PFMs with an anal plug. They achieved the same results though the duration of follow-up was not always reported; good results were found also for encopresis (75% healed or ameliorated) although the children were very young. Some authors agree that BFB can be applied to younger children [13, 36], while others have found that younger children aged less than 5 years [10], 7 years [28], or 10 years [24]—or even preadolescents [37]—were not good candidates for BFB training because of insufficient cooperation and anxiety. In conclusion, younger age is a relative contraindication to pediatric BFB, and it is better to consider the maturity and motivation in each child.

A randomized study compared two groups of children with DV where one group of 43 were treated with behavioral modifications and pelvic floor training without BFB, and the other group of 32 children were treated only with behavioral modifications [38]. Two thirds of the children were girls, and the mean age was 7 years in both groups. Treatment and follow-up lasted 12 months. More than 50% of the children also received pharmacotherapy with anticholinergics, desmopressin, and antibiotics in both groups, equally distributed. The results were significantly better in the group given pelvic floor exercises (83% versus 11% cured of incontinence, 66% versus 33% cured of enuresis, 100% versus 60% cured of constipation, and 68% versus 40% cured of UTI). The good results obtained for enuresis might have been attributable to the concomitant drug treatment.

Two groups of children with voiding dysfunction and a mean age of 10–11 years, with a prevalence of girls (two thirds), were randomized to learn pelvic floor exercises with or without BFB [39]. Bladder and sphincter behavior were evaluated by dynamic ultrasound of the urinary tract. There was a significant decrease in episodes of daytime incontinence and UTI in both groups, with no difference between the two techniques, but only the group treated with BFB exhibited a significant reduction in postvoid residual urine (PVR). This difference can be explained by the easier way of learning how to relax the PFMs using BFB. No significant effects on nocturnal incontinence and constipation were noticed. No data on urodynamic parameters were reported.

An interesting uncontrolled nonrandomized study presented the results of two different types of BFB in 102 children with voiding dysfunction [40]. A group was trained in front of a uroflowmeter for 6 h during each session with 3–4 patients, trying to obtain normal bell-shaped flow with a minimum of four voids. Another group was taught PFM relaxation techniques using a displayed electromyogram for 45–90 min and then voided without electrodes, and a third group used both methods. The success rates varied from 80% to 100% for daytime wetting and from 69% to 75% for resolution of UTI without a significant difference between the types of BFB used. As stated before, BFB is more effective if the child controls the PFMs during micturition and not without voiding or by watching the flow curve alone.

Since 1999, BFB has been applied in computer games [11, 17, 41, 42]. In the largest study, 168 children (80% of whom were girls) with voiding dysfunction were enrolled [43]. Two percent were noncompliant, because of poor motivation, and 13% had no improvement of their symptoms. Factors that predicted failure included bladder capacity less than 70% of predicted capacity and noncompliance with the treatment program. Of the 22 children who had no improvement, 12 were treated with oxybutynin and 83% of them had significant subjective improvement, two with a persistent low flow rate even after achieving normal PFM relaxation were treated with alpha-blockers, and seven underwent urodynamic study and/or magnetic resonance imaging for severe persistent symptoms. In none of these was any neurological lesion found. In a comparison of two groups of 60 girls with DV, animated BFB yielded results similar to those seen with nonanimated BFB but in a significantly shorter time (mean 3.6 versus 7.6 sessions, $p < 0.05$) [44].

Other researchers have pointed to a more psychological approach to increase motivation and achieve maximal cooperation with the BFB program, including appropriate explanations, externalization of the voiding problem, empowerment, homework, and praise [36]. This approach needs special motivation from the clinician, who must establish a collaborative relationship with the child and the family, and must enhance the child's self-esteem and sense of mastery of the problem. Of 87 children (including only seven boys) aged between 3 and 17 years (mean age 7.8 years), 77 completed the program, with an average of 4.7 sessions. Subjectively, 47 (61%) reported pronounced improvement in urinary symptoms, while 24 reported only moderate improvement. Objectively, 47 (61%) had normal flow and PVR of less than 20% of the voided volume. In 28 (36%) the flow curve improved, but residual urine remained elevated. Those with more than a 2-year history of symptoms, spinal dysraphism, poor bladder emptying, and severe constipation had only moderate improvement.

In order to find a cost–benefit approach, half-day urotherapy has been proposed, training children in pairs with voiding EMG/BFB, demonstrating recruitment and relaxation of the perineal muscles through surface or anal plug EMG electrodes [45]. This intensive and short-duration treatment was sufficient to obtain good results for voiding efficiency and improved uroflow curves after only 3-month follow-up. No data on symptoms were reported. While a short training course can be sufficient for many children, we believe that too-standardized and too-short training and follow-up could not achieve the same results in the majority of children.

Long-term studies of BFB show that the results are durable for 3–4 years [28, 34], and relapse generally develops within 3 months after the completion of the training [10].

In an interesting study, 24 of 28 children with DV were randomized to treatment with either visual and auditory BFB (which was not further described; median 10 sessions, range 6–16 sessions) or off-label treatment with an alpha blocker (doxazosin; daily dose 0.5–2 mg). No difference in results was found between the two treatment arms, and in refractory cases, both treatments were offered, obtaining good results [46]. The real difference is that BFB is a definitive therapy with a demonstrated long-term lasting effect, while alpha blocker treatment needs to be continued for a long time and there are no available data on outcomes after its discontinuation.

A recent systematic review selected and analyzed 27 publications on the effectiveness of BFB (using a visualized EMG tracing) for relaxation of the PFMs during bladder contraction in dysfunctional elimination syndrome [47]. Only one article described a randomized study, performed by Klijn et al. [48], which favored BFB with home uroflowmetry over standard therapy and videotaped instructions, but the results were not statistically significant, because of the small sample size (only 56 children). The other 26 case series analysis showed a pooled estimate of 80% for improvement of daytime incontinence, with high heterogeneity across the study results. Other outcomes analyzed were improvements in frequency (from 67% to 100%), urgency (from 71% to 88%), PVR, and flow. It was not clear if the variability in the results was due to unequal groups of patients and/or differences in training protocols and levels of motivation of the patients, parents, and trainers.

A recent randomized controlled study in two groups of 40 children with dysfunctional elimination syndrome compared the results of behavioral modification only and animated uroflowmetry/EMG/BFB along with PFM exercises and behavioral modification. Animated BFB was more effective than non-BFB management with regard to objective and subjective voiding problems and bowel dysfunction [42].

A recently published study analyzed the long-term effects of voiding school (VS) for mixed lower urinary tract conditions [49].The training program consisted of inpatient training for 2 weeks (VS) with a 2-week break, followed by another 2 weeks of inpatient training. In this intensive training, static PFM, EMG, BFB, and voiding uroflow were included. The short-term results were published in 2011 [50]. Significant improvements in continence status were noted between the start of VS and 6-month follow-up, and between the start of VS and 2-year follow-up. However, the overall continence status did not significantly differ between 6-month and 2-year follow-up. Individual shifts could be determined because of relapse. Further improvements from 6 months to 2 years were noted only in children suffering from OAB. Children who relapsed after being dry at 6-month follow-up also showed relapses in adequate fluid intake, pelvic floor tone, or soiling. This study clearly showed that adopting an intensive and identical protocol for mixed LUTDs produces different results and relapse on long-term follow-up. Therefore, rehabilitative treatment should be individualized using different escalating modalities in resistant cases and long follow-up in order to treat relapses early.

26.8 Rehabilitation and Urinary Tract Infections

All of the publications regarding pelvic floor rehabilitation in children have shown reductions in the incidence of UTI. It is difficult to differentiate the contributions to these results of behavioral and rehabilitative programs, prolonged antibiotic prophylaxis, and sometimes antimuscarinic drug treatment. It is also true that in many studies, prophylactic treatment is often dismissed after evidence of satisfactory and durable improvements in symptoms and uroflow patterns. The reductions in UTI have been around 80% in the majority of the reported papers [11, 35, 36, 39, 40, 41, 51] or even greater [13, 44, 52]. Some papers have reported lower success rates of 69% [34], 63% [10], and 56% [53]. A recent systematic review found a pooled estimate of 83% for improvement in UTI [46]. A recent randomized controlled study in children with dysfunctional elimination syndrome found better results for resolution of UTI after 1-year follow-up in a group treated with animated uroflow/EMG/BFB plus pelvic floor exercises and behavioral modification than in those who received behavioral treatment only (71% versus 55%), but the difference was not significant ($p = 0.3$) [42].

26.9 Rehabilitation and Vesicoureteral Reflux

The first paper that described an in-depth evaluation of the effect of voiding EMG/BFB on VUR was published in 2002 [54]. Twenty-five girls aged 6–10 years (mean age 9 years) underwent an average of seven sessions of BFB. Antimuscarinic drugs were not used. At 1-year follow-up, vesicoureteral reflux had resolved in 17 units (55%), improved in 5 (16%), and remained unchanged in 9 (29%). The refluxes that resolved better were grade I (80%) and grade II (60%). Overall, 14 (56%) of the 25 children were cured at 1 year, and four children underwent reimplantation because of either persistent moderate-grade reflux or parental decision. The resolution rate 1 year after BFB was markedly greater than the expected spontaneous resolution rate. Furthermore, because of the unsatisfactory surgical results in children with DV, after correction of the voiding problem prior to surgery, the outcome would more likely be successful.

Another paper reported similar results after voiding surface EMG/BFB in 78 children (98 units) with DV. After only 6 months of follow-up, resolution was observed in 63% and improvement in 29% [55]. No worsening of VUR was observed.

In many papers, spontaneous resolution of reflux has also been reported, sometimes regardless of its degree. The resolution rate has ranged from 21% [11] to 45%

[10], 47% [36], 50% [17], and 70% [1]. Actually a recent systematic review found improvement of VUR in a range from 21% to 100% [47]. A more recent randomized controlled study found better results for resolution of VUR after 1-year follow-up in a group treated with animated BFB (78% versus 12.5%, p 0.001) [42].

Therefore, before surgical correction, all children should undergo evaluation of the voiding pattern and undergo urotherapy and BFB if needed. This statement was highlighted in the 2010 American Urological Association (AUA) guidelines on management and screening of primary vesicoureteral reflux in children.

26.10 Rehabilitation and Constipation

The results for constipation are often obtained in association with a high-fiber diet and the use of laxatives. On the other hand, learning how to relax the perineal muscles can be useful to reduce fecal retention. Bowel control was reported by Kibar et al. [55] (success rate 78%) and De Paepe et al. [35] (success rate 62.5%), and a pronounced improvement in 29% of cases and moderate improvement in 61% were reported by Chin-Peuckert and Pippi Salle [36].

A randomized study using BFB showed no beneficial effect of the BFB modality [56]. A recent systematic review found improvements in constipation ranging from 18% to 100% after EMG/BFB [47]. A more recent randomized controlled study found better results for constipation after 1-year follow-up in a group treated with animated BFB (68% versus 40%, p 0.009) [42].

26.11 Rehabilitation and Pain

Chin-Peuckert and Pippi Salle [36] reported a dramatic improvement in dysuria in 12 children, including seven in whom it was not associated with UTI, after pelvic floor BFB. Hoebeke et al. [57] used BFB pelvic floor relaxation therapy in 21 children seen for nighttime pelvic pain. Such children typically wake up in the middle of the night with severe abdominal or perineal pain, and during the day some of them suffer urge syndrome. During urodynamic investigation, extremely high pelvic floor activity was recorded. The mean duration of the treatment, with one weekly session, was 3 months, and success was obtained in 17 (81%). Relapse was observed in three cases after long-term follow-up.

26.12 Rehabilitation After Posterior Urethral Valve Ablation

Despite successful valve ablation, a significant proportion of children still present with voiding disorders due to detrusor overactivity or poor compliance or increased activity of the perineal floor that mimics DV. As already mentioned in relation to rehabilitation in DV, one case we treated with EMG and uroflow BFB after urethral valve ablation was then able to relax the perineal floor and avoid abdominal contraction during voiding, but still had fractionated flow due to detrusor underactivity [12]. In a recent study, 30 children with LUTS due to posterior urethral valves—whose urodynamic evaluations showed detrusor overactivity or poor compliance in 77%, a nonrelaxing perineal floor in 23%, and obstructed bladder neck in 7%—were treated with bladder and PFM BFB [58]. The children were instructed to interrupt detrusor pressure increments by tensing the perineal muscles, and in the presence of nonrelaxing PFMs, they were instructed to tighten and then relax these muscles. An overall consistent response was achieved in 70% of the children, of whom 52% no longer required antimuscarinics and 71% no longer required intermittent catheterization at a mean follow-up of 11 months.

26.13 Rehabilitation and Underactive Bladder

In accordance with the standardization in the ICCS update in 2006 [3], the term "underactive bladder" (UB) (once called "lazy bladder") refers to a voiding dysfunction with decreased frequency, hesitancy, urge or overflow incontinence, and need for the abdominal muscles to initiate, maintain, or complete voiding. Impaired detrusor contractility is evident on urodynamic evaluation. A recent randomized controlled trial evaluated 50 children with UB, who were randomly allocated to two equal treatment groups receiving standard urotherapy with or without animated BFB and PFM exercise [59]. Animated BFB was performed with surface EMG of the perineum and of the rectus abdominis muscles once a week for a minimum of 10 sessions and a maximum of 15 sessions. With PFM exercise and BFB, the children learned adequate relaxation of the PFMs and the abdominal muscles, avoiding an increase in intra-abdominal pressure to initiate voiding. At 1-year follow-up, a significant increase in the mean number of voiding episodes, a reduction in relapses of UTI, an increase in Q_{max}, and decreases in voiding time and postvoid residual volume were found in the group treated with BFB. The conclusion was that animated BFB and PFM exercise effectively improve the sensation of bladder fullness and contractility in children with UB.

Conclusions

PFM training and BFB for those children who are refractory to a behavioral program are a proven modality to effectively treat OAB and DV in children. This treatment sometimes goes in parallel with more appropriate diagnosis using noninvasive urodynamics and, if it fails, it allows recognition of more difficult situations that need invasive diagnostic procedures such as video urodynamics or neurophysiological tests, while in the meantime, the majority of children benefit from simpler and noninvasive therapy. We have examined different types of BFB that should be chosen after precise selection of the children. To use the same BFB for different situations means a reduction in the expected success rate [52].

A bladder capacity of 70% or less of the expected bladder capacity has been shown to be a predictor of failure [43].

Children with neurogenic bladder are poor candidates for BFB even with an incomplete lesion. Antibiotic prophylaxis and sometimes antimuscarinic medication can be useful in the initial approach to obtain earlier good results and improve motivation, but should then be discontinued during follow-up. Some authors prefer a labor-intensive program, even on an inpatient basis; others prefer short sessions and homework. It should be stressed that the duration of the teaching program should not be fixed but individualized for the patient, depending on age, sex, and ability to learn a new behavior. Motivation from the child, the family and—last but not least—the therapist are important in order to achieve the best results. A training program has been shown to resolve not only symptoms but also complications or comorbidities such as UTI, reflux, and constipation—and, at the same time, to better select those few children who need more aggressive treatments. Follow-up is fundamental because initial improvements can be reduced after time. Starting a new and usually shorter program can re-establish previous good results. An algorithm of the consequential steps that can be taken is suggested in Fig. 26.4.

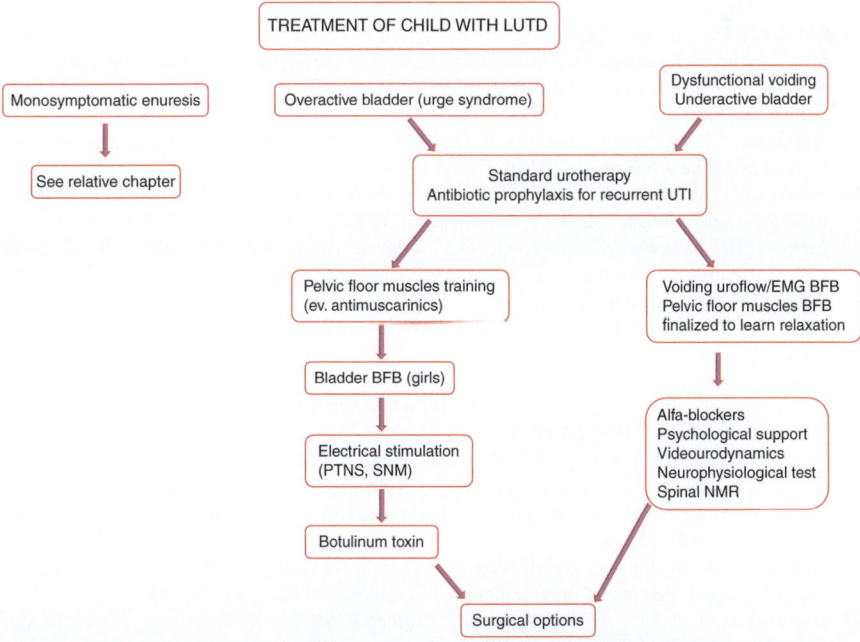

Fig. 26.4 Algorithm for treatment of a child with lower urinary tract dysfunction

References

1. Combs AJ, Glassberg AD, Gerdes D, Horowitz M. Biofeedback therapy for children with dysfunctional voiding. Urology. 1998;52(2):312–5.
2. Chase J, Austin P, McKenna P. The management of dysfunctional voiding in children: a report from the Standardization Committee of the International Children's Continence Society. J Urol. 2010;183:1296–302.
3. Neveus T, von Gontard A, Hoebeke P, Hjiälmås K, Bauer S, Bower W, Jørgensen TM, Rittig S, Vande Valle J, Yeung C-K, Djurhuus JC. The standardization of terminology of lower urinary tract function in children and adolescents: report from the Standardization Committee of the International Children's Continence Society. J Urol. 2006;176:314–24.
4. Sandri SD, Colletta F, Zanollo L. Normal perineal behavior in pediatric age. Urodinamica. 1997;7(4):223–4.
5. Ab E, Schoenmaker M, van Empelen R, Klijn AJ, de Jong TPVM. Paradoxical movement of the pelvic floor in dysfunctional voiding and the results of biofeedback. BJU Int. 2002;89(Suppl 2):48.
6. Thompson JA, O'Sullivan PB. Levator plate movement during voluntary pelvic floor muscle contraction in subjects with incontinence and prolapse: a cross sectional study and review. Int Urogynecol J. 2001;12(suppl 3):61.
7. Bower WF, Chase JW, Stillman BC. Normative pelvic floor parameters in children assessed by transabdominal ultrasound. J Urol. 2006;176:337–41.
8. Sandri SD. Are children with urinary incontinence able to learn how to contract perineal floor muscles? Urodinamica. 1997;7(4):225–6.
9. Birk L. Biofeedback: furor therapeutics. Semin Psychiatry. 1973;5:362.
10. Jerkins GR, Noe HN, Vaughn WR, Roberts E. Biofeedback training for children with bladder sphincter incoordination. J Urol. 1987;138:1113–5.
11. Mc Kenna PH, Herndon CDA, Connery S, Ferrer FA. Pelvic floor muscle retraining for pediatric voiding dysfunction using interactive computer games. J Urol. 1999;162:1056–63.
12. Sandri SD, Fanciullacci F, Politi P, Zanollo A. Applicazione del "biofeedback" nei disturbi della minzione e della continenza in età pediatrica. Urologia. 1988;55(1):42–8.
13. Hellström A-L, Hjälmas K, Jodal U. Rehabilitation of the dysfunctional bladder in children: method and 3-year follow-up. J Urol. 1987;138:847–9.
14. Sandri SD. The treatment of paediatric urge incontinence with pelvic floor training: further experience and a longer follow up. Urodinamica. 1999;9(1):42–3.
15. Meijer EFJ, Nieuwhof-Leppink AJ, Dekker-Vasse E, de Joode Smink GCJ, de Jong TPVM. Central inhibition of refractory OAB complaints, results of an inpatient training program. J Pediatr Urol. 2015;11:21e1–5.
16. Schneider MS, King LR, Surwitt RS. Kegel exercise and childhood incontinence: a new role for an old treatment. J Pediatr. 1994;124:91.
17. Pfister C, Dacher JN, Gaucher S, Liard-Zmuda A, Grise P, Mitrofanoff P. The usefulness of a minimal urodynamic evaluation and pelvic floor biofeedback in children with chronic voiding dysfunction. BJU Int. 1999;84:1054–7.
18. Wiener JS, Scales MT, Hampton J, King LR, Surwit R, Edwards CL. Long-term efficacy of simple behavioral therapy for daytime wetting in children. J. Urology. 2000;164:786–90.
19. Cardozo L, Stanton SL, Hafner J, Allan V. Biofeedback in the treatment of detrusor instability. Br J Urol. 1978;50:250–4.
20. Hjälmas K, Hellström A-L. Habilitation of dysfunctional bladder in children. Proceedings of the 11th Annual Meeting of the International Continence Society; 1981. p. 48.
21. Bael A, Lax H, de Jong TPVM, Hoebeke P, Nijman RJM, Sixt R, Verlhurst J, Hirche H, van Gool JD, on behalf of the European Bladder Dysfunction Study. The relevance of urodynamic studies for urge syndrome and dysfunctional voiding: a multicenter controlled trial in children. J Urol. 2008;180:1486–95.

22. Millard RJ, Oldenburg BF. The symptomatic, urodynamic and psychodynamic results of bladder re-education programs. J Urol. 1983;130:715–9.
23. Maizels M, King LR, Firlit CF. Urodynamic biofeedback: a new approach to treat vesical sphincter dyssynergia. J Urol. 1979;122:205–9.
24. Sugar EC, Firlit CF. Urodynamic biofeedback: a new therapeutic approach for childhood incontinence/infection (vesical voluntary sphincter dyssynergia). J Urol. 1982;128:1253.
25. Norgaard JP, Djurhuus JC. Treatment of detrusor–sphincter dyssynergia by bio-feedback. Urol Int. 1982;37:236–9.
26. Wennergren H, Larsson LE, Sandstedt P. Surface electromyography of pelvic floor muscles in healthy children: methodological study. Scand J Caring Sci. 1989;3(2):63–9.
27. Wennergren H, Öberg BE, Sandstedt P. The importance of leg support for relaxation of the pelvic floor muscles. Scand J Urol Nephrol. 1991;25:205–13.
28. Kjølseth D, Knudsen LM, Madsen B, Norgaard JP, Djuurhuus JC. Urodynamic biofeedback training for children with bladder–sphincter dyscoordination during voiding. Neurourol Urodyn. 1993;12:211–21.
29. Hoebeke P, Vande Walle J, Theunis M, De Paepe H, Oosterlink W, Renson C. Outpatients pelvic-floor therapy in girls with daytime incontinence and dysfunctional voiding. Urology. 1996;48(6):923–7.
30. Sureshkumar P, Bower W, Craig JC, Knight JF. Treatment of daytime urinary incontinence in children: a systematic review of randomized controlled trials. J Urol. 2003;170:196–200.
31. van Gool JD, de Jong TPV, Winkler-Seinstra P, Tamminen Mobius T, Lax-Gross H, Hirche H. Comparison of standard therapy, bladder rehabilitation with biofeedback and pharmacotherapy in children with non-neuropathic bladder-sphincter dysfunction. Neurourol Urodyn. 1999;18:261.
32. van Gool JD, de Jong TPVM, Winkler-Seinstra P, Tamminen Mobius T, Lax-Gross H, Hirche H, Nijman RJ, Hjälmas K, Jodal U, Bachmann H, Hoebeke P, Walle JV, Misselwitz J, John U, Bael A, on behalf of the European Bladder Dysfunction Study. Multi-center randomized controlled trial of cognitive treatment, placebo, oxybutynin, bladder training, and pelvic floor training in children with functional urinary incontinence. Neurourol Urodyn. 2014;33(5):482–7.
33. Wennergren H, Öberg BE. Pelvic floor muscle exercise for girls. Child adapted method. Neurourol Urodyn. 1991;10:387–8.
34. Wennergren H, Öberg BE. Pelvic floor exercises for children: a method of treating dysfunctional voiding. Brit. J Urol. 1995;76:9–15.
35. De Paepe H, Renson C, Van Laecke E, Raes A, Vande WJ, Hoebeke P. Pelvic-floor therapy and toilet training in young children with dysfunctional voiding and obstipation. BJU Int. 2000;85:889–93.
36. Chin-Peuckert L, Pippi Salle JL. A modified biofeedback program for children with detrusor-sphincter dyssynergia: 5-year experience. J Urol. 2001;166:1470–5.
37. Sugar E. Bladder control through biofeedback. Am J Nurs. 1983;83:1152–4.
38. Zivkovic V, Lazovic M, Vlajkovic M, Slavkovic A, Dimitrijevic L. Correlation between uroflowmetry parameters and treatment outcome in children with dysfunctional voiding. J Pediatr Urol. 2010;6:396–402.
39. Vasconcelos M, Lima E, Caiafa L, Noronha A, Cangussu R, Gomes S, Freire R, Filgueiras MT, Araùjo J, Magnus G, Cunha C, Colozimo E. Voiding dysfunction in children. Pelvic-floor exercises or biofeedback therapy: a randomized study. Pediatr Nephrol. 2006;21:1858–64.
40. Schulman SL, von Zuben FC, Plachter N, Kodman-Jones C. Biofeedback methodology: does it matter how we teach children how to relax the pelvic floor during voiding? J Urol. 2001;166:2423–6.
41. Nelson JD, Cooper CS, Boyt MA, Hawtrey CE, Austin JC. Improved uroflow parameters and post-void residual following biofeedback therapy in pediatric patients with dysfunctional voiding does not correspond to outcome. J Urol. 2004;172:1653–6.

42. Kajbafzadeh A-M, Sharifi-Rad L, Ghahestani SM, Ahmadi H, Kajbafzadeh M, Mahboubi AH. Animated biofeedback: an ideal treatment for children with dysfunctional elimination syndrome. J Urol. 2011;186:2379–85.
43. Herndon CDA, Decambre M, Mc Kenna PH. Interactive computer games for treatment of pelvic floor dysfunction. J Urol. 2001;166:1893–8.
44. Kaye JD, Palmer LS. Animated biofeedback yields more rapid results than nonanimated biofeedback in the treatment of dysfunctional voiding in girls. J Urol. 2008;180:300–5.
45. Bower WF, Yew SY, Sit KYF, Yeung CK. Half-day urotherapy improves voiding parameters in children with dysfunctional emptying. Eur Urol. 2006;49:570–4.
46. Yucel S, Akkaya E, Guntekin E, Akman S, Melikoglu M, Baykara M. Can alpha-blocker therapy be an alternative to biofeedback for dysfunctional voiding and urinary retention? A prospective study. J Urol. 2005;174:1612–5.
47. Desantis DJ, Leonard MP, Preston MA, Barrowman NJ, Guerra LA. Effectiveness of biofeedback for dysfunctional elimination syndrome in pediatrics: a systematic review. J Pediatr Urol. 2011;7:342–8.
48. Klijn AJ, Uiterwaal CSPM, Vijverberg MAW, Winkler PLH, Dik P, de Jong TPVM. Home uroflowmetry biofeedback in behavioral training for dysfunctional voiding in school-age children: a randomized controlled study. J Urol. 2006;175:2263–8.
49. Van den Broeck C, Roman de Mettelinge T, Deschepper E, Van Laecke E, Renson C, Samijn B, Hoebecke P. Prospective evaluation of the long-term effects of clinical voiding reeducation or voiding school for lower urinary tract conditions in children. J Pediatr Urol. 2016;12:37e1–6.
50. Hoebeke P, Renson C, De Schryver M, De Schryver L, Leenaerts E, Schoenaers A, Deschepper E, Walle VJ, Van den Broeck C. Prospective evaluation of clinical voiding reeducation or voiding school for lower urinary tract conditions in children. J Urol. 2011;186:648–54.
51. De Paepe H, Hoebeke P, Renson C, Van Laecke E, Raes E, Van Hoeke E, Van Daele J, Van de Walle J. Pelvic-floor therapy in girls with recurrent urinary tract infections and dysfunctional voiding. Br J Urol. 1998;81:109–13.
52. Yagci S, Kibar Y, Akay O, Kilic S, Erdemir F, Gok F, Dayanc M. The effect of biofeedback treatment on voiding and urodynamic parameters in children with voiding dysfunctions. J Urol. 2005;174:1994–8.
53. Wiener JS, Scales MT, Hampton J, King LR, Surwit R, Edwards CL. Long-term efficacy of simple behavioral therapy for daytime wetting in children. J Urol. 2000;164:786–90.
54. Palmer LS, Franco I, Rotario P, Reda EF, Friedman SC, Kolligian ME, Brock WA, Levitt SB. Biofeedback therapy expedites the resolution of reflux in older children. J Urol. 2002;168: 1699–703.
55. Kibar Y, Ors O, Demir E, Kalman S, Sakallioglu O, Dayanc M. Results of biofeedback treatment on reflux resolution rates in children with dysfunctional voiding and vesicoureteral reflux. Urology. 2007;70(3):563–6.
56. van der Plas RN, Benninga MA, Buller HA, Bossuyt PM, Akkermans LM, Redekop WK, et al. Biofeedback training in treatment of childhood constipation: a randomized control study. Lancet. 1996;348:776.
57. Hoebeke PBB, Van Laecke E, Renson C, Raes A, Dehoorne J, Vermeiren P, Walle VJ. Pelvic floor spasm in children: an unknown condition responding well to pelvic floor therapy. Eur Urol. 2004;46(5):651–4.
58. Ansari MS, Srivastava A, Kapoor R, Dubey D, Mandani A, Kumar A. Biofeedback therapy and home pelvic floor exercises for lower urinary tract dysfunction after posterior urethral valve ablation. J Urol. 2008;179:708–11.
59. Ladi-Seyedian S, Kajbafzadeh A-M, Sharifi-Had L, Shadgan B, Fan E. Management of non-neuropathic underactive bladder in children with voiding dysfunction by animated biofeedback: a randomized clinical trial. Urology. 2015;85(1):205–10.

Pharmacological Therapy

27

John Weaver and Paul Austin

27.1 Introduction

Urologists utilize clinical history, elimination diaries, noninvasive urodynamics, and conventional urodynamics to help gain an understanding of each patient's unique bladder characteristics. It is from this information that urologists can determine whether implementing pharmacologic therapy will benefit a patient; furthermore, this information helps the physician tailor the correct pharmacotherapy to each patient based on their individual bladder physiology. Figure 28.1 shows a treatment algorithm which includes the optimal time to initiate pharmacotherapy for two common urologic issues: frequency and incontinence. There is a multitude of pharmacotherapy agents in an urologist's armamentarium, and having an in-depth understanding of each agent is key in helping to determine the correct drug needed for each clinical scenario.

27.2 Anticholinergics

The most commonly prescribed pharmacotherapy for bladder dysfunction in pediatric patients is anticholinergics. Anticholinergics act on muscarinic receptors which are found in the detrusor muscle of the bladder. Bladder contractions are initiated by stimulation of these receptors with the release of acetylcholine from cholinergic nerves. The bladder consists of primarily M2 and M3 muscarinic receptor subtypes that the anticholinergics will selectively target. Anticholinergics competitively inhibit the binding of acetylcholine to muscarinic receptors at the neuromuscular junction thereby reducing the frequency and intensity of detrusor contractions

---

J. Weaver, M.D. • P. Austin, M.D. (✉)
Division of Urologic Surgery, St. Louis Children's Hospital, Washington University School, St. Louis, MO, USA
e-mail: Austinp@wustl.edu

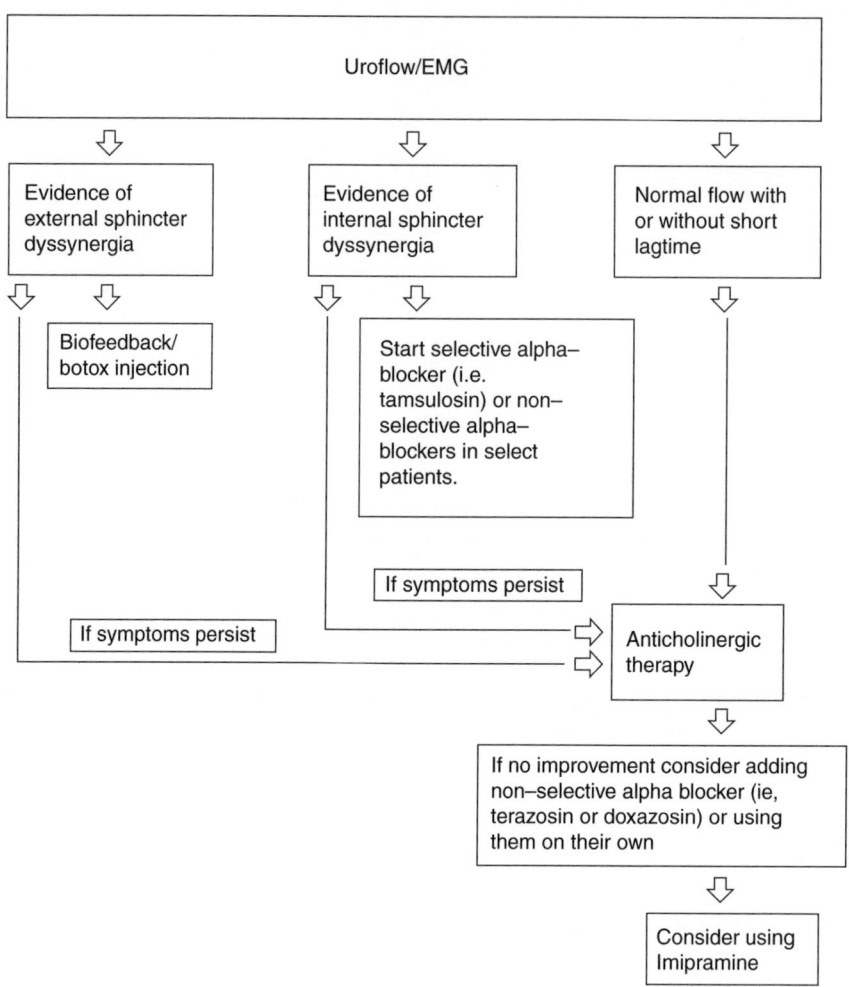

Fig. 27.1 Treatment algorithm for urinary frequency and/or urinary incontinence

during the filling phase of the bladder. This subsequently results in an increase in the functional capacity of the bladder and compliance [1, 2]. By increasing bladder compliance, anticholinergics also decrease pressures in noncompliant neurogenic bladders thereby helping to protect the upper tracts in these patients. Anticholinergics are also particularly useful in decreasing the uninhibited, pathologic contractions associated with overactive bladders. By decreasing unwanted contractions, and increasing bladder capacity and compliance, anticholinergics are effective in decreasing incontinence in the setting of neurogenic bladders [3].

Five anticholinergic agents are currently approved in the United States for the treatment of overactive bladder (darifenacin, oxybutynin, solifenacin, tolterodine, and trospium), with only two of these (oxybutynin and tolterodine) having formally achieved approval for use in children. The most commonly used antimuscarinic agent in children is oxybutynin. Oxybutynin has been extensively studied in the pediatric neurogenic bladder population and has both FDA and EMA labeling for this purpose. However, clinical trials performed in children have generally utilized patients with neurogenic voiding problems and have not concentrated on the non-neurogenic patients [4]. Nevertheless, oxybutynin is the prototype anticholinergic that targets detrusor overactivity, and there is level 1 evidence of the efficacy of anticholinergics in treating overactive bladder [5]. For overactive bladder in neurologically intact children, the usage is considered off-label but nevertheless has an extensive track record in the published literature.

Oxybutynin is a tertiary amine that has primary affinity for M3 receptors in the bladder. It is metabolized to desethyloxybutynin after passage through the hepatobiliary system. Desethyloxybutynin targets muscarinic receptor subtypes located in the salivary glands, skin, and brain. Dry mouth is the most common side effect, but constipation, gastroesophageal reflux, blurry vision, and urinary retention can all occur in children. Oxybutynin is lipid soluble and therefore likely to cross the blood-brain barrier, and in adults it has been reported to interfere with cognition. The potential for adverse cognitive effects and delirium due to antimuscarinic drugs can occur in children, but it is generally limited to overdosing situations. In a nonrandomized trial of 25 children, Sommer et al. found that treatment with oxybutynin was not associated with cognitive impairment [6]. Additionally, in a recent study by Veenboer et al., no significant differences in behavior were found between children with spinal dysraphism with and without long-term use of antimuscarinics [7].

The longer-acting extended-release formulation (oxybutynin XL) is also approved by the US Food and Drug Administration (FDA) for use in children and uses a novel delivery system resulting in absorption in the large intestine [8]. This avoids the first-pass metabolism in the liver, leading to a decrease in the active metabolite N-desethyloxybutynin.

In addition to oxybutynin, tolterodine is another anticholinergic that has been studied in children and has gained approval for use in this population. It is also a tertiary amine and selectively inhibits detrusor overactivity, as well as the amplitude of voiding contractions due to its affinity for M3 receptors [9]. Studies have shown that tolterodine increases functional bladder capacity in children less than 10 years of age with a decrease in the mean number of incontinence episodes with long-term (1 year) use [10]. However, unlike oxybutynin, tolterodine does not cross the blood-brain barrier so does not possess the same risk of cognitive disturbances that can be associated with oxybutynin at high doses. While tolterodine does have the potential to cause dry mouth and constipation similar to oxybutynin, in a study by Ayan et al. using the dysfunctional voiding symptom score, there was found to be a statistically significant decrease in the score with fewer side effects (mostly dry mouth 31% and headache 4%) when comparing tolterodine to oxybutynin [11].

27.3 Alpha-Adrenergic Antagonists (Alpha-Blockers)

Alpha-adrenoreceptors are highly concentrated at the bladder neck and urethra, and alpha-adrenergic blockade is known to result in smooth muscle relaxation and decreased bladder outlet resistance [12]. Currently, alpha-blockers are a mainstay drug used to facilitate bladder emptying in the adult population, particularly in adult males with benign prostatic hyperplasia. In addition to their known role in the adult population, alpha-adrenergic antagonists have also been studied in detail in other populations. Over 40 years ago, Krane and Olsson demonstrated that nonselective alpha-blocker therapy can significantly improve bladder emptying in patients with neurogenic bladders [13]. They found that alpha-blockers improve bladder emptying, decrease detrusor pressure, and aid in the resolution of upper tract changes with improved vesicoureteral reflux and hydronephrosis; however, these studies were limited because only nonselective alpha-blockers were available at the time of the study. Nonselective alpha-blockers antagonize both the alpha-1- and alpha-2 adrenergic receptors, which can produce a profound hypotensive effect.

Subsequently in the 1980s, selective alpha-blockers were created and resulted in a reemergence of alpha-blockers in the clinical management of pediatric neurogenic bladders that target the alpha-1 adrenergic receptors at the bladder outlet and along the proximal urethra [14–16]. An uncontrolled, selected group of 17 children with neurogenic bladder, treated with alfuzosin, resulted in a significant decrease in the detrusor leak point pressure and an increase in the detrusor wall compliance values [16]. However, no efficacy was seen using tamsulosin in a double-blind, randomized, placebo-controlled trial in children with neurogenic bladders and detrusor leak point pressure 40 cm H_2O or greater [15]. Given the limitations and the paucity of overall data in the literature, alpha-blockers are considered investigational in the pediatric neurogenic population.

Early work on the benefits of alpha-blockers on pediatric lower urinary tract dysfunction by Austin et al. pioneered the introduction of alpha-blockers into the armamentarium of drugs that can be used to treat voiding issues in children with non-neurogenic bladders [14]. In this pilot report, there was an 82% improvement in the measured parameters of 17 patients treated with alpha-blocker therapy. In a follow-up of their initial study, the group continued to see improvement in multiple lower urinary tract symptoms, daytime incontinence episodes, and post-void residual measurements in 55 children treated with doxazosin for dysfunctional voiding [17]. Further studies have also found alpha-blockers to be useful in treating urgency and urge incontinence [18]. There are known to be alpha-1D receptors in the bladder that can modulate sensory signals from the bladder [19]. Nonselective alpha-blockers can bind presynaptically and inhibit acetylcholine release, reducing instability [20, 21]. Selective alpha-blockers have also been documented to relieve symptoms of instability as well in adult studies [22].

Researchers are still attempting to delineate the optimal role for alpha-blockers for each pediatric population. An uroflow finding of a prolonged "EMG lag time" is associated with bladder neck and internal urethral sphincter discoordination and may be used to select patients for alpha-blocker therapy [23, 24]. The EMG lag time is the time duration after the external sphincter relaxes and the flow of urine. A prolonged lag time of greater than 6 s is suggested as a reliable indicator of tailoring lower urinary tract dysfunction treatment with alpha-blocker therapy [24].

27.4 Beta-3 Adrenergic Receptor Agonists

In recent years beta-3 adrenergic receptor agonists have been found in numerous randomized placebo-controlled studies to significantly reduce incontinence episodes, urgency incontinence, nocturia, and mean number of micturitions per 24 h in patients with overactive bladder. Additionally, the beta-3 agonists improve bladder compliance and increase bladder capacity, and following beta-3 agonist use residual urine was not statistically increased nor was urinary retention reported in anyone, even in adult males with symptoms of bladder outlet obstruction [25–27].

There are three types of beta-adrenergic receptors: labeled beta-1, beta-2, and beta-3. Beta-3 receptors are thought to be the main bladder subtype, accounting for 97% of the beta-receptors, and when stimulated elicit relaxation of the detrusor muscle by activating adenylate cyclase causing increases in the intracellular levels of cyclic AMP and calcium [28–30]. Mirabegron is the beta-3 agonist with FDA, EMA, and Japanese labeling for adult indication and usage in the treatment of overactive bladder [25]. Pediatric usage for overactive bladder is off-label.

Mirabegron has a favorable side effect profile. Beta-3 receptors are found in the heart so there were initially concerns that beta-3 receptor agonists would result in significant cardiac side effects. However, bladder efficacy trials have found only slight dose-dependent increases in heart rate from baseline, and the maximum blood pressure increases noted were 4 mm Hg (systolic). There have not been any significant EKG changes or substantial cardiac adverse events related to mirabegron [25, 26]. Other side effects include dry mouth, constipation, and headache, but these occur in less than 3% of patients and are much less common when compared to antimuscarinics. Thus, beta-3 receptors are safe in adults; however, their side effect profiles have not yet been studied in children [26, 27].

References

1. Finney SM, Andersson KE, Gillespie JI, et al. Antimuscarinic drugs in detrusor overactivity and the overactive bladder syndrome: motor or sensory actions? BJU Int. 2006;98:503–7.
2. Nijman RJ. Role of antimuscarinics in the treatment of nonneurogenic daytime urinary incontinence in children. Urology. 2004;63:45–50.
3. Austin PF, Vricella GJ. Functional disorders of lower urinary tract in children. In: Campbell-walsh urology tenth edition. Part XV Pediatric urology. 2012. pp. 3297–316.
4. Austin PF, Franco I. Chapter 15: Pharmacotherapy of the child with functional incontinence retention. In: Pediatric incontinence: evaluation and clinical management. Chichester: John Wiley and Sons, Ltd; 2015. https://doi.org/10.1002/9781118814789.ch15.
5. Andersson KE, Chapple CR, Cardozo L, Cruz F, Hashim H, Michel MC, et al. Pharmacological treatment of overactive bladder: report from the international consultation on incontinence. Curr Opin Urol. 2009;19(4):380–94.
6. Sommer BR, O'Hara R, Askari N, et al. The effect of oxybutynin treatment on cognition in children with diurnal incontinence. J Urol. 2005;173:2125–7.
7. Veenboer PW, Huisman J, Chrzan RJ. Behavioral effects of long-term antimuscarinic use in patients with spinal dysraphism: a case control study. J Urol. 2013;190:2228–32.
8. Youdim K, Kogan BA. Preliminary study of the safety and efficacy of extended-release oxybutynin in children. Urology. 2002;59:428–32.

9. Gillespie JI, Palea S, Guilloteau V, Guerard M, Lluel P, Korstanje C. Modulation of non-voiding activity by the muscarinergic antagonist tolterodine and the beta(3)-adrenoceptor agonist mirabegron in conscious rats with partial outflow obstruction. BJU Int. 2012;110(2 Pt 2):E132–42.
10. Reddy PP, Borgstein NG, Nijman RJ, Ellsworth PI. Long-term efficacy and safety of tolterodine in children with neurogenic detrusor overactivity. J Pediatr Urol. 2008;4(6):428–33.
11. Ayan S, Kaya K, Topsakal K, Kilicarslan H, Gokce G, Gultekin Y. Efficacy of tolterodine as a first-line treatment for non-neurogenic voiding dysfunction in children. BJU Int. 2005;96(3):411–4.
12. Ek A. Adrenergic innervation and adrenergic mechanisms: a study of the human urethra. Acta Pharmacol Toxicol (Copenh). 1978;43:35–40.
13. Krane RJ, Olsson CA. Phenoxybenzamine in neurogenic bladder dysfunction. II. Clinical considerations. J Urol. 1973;110(6):653–6.
14. Austin PF, Homsy YL, Masel JL, Cain MP, Casale AJ, Rink RC. Alpha-adrenergic blockade in children with neuropathic and nonneuropathic voiding dysfunction. J Urol. 1999;162(3 Pt 2):1064–7.
15. Homsy Y, Arnold P, Zhang W. Phase IIb/III dose ranging study of tamsulosin as treatment for children with neuropathic bladder. J Urol. 2011;186(5):2033–9.
16. Schulte-Baukloh H, Michael T, Miller K, Knispel HH. Alfuzosin in the treatment of high leak-point pressure in children with neurogenic bladder. BJU Int. 2002;90(7):716–20.
17. Cain MP, Wu SD, Austin PF, et al. Alpha blocker therapy for children with dysfunctional voiding and urinary retention. J Urol. 2003;170:1514–5.
18. Franco I, Cagliostro S, Collett T, Reda E. The use of alpha blockers to treat urgency/frequency syndrome in children. San Francisco, CA: American Acadamey of Pediatrics Meeting; 2007.
19. Ishihama H, Momota Y, Yanase H, Wang X, de Groat WC, Kawatani M. Activation of alpha1D adrenergic receptors in the rat urothelium facilitates the micturition reflex. J Urol. 2006;175(1):358–64.
20. Somogyi GT, Tanowitz M, de Groat WC. Prejunctional facilitatory alpha 1-adrenoceptors in the rat urinary bladder. Br J Pharmacol. 1995;114(8):1710–6.
21. Szell EA, Yamamoto T, de Groat WC, Somogyi GT. Smooth muscle and parasympathetic nerve terminals in the rat urinary bladder have different subtypes of alpha(1) adrenoceptors. Br J Pharmacol. 2000;130(7):1685–91.
22. Athanasopoulos A, Gyftopoulos K, Giannitsas K, Fisfis J, Perimenis P, Barbalias G. Combination treatment with an alpha-blocker plus an anticholinergic for bladder outlet obstruction: a prospective, randomized, controlled study. J Urol. 2003;169(6):2253–6.
23. Van Batavia JP, Combs AJ, Horowitz M, et al. Primary bladder neck dysfunction in children and adolescents III: results of long-term alpha-blocker therapy. J Urol. 2010;183:724–30.
24. Van Batavia JP, Combs AJ, Hyun G, et al. Simplifying the diagnosis of 4 common voiding conditions using uroflow/electromyography, electromyography lag time and voiding history. J Urol. 2011;186(Suppl. 4):1721–6.
25. Andersson KE, Martin N, Nitti V. Selective beta(3)-adrenoceptor agonists for the treatment of overactive bladder. J Urol. 2013;190(4):1173–80.
26. Chapple CR, Cardozo L, Nitti VW, Siddiqui E, Michel MC. Mirabegron in overactive bladder: a review of efficacy, safety, and tolerability. Neurourol Urodyn. 2014;33(1):17–30.
27. Yamaguchi O, Marui E, Kakizaki H, Homma Y, Igawa Y, Takeda M, et al. Phase III, randomised, double-blind, placebo-controlled study of the beta3 -adrenoceptor agonist mirabegron, 50 mg once daily, in Japanese patients with overactive bladder. BJU Int. 2014;113(6):951–60.
28. Austin PF, Bauer SB. Chapter 27: Medical management of the neurogenic bladder. In: Pediatric incontinence; evaluation and clinical management. Chichester: John Wiley and Sons, Ltd; 2015. https://doi.org/10.1002/9781118814789.ch27.
29. Chase J, Austin PF, Hoebeke P, et al. The management of dysfunctional voiding in children: a report from the standardisation committee of the International children's continence society. J Urol. 2010;183:1296–302.
30. Thom M, Campigotto M, Vemulakonda V, et al. Management of lower urinary tract dysfunction: a stepwise approach. J Pediatr Urol. 2012;8:20–93.

Sacral Neuromodulation in Children

28

Ilaria Jansen, Ana Ludy Lopes Mendes,
Francesco Cappellano, Mario De Gennaro,
and Giovanni Mosiello

28.1 Introduction

The beneficial use of electrical current on central nervous system to activate neural structures facilitating neural plasticity and normative afferent and efferent activity of the lower urinary tract is well established. Different modalities of neuromodulation have been used in children, and the level of interest for treating bladder and bowel dysfunction (BBD) is increasing during time especially for sacral neuromodulation (SNM) [1, 2].

In fact stimulation of the parasympathetic nerves via the sacral micturition centre (spinal levels S2–S4) travels in the pelvic nerve resulting in contraction of the detrusor muscle (via release of the predominantly cholinergic transmitter) and relaxation of the sphincter thereby facilitating micturition.

I. Jansen
Department of Urology, AMC, Amsterdam, Netherlands

Department of Biomedical Engineering and Physics, AMC, Amsterdam, Netherlands

A.L. Lopes Mendes
Division of Urology, Surgery for Continence and Neuro-Urology, Bambino Gesù Pediatric Hospital, Rome, Italy
e-mail: olalu@hotmail.it

F. Cappellano
Department of Urologist, Nation Hospital, Abu Dhabi, UAE

Department of Neuro-Urology, Verona University, Verona, Italy

M. De Gennaro
Robotic and Urology Unit, Bambino Gesù Pediatric Hospital, Rome, Italy

G. Mosiello (✉)
Pediatric NeuroUrology Research and Clinic, Bambino Gesù Pediatric Hospital, Rome, Italy
e-mail: giovanni.mosiello@opbg.net

From the first description in 1988, a significant number of reports have been published, and SNM became rapidly a well-accepted treatment in adults. The Food and Drug Administration (FDA) in 1997 firstly approved the use of SNM in urological patients for the treatment of urge urinary incontinence. Successively, in 1999 SNM was approved for the treatment of urinary urgency-frequency and nonobstructive urinary retention and in 2012 for the treatment of adults with constipation and faecal incontinence [3–8]. Nowadays, SNM is also used in neurogenic bladder dysfunction (NBD). A systematic review, published by Kessler et al., analysed 26 independent studies stating that there is evidence that SNM may be effective in adults with neurogenic bladder (NB), even if it is still not possible to draw definitive conclusion [9]. On the 565 evaluated reports, 34 papers only were assessed for eligibility, because the other 531 were not referred to neurogenic LUTS. The obvious conclusion is that SNM is widely accepted and used in adults for refractory nonobstructive chronic urinary retention (NOUR), urge incontinence and urgency-frequency syndrome and in some cases could be successfully used in NBD. For these reasons it is surprising that the first prospective randomized controlled study evaluating the possible benefits of SNM in children has been performed in 2004 by Guys in NBD, because before that, only few paediatric cases have been reported in adults' series [10, 11].

The Guys' experience has been very important even if results showed a comparable results in terms of efficacy between patients treated with SNM and control group [10]. This paper stated SNM safety in paediatric age and suggested some critical points for increasing results, such as patient selection especially regarding severity of lesions and prospects for bringing to further successful experiences. Actually SNM is not a first-line treatment but rather a second or better third-line treatment for patients in which the conservative treatments have failed. During the past years, the technique of SNM has become less invasive, safer, reliable and effective thanks to technical improvements. The reoperation and complication rates decreased significantly, and the improved clinical results have expanded the possible indications. SNM is mainly used in children and young adults for overactive bladder (OAB), nonobstructive urinary retention (NOUR), pelvic pain and NBD.

28.2 Indications

In children presenting various degrees of LUTD including incontinence, overactive bladder and urinary retention not responding to conventional therapies, SNM provides an attractive option. Different neuroanatomical pathways have been described as targets for neuromodulation. The third sacral (S3) nerve root remains the main access point used for neuromodulation treatment. Anyway in the United States, the FDA has approved SNS and PTNS for the treatment of urological diseases, but SNM is not approved in children younger than 16 years. In Europe the age limits are not so strictly defined as in the United States, but the majority of experiences are mainly referred to post-puberal patients. For this reason failure to have relief of symptoms, after a trial of behavioural therapy and anticholinergic medications, is not sufficient to consider neuromodulation therapy in children as in adults [12]. Implantation in very young patient is generally avoided for several reasons such as the risk of electrode dislocation with stature growth during time, the reduced collaboration and the lack of a correct time to evaluate the efficacy of other treatments.

Inclusion criteria are age greater than 6 years old (school age), urinary incontinence requiring pads, continence status <90 min, post-void residual greater 50% than bladder capacity and filling pressure or leak point pressure or detrusor overactivity >40 cm H_2O, motivation of patient and caregivers.

Exclusion criteria for neuromodulation have still not clearly defined but include: sacral agenesis or severe sacral malformations, severe psychological problems and lack of motivation. Locating the nerve in obese patient is technically challenging; likewise, skeleton deformity could present similar challenges as well as scoliosis. Anyway a recent retrospective study showed similar results (progression to stage II implant) between obese and nonobese patients [13]. Older patients have been shown to be associated with a lower cure rate, but this means that they will be treated in adult age with theoretically a reduced percentage of success [14, 15].

Currently, MRI of the abdomen or pelvis is contraindicated with neuromodulation owing to concerns regarding dislocation of the device, changes to the programme caused by the magnetic fields and heating of the metal electrodes. The findings of recent studies suggest that MRI can be safely performed outside of the pelvis. In young female adults, pregnancy must be considered, because pregnant women should not undergo neuromodulation treatment owing to the theoretical risk of foetal loss or preterm labour [16, 17]. If pregnancy is detected after a device has been placed, it should be turned off during pregnancy and restarted after the delivery [18].

28.3 Patients Selection

All the patients must be assessed through history taken and physical examination, including genitalia, anus, rectum and neurological examination. Also an accurate records of 3–7 days voiding diary, urodynamics and neurophysiological measurement in order to confirm the diagnosis and determine whether to accept the preliminary suitable candidates for SNS therapy are generally done in several centres. Video urodynamics has more advantages than conventional urodynamics in choosing whether to propose the SNM. In addition, urinalysis, urine culture, urinary tract ultrasonography, cystoscopy urethra and bladder wash cytology examination should be taken before the treatment to rule out other diseases. In our experience, started in 2008, we used to perform in all patients a psychological evaluation, either in NBD or in non-neurogenic LUTD. Psychological evaluation seems to be useful evaluating the psychological status of patients and helps as well to define in adolescents the choice to perform the surgical procedure in general or local anaesthesia. In neurological condition or NOUR, we have always performed preoperatively neurophysiologic tests (somatosensory evoked potentials) and the evaluation of ASIA impairment scale in order to determine the less neurologically involved side, if present. This data is useful in children, because during the surgical procedure, we prefer to start to stimulate the S3 side according to the preoperative evaluation, considering always the less-damaged side as first choice. The clinical and urodynamic evaluation are useful to assess sensation of bladder filling, end-filling detrusor pressure (EFDP), detrusor pressure at maximum flow (DPM), voided volume (VVol), maximum flow (Qmax), post-voided residue (PVR), urinary frequency (Freq), urinary incontinence (Leak) and number of pads and catheterizations/day (CIC). The clinical response, defining responders from nonresponders, will be more useful at first step of treatment, during two-stage implant: patient and caregivers' satisfaction and one or more of the following criteria: <50% incontinence episodes, <50% post-voiding residual, <50% of necessity for CIC, >50% voided volume or presence of bladder sensation [19].

28.4 Surgical Technique

In adults the SNM procedure is performed generally in two stages: the acute stimulation stage I to elicited appropriate responses and a subsequent definitive implant stage II. In paediatric series some authors performed the two stages in the same general anaesthesia, resulting in one-stage procedure. Our choice has been always for the two stages SNM procedure, as in adult series.

Generally children above 12 years old or older underwent stimulation test phase I (first stage), under local anaesthesia. This permits to consider either motor responses (great toe flexion and anus contraction), either sensory response as paraesthesia in genital or anal area. General anaesthesia is considered especially in younger children or less collaborative, according to preoperative evaluation.

Patients are placed in prone position with hips and knees folded in order to have the sacrum horizontally and the best image of contractions (Fig. 28.1a).

The anatomic borders and landmarks of the sacrum are marked: the base (by following the iliac crest medially), the apex (with the sacrococcygeal articulation), the medial sacral crest (in the dorsal midline) and the sacral hiatus. Using a foramen needle, the third sacral foramen is located percutaneously using the previous

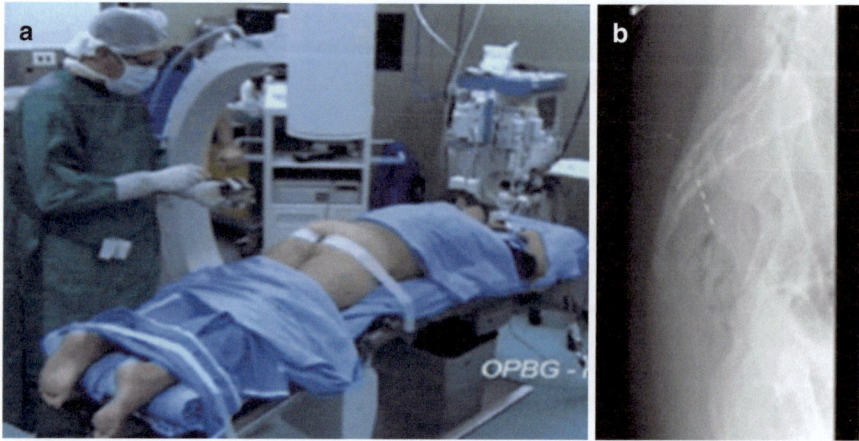

Fig. 28.1 Implant of SNM. (**a**) Patient in prone position with folded hips. (**b**) Third sacral foramen is located and the lead is left in place

described landmarks or with the help of an anterior-posterior fluoroscopy (Fig. 28.1b). The S3 nerve is then located by moving the needle with 60% inclination. The test of the nerve response is than performed with increasing the intensity of the stimulation. We always have used tined quadripolar lead (Medtronic 3889 model, Minneapolis MN, USA) instead of temporary wire (Medtronic 3057 model, Minneapolis, MN, USA) because: reduced risk of migration or displacement, possible longer testing period, not change of the electrode during the second step, reducing operative time, and performing permanent stimulation in the same position. During operation in the different steps (needle insertion, dilation, insertion of quadripolar electrode), again fluoroscopic control can be useful, in lateral vision, in order to define and maintain the correct needle depth for the correct placement during all the implant steps.

During operation we evaluated the intraoperative response in order to decide if proceed with the implant of electrode and in which side. We never performed a bilateral implant. We always started with the side selected preoperatively, and if the motor and/or sensitive answer is not satisficing, we usually proceed evaluating the contralateral.

The external pulse generator, used during the test phase, is connected to the electrode with a temporary extension and is usually activated 1–6 h after implantation.

Usually patients are discharged home 12–24 h after the procedure, depending on general status and postoperative pain level. In our experience the test phase ranges from 15 days up to 3 months, on average of 4 weeks. Continuous stimulation is generally started at 210 ms, 16 Hz frequency and 2 V amplitude and during the follow-up period is set, especially for amplitude 1–10 V and frequency 10–20 Hz.

During the test phase, patients underwent urodynamic test are asked to fill out a valuation diary, bladder and bowel and a QoL questionnaire. Patients are then evaluated based on satisfaction and one or more of the following criteria: <50% incontinence episodes, <50% post-voiding residual, <50% of necessity for CIC and >50% of increased voided volume. Urodynamic test is considered for decision in controversial clinical situation. The patients who successfully passed the test phase, according to the criteria listed above, and who were compliant with the therapy proceeded to the second phase during which the extension is removed and the same electrode is connected to the definitive permanent stimulator (Interstim II, Medtronic, Minneapolis MN, USA) (Fig. 28.2).

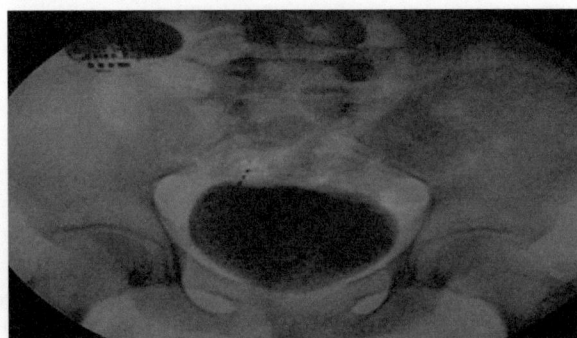

Fig. 28.2 Evidence of SNM in patient during urinary cystography

The follow-up is taken at 2 weeks, 3 months, 6 months and then once every 6 months after the implant of SNM for the first 3 years than ones a years. At the moment no consensus is reported for the follow-up time.

Each follow-up consultation should cover physical examination, voiding diary, programmed stimulation parameters detected and/or adjustment.

28.5 Discussion

The first published study on sacral neuromodulation in children with NBD was done by Guys et al. [10]. A prospective randomized study was performed, and 42 patients were enrolled, mainly with spina bifida (SB), where they compared urodynamic outcomes and incontinence. Various treatments have been used before inclusion in the study. Statistical analysis of the two patient groups included in the study and demonstrated no difference regarding gender, median age and urodynamic variables such as compliance, functional bladder capacity, bladder filling, leak point pressure, bladder activity and PVR. Twenty-one children received an implant, and 21 children were in the control group. All patients in the control group were treated with oxybutynin with dosage adjusted according to age and a maximal dose of 15 mg daily.

Comparison of urodynamic variables at each study time disclosed no statistical difference between the implant and control groups, regarding the compliance, bladder filling pressure and PVR. A significant increase ($p < 0.05$) in leak point pressure was noted in patients treated with SNM at 3, 6, 9 and 12 months. Controversially at the end of the study, functional bladder capacity was significantly greater in the control group.

Evaluation of interindividual variations in the implant group disclosed that compliance and functional bladder capacity were significantly greater at 6 and 9 months but not at 12 months. Total bladder capacity also increased significantly. However, there was no measurable improvement in bladder filling pressure and PVR. Nine patients in the implant group reported improvement in intestinal transit (evaluated from diary data), five total disappearance of urinary infection and six sensation of a full bladder. No patient in the control group reported subjective improvement.

Further experiences reported successful results in non-neurogenic lower urinary tract dysfunction [19]. Humphreys et al. reported in a group of 23 patients an improvement ranging between 60 and 83% in urinary symptoms and an 80% in bowel dysfunction [20]. Later, analysing 105 patients, the results continue to be encouraging with 66–88% improvement note for the above conditions [21]. Roth in 2008 reported improvement of 88% of incontinence, 69% of urgency, 89% of frequency in nocturnal enuresis and 71% of constipation in 20 patients. Complications were seen in 20% of cases [22].

In 2010 Haddad M et al. published a prospective, randomized, open-label, crossover study on sacral neuromodulation in children older than 5 years old with urinary and faecal incontinence [23]. The neuromodulators were implanted in a total of 33 patients, and the children were randomly divided in two groups. The neuromodulators group A were 6 months ON, followed by 6 months OFF, and the neuromodulator group B had the opposite sequence. The two phases were separated by 45 days to return to baseline status. Nineteen patients presented both faecal and urinary incontinence, nine patients urinary incontinence only and in five cases faecal incontinence only. Patients were classified as responders or nonresponders regarding urinary and faecal performance after each phase of the ON and OFF sequence. Response was defined as resolution of urinary leakage and/or faecal soiling with no need for pads or a decrease of more than 50% in the number of leaks and/or soiling with minimum protection needed between the beginning and end of each sequence. Overall positive response rate was more than 75% for urinary (81%) and bowel (81%) function. They concluded that sacral neuromodulation is more effective than conservative treatment for both types of incontinence [23].

A retrospective study performed in Gent University group reported by Groen et al. includes 18 patients, of which, 5 children presented neurogenic bladder. The SNM was introduced to treat dysfunctional elimination syndrome, neurogenic bladder, bladder overactivity and even for Fowler's syndrome [19].

Criteria for IPG placement were 50% reduction of incontinence episodes, 50% PVR volume, 50% reduction of necessity for CIC and 50% improvement in urinary frequency.

Outcome was defined as: full response, in case of 100% patient satisfaction and greater than 90% objective improvement for at least one implantation criterion; partial response, if patient were satisfied and 50–90% objective improvement has seen for at least one implantation criterion and, failure, if less than 50% objective improvement or no patient satisfaction were reported. The initial full response was achieved in 50% of patients and partial response in 28%.

The patient with anal atresia had a full response, with greater than 90% decrease in incontinence episodes, and the patient with Guillain-Barré syndrome had less urgency, incontinence and enuresis [19].

Van Wunnik et al. in 2012 presented their results in 13 girls aged between 10 and 18 years old, all presenting functional constipation according to Rome III criteria and not responding to oral and rectal treatment. After implantation 11/13 presented spontaneous defecation (none before treatment) [24].

The implant of SNM is not devoid of complications, in fact, the most common complication reported in literature are pain in the implantation side, wound infections, generator problems, migrations of the device, battery depletion and bowel problems [10, 19, 21, 23].

In conclusion, SNM up to now has been reported mostly in small series, as a second- or third-line treatment in patients not responding to conventional treatment. SNM seems to be a safe reversible treatment, with reduced invasiveness and effective in a high percentage of well-selected patients. Reported changes on bladder function with neuromodulation include significantly increased bladder capacity, decreased severity of urgency, improved continence and decreased frequency of urinary tract infection. Significant improvement in urodynamic parameters such us bladder compliance, number of involuntary contractions and bladder volume at first detrusor contraction have also been noted. For bowel dysfunction, a very high percentage of patients presented improvement of symptoms. General limits in these studies are the minimal standardization of populations and different clinical protocol, including implant technique and outcome measures. For these reasons, SNM in children needs further controlled and randomized studies, evaluating the possibility of introducing this treatment as a first-line choice in children with bladder-bowel dysfunction and define criteria for optimal indications and predict efficacy.

References

1. Barroso U Jr, Tourinho R, Lordelo P, Hoebeke P, Chase J. Electrical stimulation for lower urinary tract dysfunction in children: a systematic review of the literature. Neurourol Urodyn. 2011;30(8):1429–36. PubMed PMID: 21717502
2. De Gennaro M, Capitanucci ML, Mosiello G, Zaccara A. Current state of nerve stimulation technique for lower urinary tract dysfunction in children. J Urol. 2011;185(5):1571–7. PubMed PMID: 21419450
3. Tanagho EA. Neural stimulation for bladder control. Semin Neurol. 1988;8(2):170–3. PubMed PMID: 3055124
4. Herbison GP, Arnold EP. Sacral neuromodulation with implanted devices for urinary storage and voiding dysfunction in adults. Cochrane Database Syst Rev. 2009;2:CD004202. PubMed PMID: 19370596
5. Kessler TM, Buchser E, Meyer S, Engeler DS, Al-Khodairy AW, Bersch U, et al. Sacral neuromodulation for refractory lower urinary tract dysfunction: results of a nationwide registry in Switzerland. Eur Urol. 2007;51(5):1357–63. PubMed PMID: 17113216
6. van Kerrebroeck PE, van Voskuilen AC, Heesakkers JP, Lycklama a Nijholt AA, Siegel S, Jonas U, et al. Results of sacral neuromodulation therapy for urinary voiding dysfunction: outcomes of a prospective, worldwide clinical study. J Urol. 2007;178(5):2029–34. PubMed PMID: 17869298
7. Thomas GP, Dudding TC, Rahbour G, Nicholls RJ, Vaizey CJ. Sacral nerve stimulation for constipation. Br J Surg. 2013;100(2):174–81. PubMed PMID: 23124687
8. Weil EH, Ruiz-Cerda JL, Eerdmans PH, Janknegt RA, Bemelmans BL, van Kerrebroeck PE. Sacral root neuromodulation in the treatment of refractory urinary urge incontinence: a prospective randomized clinical trial. Eur Urol. 2000;37(2):161–71. PubMed PMID: 10705194
9. Kessler TM, La Framboise D, Trelle S, Fowler CJ, Kiss G, Pannek J, et al. Sacral neuromodulation for neurogenic lower urinary tract dysfunction: systematic review and meta-analysis. Eur Urol. 2010;58(6):865–74. PubMed PMID: 20934242
10. Guys JM, Haddad M, Planche D, Torre M, Louis-Borrione C, Breaud J. Sacral neuromodulation for neurogenic bladder dysfunction in children. J Urol. 2004;172(4 Pt 2):1673–6. PubMed PMID: 15371787
11. Tanagho EA. Neuromodulation in the management of voiding dysfunction in children. J Urol. 1992;148(2 Pt 2):655–7. PubMed PMID: 1640540
12. Fulton M, Peters KM. Neuromodulation for voiding dysfunction and fecal incontinence: a urology perspective. Urol Clin North Am. 2012;39(3):405–12. PubMed PMID: 22877724
13. Levin PJ, Wu JM, Siddiqui NY, Amundsen CL. Does obesity impact the success of an InterStim test phase for the treatment of refractory urge urinary incontinence in female patients? Female Pelvic Med Reconstr Surg. 2012;18(4):243–6. PubMed PMID: 22777375
14. Amundsen CL, Romero AA, Jamison MG, Webster GD. Sacral neuromodulation for intractable urge incontinence: are there factors associated with cure? Urology. 2005;66(4):746–50. PubMed PMID: 16230129
15. Lombardi G, Del Popolo G. Clinical outcome of sacral neuromodulation in incomplete spinal cord injured patients suffering from neurogenic lower urinary tract symptoms. Spinal Cord. 2009;47(6):486–91. PubMed PMID: 19238164

16. Chermansky CJ, Krlin RM, Holley TD, Woo HH, Winters JC. Magnetic resonance imaging following InterStim(R): an institutional experience with imaging safety and patient satisfaction. Neurourol Urodyn. 2011;30(8):1486–8. PubMed PMID: 21780166
17. van der Jagt PK, Dik P, Froeling M, Kwee TC, Nievelstein RA, ten Haken B, et al. Architectural configuration and microstructural properties of the sacral plexus: a diffusion tensor MRI and fiber tractography study. NeuroImage. 2012;62(3):1792–9. PubMed PMID: 22705377
18. Bartley J, Gilleran J, Peters K. Neuromodulation for overactive bladder. Nat Rev Urol. 2013;10(9):513–21. PubMed PMID: 23817408
19. Groen LA, Hoebeke P, Loret N, Van Praet C, Van Laecke E, Ann R, et al. Sacral neuromodulation with an implantable pulse generator in children with lower urinary tract symptoms: 15-year experience. J Urol. 2012;188(4):1313–7. PubMed PMID: 22902022
20. Humphreys MR, Vandersteen DR, Slezak JM, Hollatz P, Smith CA, Smith JE, et al. Preliminary results of sacral neuromodulation in 23 children. J Urol. 2006;176(5):2227–31. PubMed PMID: 17070300
21. Dwyer ME, Vandersteen DR, Hollatz P, Reinberg YE. Sacral neuromodulation for the dysfunctional elimination syndrome: a 10-year single-center experience with 105 consecutive children. Urology. 2014;84(4):911–7. PubMed PMID: 25096339
22. Roth TJ, Vandersteen DR, Hollatz P, Inman BA, Reinberg YE. Sacral neuromodulation for the dysfunctional elimination syndrome: a single center experience with 20 children. J Urol. 2008;180(1):306–11. discussion 11. PubMed PMID: 18499169
23. Haddad M, Besson R, Aubert D, Ravasse P, Lemelle J, El Ghoneimi A, et al. Sacral neuromodulation in children with urinary and fecal incontinence: a multicenter, open label, randomized, crossover study. J Urol. 2010;184(2):696–701. PubMed PMID: 20561645
24. van Wunnik BP, Peeters B, Govaert B, Nieman FH, Benninga MA, Baeten CG. Sacral neuromodulation therapy: a promising treatment for adolescents with refractory functional constipation. Dis Colon Rectum. 2012;55(3):278–85. PubMed PMID: 22469794

Bowel Dysfunction Management

29

Giuseppe Masnata, Valeria Manca, Laura Chia, and Francesca Esu

The term "bowel dysfunction" includes constipation, diarrhoea, faecal incontinence, inability to control bowel movements and rectal bleeding. The gastrointestinal and genito-urinary tract share several aspects, including the same embryonic origin, the same pelvic position, the same innervation and the same relation between pelvic floor and levator ani muscle.

The frequency of bowel movements in childhood decreases by an average of four per day in the first week of life, to 1.7 per day from the age of 2. During this period the stool volume increases up to ten times or more [1].

Respectively in the UK only the 34% of toddlers and in Brazil the 37% of children younger than 12 years old were defined constipated by their parents [2].

In absence of painful symptoms, parents often don't take into account the bowel habits of children older than 4/5 years, and they pay less attention to the frequency of their children's bowel movements while more to the urinary and faecal incontinence episodes [3].

Bladder bowel dysfunction (BBD) is a generic expression to describe children with lower urinary tract symptoms (LUTS) associated with intestinal dysfunction. In this clinical condition, bladder symptoms, such as urinary urgency, incontinence and urinary tract infections (UTI), are related to problems in bladder voiding. Commonly, constipation with or without faecal incontinence coexists with dysfunctional voiding as a result of non-relaxation of the pelvic muscle floor [3].

The International Children's Continence Society (ICCS) recommends the use of the Rome III Criteria for the diagnosis of functional disorders of evacuation in children (Table 29.1).

G. Masnata (✉) • V. Manca • L. Chia • F. Esu
Pediatric Urology Unit and Spina Bifida Center, Brotzu Hospital, Cagliari, Italy
e-mail: giuseppemasnata@gmail.com; valeria.manca@gmail.com; lauretta.chia@gmail.com; franci.esu@libero.it

© Springer International Publishing AG, part of Springer Nature 2018
G. Mosiello et al. (eds.), *Clinical Urodynamics in Childhood and Adolescence*, Urodynamics, Neurourology and Pelvic Floor Dysfunctions,
https://doi.org/10.1007/978-3-319-42193-3_29

Table 29.1 Rome III functional constipation diagnostic criteria in children

Diagnostic criteria[a] must include two or more of the following in a child with a developmental age of at least 4 years with insufficient criteria for diagnosis of IBS:
- Two or fewer defecations in the toilet per week
- At least one episode of faecal incontinence per week
- History of retentive posturing or excessive volitional stool retention
- History of painful or hard bowel movements
- Presence of a large faecal mass in the rectum
- History of large diameter stools which may obstruct the toilet

[a]Criteria fulfilled at least once per week for at least 2 months prior to diagnosis

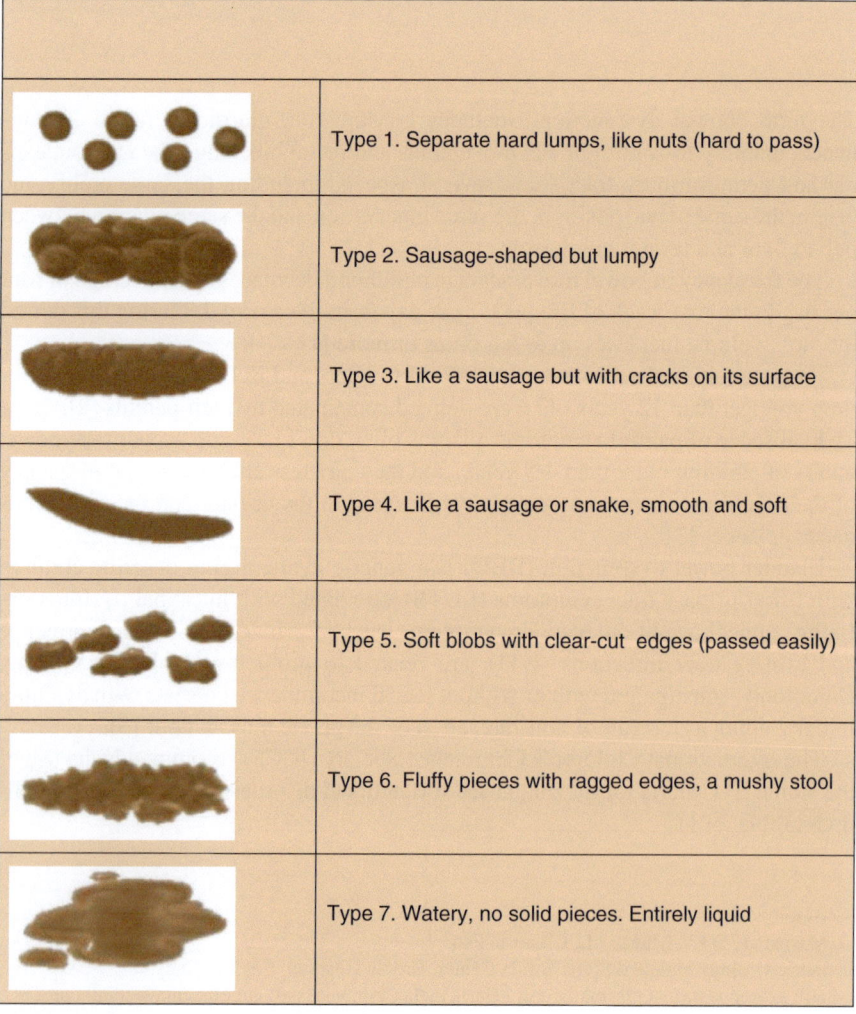

Fig. 29.1 Bristol Stool Form Scale

We define constipation when the bowel movements are less than three per week, stools are hard and the evacuation is irregular and painful [4].

The Bristol Stool Form Scale (BSFS) represents a practical instrument extremely useful for the diagnosis and for the evaluation of the therapy response (Fig. 29.1).

In most children constipation is caused by bad eating habits. The result is the creation of hard stools, the reduction in frequency of bowel movements and abdominal pain that brings to voluntary refusal of evacuation. In other cases constipation is a chronic process in which the child, who is approaching the use of toilet and a voluntary faecal continence, has the tendency to retain the stools because of the unavailability of toilet or because occupied by games [5, 6].

Faecal incontinence usually is the result of leakage of loose stool that pass sideways to the hard stools present in the rectum. The loss occurs every time the child try to expel gases, and the muscles used to retain the stools do not ensure continence. Faecal incontinence is from three to six times more common among male than in female children. It has a significant impact in children's quality of life (QoL) with a resulting loss of self-esteem, social isolation and depression [1].

The dilation of the rectum is caused by the presence of hard stools, which compress also the bladder. Furthermore, frequent pelvic spasms prevent full relaxation during urination and lead to an early termination of it with post-void residual. Klijn M et al. highlighted as in children with constipation and LUTS the average diameter of the rectal ampulla is 4.9 cm while in the control group is 2.1 cm [7]. Chronic constipation occurs in neurogenic bowel dysfunction (NBD), peripheral or central, such as spina bifida and spinal cord injuries. Faecal incontinence and constipation associated with myelomeningocele, anorectal malformations and Hirschsprung's disease are common, debilitating and difficult to treat.

29.1 Bowel Dysfunction Management in Children

The treatment of constipation is different in infants and children. The European Society for Paediatric Gastroenterology Hepatology and Nutrition (ESPGHAN) developed the guidelines and suggested to standardize the quality of health care, improving the evaluation and treatment of children with functional constipation. They also developed two algorithms: one for children <6 months of age and one for older children. The ESPGHAN insists on using the Rome III Criteria for classifying functional constipation. Children under 4 years should satisfy two of the criteria for at least 1 month, while those with more than 4 years should satisfy two of the criteria for at least 2 months. Abdominal pain, which is often associated, is not considered a criterion of functional constipation [8].

Functional constipation is often treated in infant with a high-fibre diet and regularization of water intake. If these measures are not successful, it is suggested the occasional administration of glycerin suppositories, which should be used carefully because they can cause anal irritation.

The treatment of chronic constipation and faecal incontinence in children requires a comprehensive programme, including the use of laxatives, toilet training and a proper diet [9].

The treatment of chronic constipation requires a complete voiding of the colon, in order to create a "working memory" and to make the intestine autonomous. The goal of the therapy is the passage of loose stools, preferably once per day.

During the treatment it is important to combine a diet that includes more fruits, raw vegetables, bran, whole bread, cereals and an adequate intake of liquids other than milk [8].

The use of probiotics to treat constipation in children is not supported by controlled trials in children and adults. They are defined as live microorganisms which, if given in adequate amounts, confer benefit to the host. Therapy with probiotics may be indicated together with other therapies.

Treatment with laxatives and toilet training is widely discussed in literature. Some studies support the combined use of both therapies [10, 11]. Some others support the laxative therapy as more effective than toilet training.

ESPGHAN and NASPGHAN suggest the use of polyethylene glycol (PEG without electrolytes—3350) from the first months of life. The treatment is generally effective and shows no side effects. The maintenance effective dose is about 0.8 g/kg of body weight per day [12].

The diagnostic and therapeutic approach to children with BBD should include the bladder voiding by bladder diary and the contemporary evaluation of constipation with BSFS (Fig. 29.1). Once anatomical abnormalities are excluded, behavioural therapy is generally regarded as the first-line treatment. The posture, the appropriate position on the toilet and the controlled voiding are the key points for the treatment of voiding dysfunction, associated with a proper bowel emptying [13].

Today an increasingly used technique is transanal irrigation of the bowel with appropriate devices as the Peristeen® irrigation kit (Coloplast A/S, Kokkedal, Denmark). This is particularly indicated in patients affected with neurogenic problems since their birth and all cases of chronic constipation or resistant to conventional therapy. Several studies demonstrated the effectiveness of transanal irrigation in reducing constipation, improving anal continence and improving QoL.

A randomized study compared transanal irrigation with best supportive bowel management without irrigation. As a result transanal irrigation significantly reduces the time of bowel management (47 vs. 74 min/day) and the rate of urinary tract infections and improves symptoms during and/or after defecation [14]. This procedure is relatively safe. The most severe complication is the risk of intestinal perforation, which occurs in 1 over 50,000 irrigations (0.002% of cases). Therefore transanal irrigation is not indicated in patients with bowel obstruction, inflammatory bowel disease and diverticulitis or in cases of recent abdomino-perineal surgery.

Patients with NBD can be treated in several ways. First of all, a conservative approach is suggested: the change of diet, drugs, electrical stimulation treatment, biofeedback and transanal irrigation. If conservative treatment is not effective, clinicians can suggest surgical procedures as MACE (Malone Anterograde Continence Enemas), colostomies and artificial bowel sphincters.

The antegrade delivery of cleansing solutions helps the patient to evacuate regularly the colon, avoid impaction of faeces and reduce faecal incontinence. Six open retrospective studies in children suggest how MACE can be an option in children with intractable constipation. Potential complication should be considered and examined with parents and children, as the development of granulation tissue, leakage around the tube, tube dislodgment, skin infection and stoma stenosis [8].

All these different approaches, conservatives or surgical, can be combined for better effectiveness and tailored on a single patient.

References

1. Abi-Hanna A, Lake AM. Constipation and encopresis in childhood. Pediatr Rev. 1998;19(1):23–31.
2. Loening-Baucke V. Urinary incontinence and urinary tract infection and their resolution with treatment of chronic constipation of childhood. Pediatrics. 1997;100(2, Part 1):228–32.
3. Halachmi S, Farhat WA. Interactions of constipation, dysfunctional elimination syndrome, and vesicoureteral reflux. Adv Urol. 2008;2008:828275.
4. Burgers RE, Mugie SM, Chase J, Cooper CS, von Gontard A, et al. Management of functional constipation in children with lower urinary tract symptoms: report from the standardization committee of the International children's continence society. J Urol. 2013;190:29–36.
5. Issenman RM, Filmer RB, Gorski PA. A review of bowel and bladder control development in children: how gastrointestinal and urologic conditions relate to problems in toilet training. Pediatrics. 1999;103(6, Part 2):1346–52.
6. Solzi G, Di Lorenzo C. Are constipated children different from constipated adults? Dig Dis. 1999;17(5–6):308–15.
7. Klijn AJ, Asselman M, Vijverberg MAW, Dik P, de Jong TPVM. The diameter of the rectum on ultrasonography as a diagnostic tool for constipation in children with dysfunctional voiding. J Urol. 2004;172(5, Part 1):1986–8.
8. Tabbers MM, DiLorenzo C, Berger MY, et al. Evaluation and treatment of functional constipation in infants and children: evidence-based recommendations from ESPGHAN and NASPGHAN. J Pediatr Gastroenterol Nutr. 2014;58:258.
9. Brazzelli M, Griffiths PV, Cody JD, Tappin D. Behavioural and cognitive interventions with or without other treatments for the management of faecal incontinence in children. Cochrane Database Syst Rev. 2011;12:CD002240.
10. Loening-Baucke V. Controversies in the management of chronic constipation. J Pediatr Gastroenterol Nutr. 2001;32(Suppl 1):S38.
11. Brooks RC, Copen RM, Cox DJ, et al. Review of the treatment literature for encopresis, functional constipation, and stool-toileting refusal. Ann Behav Med. 2000;22:260.
12. Abrams P, Andersson KE, Birder L, Brubaker L, Cardozo L, Chapple C, et al. Members of Committees, Fourth International Consultation on Incontinence. Fourth international consultation on incontinence recommendations of the International Scientific Committee: evaluation and treatment of urinary incontinence, pelvic organ prolapse, and fecal incontinence. Neurourol Urodyn. 2010;29:213–40.
13. Dos Santos J, Varghese A, Williams K, Koyle MA. Recommendations for the management of bladder bowel dysfunction in children. Pediat Therapeut. 2014;4:1.
14. Christensen P, Bazzocchi G, Coggrave M, et al. A randomized, controlled trial of transanal irrigation versus conservative bowel management in spinal cord-injured patients. Gastroenterology. 2006;131:738–47.

Percutaneous Tibial Nerve Stimulation (PTNS) and Transcutaneous Electrical Nerve Stimulation (TENS)

30

Maria Luisa Capitanucci, Giovanni Mosiello, and Mario De Gennaro

30.1 Introduction

Among different neuromodulation techniques, transcutaneous electrical nerve stimulation (TENS) and percutaneous tibial nerve stimulation (PTNS) offer minimally invasive, nonsurgical, and reversible second-line means to treat lower urinary tract dysfunctions (LUTD) in children [1]. Using perineal, suprapubic, or sacral surface electrodes, TENS has been widely popularized to treat refractory overactive bladder (OAB) in children [2–9]. Several nonrandomized (NRCT) and randomized controlled trials (RCT) have been done, confirming efficacy of TENS in children with OAB [10–13]. Peripheral tibial nerve stimulation was initially tested in clinical trial more than 25 years ago [14]. RCT in adult patients upgraded PTNS to level 1 of evidence [14, 15]. These landmark reports led to resurgent interest in PTNS as a potential treatment option also in children with refractory LUTD. However, since needle insertion is required to perform PTNS, few experiences have been reported with this technique in children. Published uncontrolled cohort studies seem to indicate good tolerability [16] and efficacy [17, 18] of PTNS in children with OAB and dysfunctional voiding (DV). Recently, encouraging urodynamic results were obtained with stimulation of posterior tibial nerve through surface electrodes (*transcutaneous* posterior tibial nerve stimulation) [19], offering a noninvasive alternative to the classical PTNS technique.

M.L. Capitanucci, M.D. (✉) • M. De Gennaro, M.D.
Urology, Robotic Surgery and Urodynamic Unit—Department of Surgery,
Children's Hospital Bambino Gesu', Rome, Italy
e-mail: mluisa.capitanucci@opbg.net; mario.degennaro@opbg.net

G. Mosiello, M.D.
Pediatric NeuroUrology Research and Clinic, Bambino Gesù Pediatric Hospital, Rome, Italy
e-mail: giovanni.mosiello@opbg.net

© Springer International Publishing AG, part of Springer Nature 2018
G. Mosiello et al. (eds.), *Clinical Urodynamics in Childhood and Adolescence*,
Urodynamics, Neurourology and Pelvic Floor Dysfunctions,
https://doi.org/10.1007/978-3-319-42193-3_30

30.2 Technique

Technique of PTNS was described by Stoller in the late 1990s [1]. PTNS device was approved by FDA in 2006. PTNS is performed by means of a 34 gauge needle electrode inserted 4–5 cm cephalad to the medial malleolus (Fig. 30.1). When current is applied, flexion of big toe or movement of other toes confirms correct electrode positioning. The electric current is a continuous, square wave form with a duration of 200 μs and a frequency of 20 Hz. Current intensity is the highest level tolerated by patient. Generally, sessions last for 30 min and are done once a week for 12 weeks. However, a more frequent stimulation and/or a shortened treatment program seems to guarantee similar positive results in adult patients [1]. Since needle insertion is required, PTNS is performed in outpatient clinic.

TENS may be performed using perineal, suprapubic, or sacral surface electrode. Since stimulation of anal and genital regions cannot be considered a noninvasive method in children, this technique should be used with great caution especially in non-neurogenic patients. Suprapubic technique has not been popularized as sacral one, which work through a direct stimulation of S3 region (Fig. 30.2). Frequency and duration of sacral stimulation by TENS are variable between different experiences [3–13]. However, in recent RCT [12, 13], sacral stimulation was done 20 min 3 times per week on alternate days with a frequency of 10 Hz, pulse width of 700 ms, and intensity determined by the sensitivity threshold of the child; the number of TENS sessions ranged

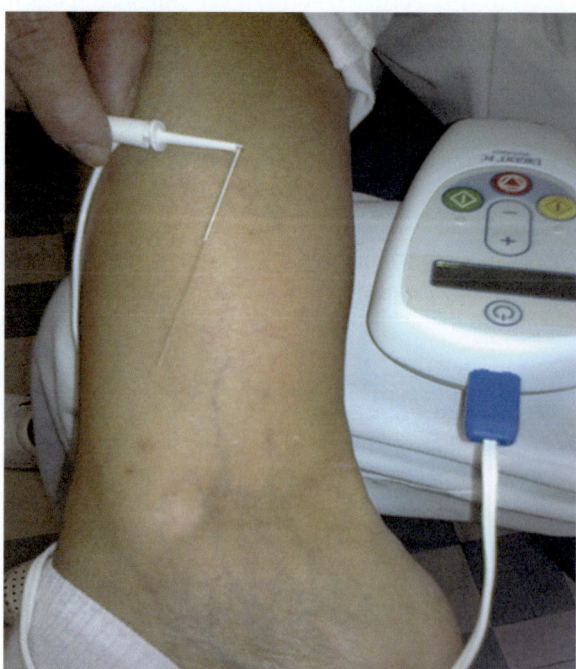

Fig. 30.1 PTNS technique: a fine needle is inserted 4–5 cm cephalad to the medial malleolus

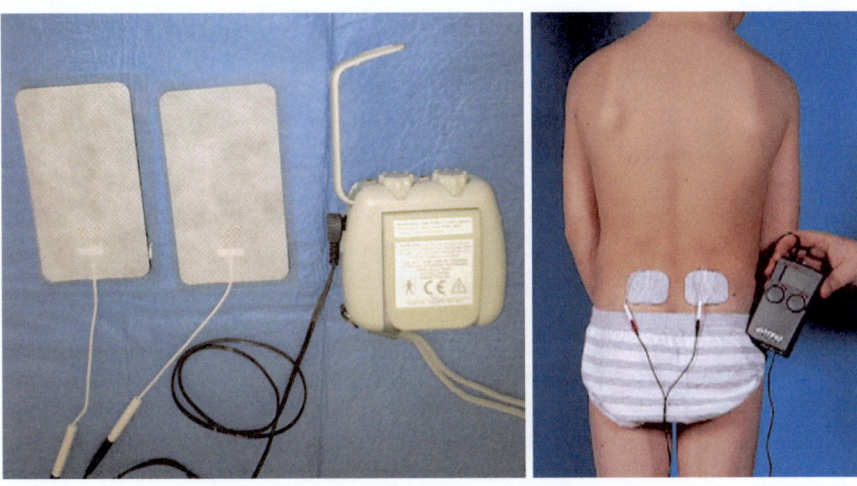

Fig. 30.2 Transcutaneous electrical nerve stimulation with sacral surface electrodes

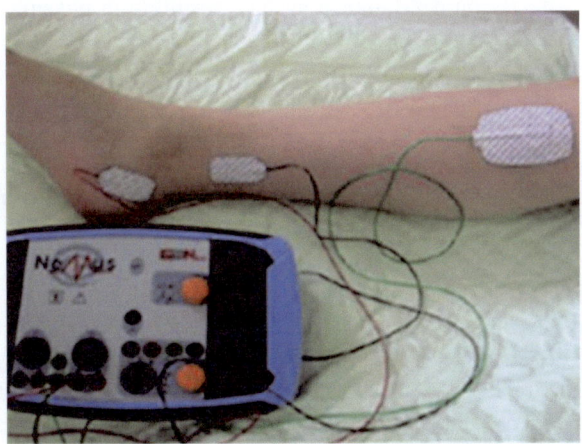

Fig. 30.3 Transcutaneous posterior tibial nerve stimulation in children. Image from Boudaud N, Binet A, Line A et al. (2015). Management of refractory overactive bladder in children by transcutaneous posterior tibial nerve stimulation: a controlled study. J Ped Urol, 11: 138e1–138e10

from 10 to 20 [12, 13]. Differently from PTNS, TENS can be easily performed at home, being a transcutaneous stimulation by means of surface electrodes.

Since transcutaneous stimulation has several advantages (simple, noninvasive, painless, and easy to use at home) with respect to percutaneous one, transcutaneous posterior tibial nerve stimulation (TPTNS) has been recently tested by Boudaud et al. [19]. TPTNS was performed through two surface electrodes placed above and below the medial malleolus; an earth surface electrode was placed over the same area (Fig. 30.3). Two 30 min sessions a week for 12 consecutive weeks were done with a continuous stimulation of 200 μs, a frequency of 10 Hz, and a current intensity below the pain threshold [19].

30.3 Mechanism of Action

Posterior tibial nerve is a peripheral mixed nerve (L4-S3), which also contributes to sensory and motor control of bladder-sphincter complex. Even if several studies have tried to better clarify mechanism of action of PTNS, it still remains unclear. The main neurophysiological mechanism of PTNS could be bladder activity modulation by depolarizing somatic sacral and lumbar afferent fibers [1]. An effect on supraspinal centers has also been demonstrated by Finazzi-Agro'et al. [20] who found significant increase in long latency somatosensory evoked potential amplitude after the end of PTNS program. This finding could reflect a modification in elaboration mechanism of sensory stimuli, suggesting a possible reorganization of cortical excitability after PTNS. A peripheral effect on the bladder has also been hypothesized by Danisman who demonstrated reduction of mast cell count in an animal model [1].

TENS acts directly on neurological system, resulting in physiological changes that lead to neural reconditioning [12]. Its therapeutic effect is achieved through the recovery of cerebral activity associated with self-regulation and attenuation of activity of the cingulated gyrus, renerving partially denervated fibers [21].

30.4 Effectiveness of PTNS and TENS in Pediatric Lower Urinary Tract Dysfunction

Only prospective NRCT (level of evidence 2–3) are available for PTNS as treatment for refractory LUTD in children (Table 30.1). In 2002, Hoebeke et al. published the first pilot study on PTNS in pediatric OAB [5]. The authors found reasonable efficacy of PTNS and patient compliance (Table 30.1). Successively, our group studied and confirmed the good tolerability of PTNS in children, evaluating level and type of pain at needle insertion and during stimulation [4]. Relevant improvement rate was found in both children with OAB

Table 30.1 PTNS in children with lower urinary tract dysfunction

Author, year	Pts.	Study type	LUTD	% Clinical outcome	% UD outcome
Hoebeke P, 2002 [17]	32	NRCT	OAB	25 cured 35 improved	– –
De Gennaro M, 2004 [16]	23	NRCT	OAB DV NB	80 improved 71 improved No improvement	62.5 normal BC 50 normal PVR No improvement
Capitanucci ML, 2009 [18]	44	NRCT	OAB DV	41 cured 71 cured	33 normal Vvol 57 normal PVR

OAB overactive bladder, *DV* dysfunctional voiding, *NB* neurogenic bladder, *NRCT* nonrandomized controlled trials, *BC* bladder capacity, *PVR* post-voiding residuum, *Vvol* voided volume

(80%) and DV (71%) who were investigated for PTNS tolerability. Recently, we analyzed long-term results of PTNS in different types of pediatric refractory LUTD, comparing neurogenic with non-neurogenic LUTD and OAB with DV cases (Table 30.1) [6]. Improvement was significantly greater ($p < 0.002$) in non-neurogenic (78%) than in neurogenic (14%) patients [6]. Improvement in some patients with neurogenic LUTD due to spinal dysraphism could be explained by the heterogeneity and incompleteness of neurological lesions. A careful selection of neurogenic patients could improve PTNS effectiveness in this patient subset. In this view, changes of amplitude of long latency somatosensory evoked potential [8] could be particularly useful to identify neuropathic children who might be responders to PTNS. Cure rate at 2-year follow-up in OAB and DV cases [6] is reported in Table 30.1: at long term, 50% of patients with OAB and in 29% of those with DV needed a chronic monthly PTNS session to maintain results. Whether such maintenance session has precise neurophysiological basis or is simply a placebo effect remains to be clarified. To avoid needle insertion, transcutaneous posterior tibial nerve stimulation (TPTNS) by means of surface electrodes has been recently tested in children with OAB by Boudaud et al. [19]. Comparing children treated with TPTNS with a control group (sham treatment), authors found a significant improvement in urodynamic parameters (voided volume during urgency, maximal cystometric capacity, volume at the onset of the first overactive detrusor contraction, and amplitude of overactive detrusor contraction) of TPTNS group [19]. Paradoxically, clinical results were better in sham than in TPTNS group, underlining the role of a possible placebo effect of any type of management in this pediatric population [19].

Following the controlled clinical trial by Bower et al. [4], who clearly showed inhibition of detrusor activity using suprapubic and sacral stimulation, several NRCT and RCT [5–13] have been published to evaluate efficacy of TENS in children, mainly with OAB (Table 30.2). Two pilot studies were published in 2001 on

Table 30.2 TENS in children with lower urinary tract dysfunction

Author, year	Pts.	Study type	LUTD	% Clinical outcome	% UD outcome
Balcom AH, 1997 [3]	29	NRCT	NB	Sensation improved	BC augmented
Hoebeke P, 2001 [6]	41	NRCT	OAB	76 improved 56 cured	BC augmented
Barroso U, 2006 [7]	36	NRCT	OAB DV	59 cured –	– PVR improved
Malm-Buatsi E, 2007 [8]	18	NRCT	OAB	60 improved 13 cured	Vvol normalized
Hagstroem S, 2009 [10]	27	RCT	OAB	61 improved	Vvol unchanged
De Oliveira L, 2013 [12]	45	RCT	PMNE	61.8 improved	–
Quintiliano F, 2014 [13]	28	RCT	OAB	46 cured	–

OAB overactive bladder, *DV* dysfunctional voiding, *NB* neurogenic bladder, *PMNE* primary monosymptomatic nocturnal enuresis, *NRCT* nonrandomized controlled trials, *RCT* randomized controlled trial, *BC* bladder capacity, *PVR* post-voiding residuum, *Vvol* voided volume idiopathic OAB in children treated with daily TENS for 1 month with electrodes placed over the S3 foramen [6] or with sacral and suprapubic stimulation [5]. The two studies showed improvement in urgency as well as a reduced number of incontinence episodes with increased voided volume. Recently, a RCT in children with OAB [13] showed a complete resolution of LUTS in 46% of patients treated with TENS versus 20% of children who received oxybutynin; constipation improved in all patients after TENS. De Oliveira et al. [12] demonstrated effectiveness of TENS in children with primary monosymptomatic nocturnal enuresis: a significantly greater increase in dry nights ($p = 0.0003$) was found in patients treated with TENS (61.8%) compared to controls (37.3%). Comparing TENS versus PTNS, Barroso et al. [22] found that TENS is more effective in resolving OAB symptoms than PTNS, which matches parental perception. However, there were no statistically significant differences in the evaluation by dysfunctional voiding symptom score or in complete resolution of urgency or diurnal incontinence between the two techniques [22].

Conclusions

Results of PTNS and TENS in children with non-neurogenic LUTD and primary monosymptomatic nocturnal enuresis indicate that these peripheral neurostimulation techniques should be a part of the pediatric urological armamentarium. Efficacy of PTNS and TENS is comparable in children with OAB while patients with DV seem beneficiate of PTNS. Further trials are needed to confirm effectiveness of transcutaneous posterior tibial nerve stimulation in children with both OAB and DV.

References

1. De Gennaro M, Capitanucci ML, Mosiello G, Zaccara A. Current state of nerve stimulation technique for lower urinary tract dysfunction in children. J Urol. 2011;185(5):1571–7.
2. Kajbafzaden AM, Sharif-Rad L, Seyedan SSL, Masoumi A. Functional electrical stimulation for management of urinary incontinence in children with myelomeningocele: a randomized trial. Pediatr Surg Int. 2014;30:663–8.
3. Balcom AH, Wiatrak M, Biefeld T, et al. Initial experience with home therapeutic electrical stimulation for continence in the myelomeningocele population. J Urol. 1997;158:1272–6.
4. Bower WF, Moore KH, Adams RD, et al. A urodynamic study of surface neuromodulation versus sham in detrusor instability and sensory urgency. J Urol. 1998;160:2133–6.
5. Bower WF, Moore KH, Adams RD. A pilot study of the home application of transcutaneous neuromodulation in children with urgency or urge incontinence. J Urol. 2001;166:2420–2.
6. Hoebeke P, Van Laecke E, Everaert K, et al. Transcutaneous neuromodulation for the urge syndrome in children: a pilot study. J Urol. 2001;166:2416–9.
7. Barroso U, Lordelo P, Lopes AA, et al. Nonpharmacological treatment of lower rinary tract dysfunction using biofeedback and transcutaneous electrical stimulation: a pilot study. BJU. 2006;98:166–71.
8. Malm-Buatsi E, Nepple KG, Boyt MA, et al. Efficacy of transcutaneous electrical nerve stimulation in children with overactive bladder refractory to pharmaco therapy. Urology. 2007;70:980.

9. Tugtepe H, Thomas DT, Ergun R, et al. The effectiveness of transcutaneous electrical neural stimulation therapy in patients with urinary incontinence resistant to initial medical treatment or biofeedback. J Pediatr Urol. 2015;11:137e1–5.
10. Hagstroem S, Mahler B, Madsen B, et al. Transcutaneous electrical nerve stimulation for refractory daytime urinary urge incontinence. J Urol. 2009;182:2072–8.
11. Lordelo P, Teles A, Veiga ML, et al. Transcutaneous electrical nerve stimulation in children with overactive bladder: a randomized clinical trial. J Urol. 2010;184(2):683–9.
12. de Oliveira LF, de Oliveira DM, da Silva de Paula LL, et al. Transcutaneous parasacral electrical neural stimulation in children with primary monosymptomatic enuresis: a prospective randomized clinical trial. J Urol. 2013;190:1359–63.
13. Quintiliano F, Veiga M, Moraes M, et al. Transcutaneous parasacral electrical stimulation vs oxybutynin for the treatment of overactive bladder in children: a randomized clinical trial. J Urol. 2014;193:1749–53.
14. Gabriele G, Topazio L, Iacovelli V, et al. Percutaneous tibial nerve stimulation (PTNS) efficacy in the treatment of lower urinary tract dysfunctions: a systematic review. BMC Urol. 2013;13:61–72.
15. Schneider MP, Gross T, Bachmann LM, et al. Tibial nerve stimulation for treating neurogenic lower urinary tract dysfunction: a systematic review. Eur Urol. 2015;68(5):859–67.
16. De Gennaro M, Capitanucci ML, Mastracci P, et al. Percutaneous tibial nerve neuromodulation is well tolerated in children and effective for treating refractory vesical dysfunction. J Urol. 2004;171:1911–3.
17. Hoebeke P, Renon C, Petillon L, et al. Percutaneous electrical nerve stimulation in children with therapy resistant non-neuropathic bladder-sphincter dysfunction. J Urol. 2002;168:2605–7.
18. Capitanucci ML, Camanni D, Demelas F, et al. Long-term efficacy of percutaneous tibial nerve stimulation for different types of lower urinary tract dysfunction in children. J Urol. 2009;182((4):2056–61.
19. Boudaud N, Binet A, Line A, et al. Management of refractory overactive bladder in children by transcutaneous posterior tibial nerve stimulation: a controlled study. J Ped Urol. 2015;11:138e1–138e10.
20. Finazzi-Agro' E, Rocchi C, Pachatz C, et al. Percutaneous tibial nerve stimulation produces effect on brain activity: study on the modifications of the long latency somatosensory evoked potentials. Neurourol Urodyn. 2009;28:320–4.
21. Dasgupta R, Critchley HD, Dolan RJ, et al. Changes in brain activity following sacral neuromodulation for urinary retention. J Urol. 2005;174:2268–72.
22. Barroso U, Viterbo V, Bittencourt J, et al. Posterior tibial nerve stimulation vs parasacral transcutaneous neuromodulation for overactive bladder in children. J Urol. 2013;190(2):673–7.

Botulinum Toxin, Endoscopy, and Mini-Invasive Treatment

31

Giovanni Palleschi, Antonio Luigi Pastore, Davide Moschese, and Antonio Carbone

31.1 Introduction

The management of urinary incontinence (UI) and voiding dysfunction in children is of utmost importance because an ineffective treatment could lead to severe complications, limiting life's expectancy and importantly reducing social interactions, with major psychological impact on patient's families. Of course, many factors can affect the success of a therapeutic approach in such a population, as described by the International Consultation on Incontinence and here reported [1]:

- Child's motivation to participate to the treatment
- Providing information and instructions about daily habits, underlining the importance of having regular fluid intake and regular voidings
- Regular review of new interventions

All the clinicians and the caregivers should convey a sense of understanding and compassion to both the child and the family [1]. When conservative (behavioral therapy, rehabilitation programs) and pharmacological treatments fail, second-line approaches should be considered. In this case, if an invasive treatment is scheduled, it is of high importance that this could be a mini-invasive one, considering the age of these patients. For this reason, today there is a strong research for standardization of

G. Palleschi (✉) • A. L. Pastore • A. Carbone
Faculty of Pharmacy and Medicine, Department of Medico-Surgical Sciences and Biotechnologies, Sapienza University of Rome, Latina, Italy

ICOT Hospital—Uroresearch Association, Latina, Italy
e-mail: giovanni.palleschi@uniroma1.it

D. Moschese
Faculty of Pharmacy and Medicine, Department of Medico-Surgical Sciences and Biotechnologies, Sapienza University of Rome, Latina, Italy

© Springer International Publishing AG, part of Springer Nature 2018
G. Mosiello et al. (eds.), *Clinical Urodynamics in Childhood and Adolescence*, Urodynamics, Neurourology and Pelvic Floor Dysfunctions, https://doi.org/10.1007/978-3-319-42193-3_31

mini-invasive procedures in pediatric age and adolescence to treat incontinence and voiding dysfunction, with special regard to endoscopic, laparoscopic, and laparoscopic robot-assisted techniques. In this chapter we focused the attention on the most important mini-invasive approaches today available to face UI and voiding dysfunction in children, usually secondary to neurogenic and congenital conditions.

31.2 Botulinum Toxin

Onabotulinum toxin A (onaBNTa) is commonly used for treating adults suffering from neurogenic detrusor overactivity (NDO) and wet idiopathic overactive bladder (OAB) [2]. This therapeutic approach has been widely practiced after it has received its regulatory approval for these specific uses in adults [3]. Therefore, the International Guidelines support the use of onaBNTa in patients refractory to oral treatment with high levels of recommendation [4]. Although the administration of onaBNTa is still considered off-label in children, some data on its efficacy and safety have already been reported, and phase III clinical trials are ongoing on this population [5]. Therefore, nowadays there is high-quality evidence for the efficacy of detrusor injections of onaBNTa in adults with NDO and in children and young people with myelodysplasia [6]. Most of the authors report promising results of treatment with onaBNTa in children with neurogenic conditions, even if they suggest that more studies need to be performed since onaBNTa is not yet registered for injection into the detrusor or into the sphincter of the pediatric population [7, 8]. Thus, further prospective trials are needed before a general recommendation could be assessed [8]. Among the studies already published, Hoebeke et al. performed an uncontrolled prospective investigation in children with NDO refractory to pharmacological treatment [9]. These authors described 70% of success in improving UI. A very limited experience shows promising results in treating UI by an electromotive administration of onaBNTa; in this trial, 15 subjects were enrolled with significant improvement of UI without side effects [10]. Other authors reported initial favorable experience to treat dysfunctional voiding by the administration of onaBNTa in urethral sphincter in children [11, 12]. A particular prospective trial has been performed by Mokhless et al. to determine if onaBNTa injection at the bladder neck could improve vesical dysfunction in 20 boys after posterior urethral valve (UV) ablation [13]. However, temporarily abolishing the effect of bladder neck by onaBNTa injection did not seem to improve the outcome in those patients. Summarizing the evidence from the experiences reported in literature, onaBNTa in children is then used either for NDO associated with UI and in subjects with non-compliant bladders without NDO, although with lower efficacy. Differently from adults, the dosage of onaBNTa in children should be based on body weight. In fact, most of the studies report that investigators administered doses of 5–12 U/kg body weight (similar to doses used in the i.m. treatment of juvenile cerebral palsy) with a total dose of 50–360 U onaBNTa, reflecting a higher dose/kg body weight than is used in adults [12]. However, no studies specifically assessed or stratified the effects of different doses or number of injection sites in children. Regarding the technique, young patients are usually treated under general anesthesia, performing injection with rigid or flexible cystoscopes, depending on the clinician's choice. The number of injections varies from 20 to 50 similarly to adult protocols, and usually the bladder trigone is spared from the injections. Considering all these evidences, a larger use of onaBNTa in the future years either in children and in adults is expected, also due to the recent publication of studies that provide suggestions about how to manage patients with NDO in their transition from childhood to the adult age [14: Adolescence transitional care in neurogenic detrusor overactivity and the use of OnabotulinumtoxinA: A clinical algorithm from an Italian consensus statement. Palleschi G, Mosiello G, Iacovelli V, Musco S, Del Popolo G, Giannantoni A, Carbone A, Carone R, Tubaro A, De Gennaro M, Marte A, Finazzi Agrò E.Neurourol Urodyn. 2017 Sep 6.].

31.3 Endoscopic Treatments

The use of endoscopy in pediatric patients is a routine practice for various urological pathologic conditions. Endoscopy represents a mini-invasive approach, and in this population it has to be preferred every time possible. Surgical endoscopy has been adopted especially for the treatment of urethral conditions, such as UV or stenosis, ureteroceles (UC), and especially for the cure of vesicoureteral reflux (VUR) and UI. The use of cold endoscopic incision of UV is widely practiced, and it has shown efficacy and safety over many years. Review articles support this approach reporting that also in rare cases of anterior urethral valve (AUV) associated with posterior urethral valves (PUV), the endoscopic management can result in improvement in renal function, reversal of obstructive changes, and improvement or resolution of voiding dysfunction [14, 15]. Current data available from the literature support the use of endoscopy to treat UC, also combined with ureteral stones. Many papers describe the endoscopic incision of UC (endoscopic puncture) as a safe and effective treatment of symptomatic children especially with single-system intravesical UC [16]. Similar data are reported regarding the endoscopic treatment of bladder neck stenosis and urethral strictures, supported by long-term outcomes about renal function, bladder output, and quality of life (QoL). Recently, the literature has provided data regarding the application of technological innovations in the treatment of these conditions. Gholdoian et al. reported a retrospective analysis of their single-center experience in the use of KTP-532 laser for treating 33 subjects suffering from UV and UC [17]. Overall, the success rate was excellent in the treatment of UV and UC, with a mean follow-up of 3 years in the PUV group, in which no urethral strictures and micturition abnormalities were observed during the follow-up. In details, the majority of UC were decompressed, and only half of patients required an additional procedure. Honestly, the authors report that the experience with urethral stricture was not as promising as expected, because all of the patients required open urethral reconstruction during the years of the follow-up. However, the desirable thermal characteristics of the KTP laser, along with minimal complications and the availability of delicate pediatric endoscopic instruments, have made this operation optimally suited for treating PUV and UC in infants. The use of laser is also reported by other authors. Particularly, a prospective study performed by

Shoukry et al. in 2016 reports the effectiveness and complications of retrograde endoscopic holmium/yttrium aluminum garnet (Ho:YAG) laser urethrotomy (HLU) for the treatment of pediatric urethral strictures in 29 young males [18]. Although these data are promising and the authors support the use of laser for urethral strictures, the advantages for treating this condition in children still remain to be established by prospective, comparative, long-term studies with larger case series. Endoscopy surely represents an important therapeutic option for VUR. In this pathologic condition, the primary goal is the preservation of the kidney and its function [19]. Endoscopic correction of VUR is an outpatient procedure associated with decreased morbidity compared with ureteral reimplantation [19]. The technique includes the ureteral hydrodistention and intraluminal submucosal injection (hydrodistention implantation technique [HIT]) and has improved the success rate in curing VUR with respect to the subureteral transurethral injection [19]. Then, further modifications of the HIT procedure include the use of proximal and distal intraluminal injections (double HIT) that result in coaptation of both the ureteral tunnel and orifice. In fact, nowadays, the endoscopic injection of dextranomer/hyaluronic acid copolymer, via the HIT and double HIT, is considered as a highly successful, minimally invasive approach to cure VUR, alternative to open surgical correction, with low morbidity [19]. In 2012, 278 pediatric urologists in the United States were contacted to complete a 15-question survey regarding Dx/HA injection technique(s) currently used in their practice. This survey showed that the double HIT method is currently the most commonly performed technique for endoscopic correction of VUR by pediatric urologists in the United States [20]. However, an interesting study by Herbst et al. from the US Pediatric Health Information System including the review of over 14,000 subjects treated for VUR from 2004 to 2011 reports that there is a trend toward decreasing intervention for primary VUR, which appears to be due to reduced use of injection therapy, because the average reimplantation rate remained stable during this time [21]. On the other side, when a therapeutic surgical approach is needed to treat VUR, endoscopic option should initially be the treatment of choice, especially for its mini-invasiveness. This is supported by a large volume of data from the literature, coming from over 100 published papers reviewed by Cosentino et al. [22]. Bulking agents are used not only in cases of VUR. In fact, these agents have been adopted in urology to improve the urethral resistance in subjects with stress urinary incontinence (SUI), even if with variable outcomes in adult population. Children with sphincteric incompetence may receive symptoms improvement by the injection of bulking agents. A careful preoperative evaluation has to be performed with the aim to assess the presence or not of low compliance and detrusor overactivity (DO) which could be responsible for treatment failure or for complications. As for the adults, the risk to develop granuloma in the site of injection and to have a migration of the bulking substance has limited the diffusion of this approach also in pediatric population [23, 24]. Various agents have been used to perform this technique (dextranomer, hyaluronic acid, polydimethylsiloxane), but most of the data available come from studies with bovine collagen with a success rate varying from 20 to 50% [25–28]. One of the most important limits of this technique is the short duration of the effect and the need for reinterventions [28].

The procedure usually consists in the injection of the bulking agent endoscopically in the bladder neck area, and usually more than one injection is necessary. Also in the case series with the best outcomes, patients need to be re-treated after some years with a success rate up to 70% [29, 30]. Although literature reports a significant variability of results and therefore this approach cannot achieve a strong grade of recommendation, many subjects prefer to receive this treatment because it is less invasive with respect to surgery (i.e., bladder neck reconstruction or artificial sphincter implantation). Recently some experienced urologists report the injection of the bulking agent by a laparoscopic approach, but this represents a procedure still under investigation [31].

31.4 Slings

The use of suburethral slings for treating SUI has been adopted worldwide with large evidence of efficacy and safety. This is an effective treatment for type III SUI secondary to poor proximal urethral sphincter function. Fascial slings, made by the fascia of the anterior rectus muscle, have been widely used to increase outlet resistance in children with neurogenic SUI starting with a preliminary experience in one patient suffering from myelodysplasia in 1986 [32]. The authors reported a complete success with total continence associated with intermittent postoperative catheterization. The fascial sling may be represented by a graft or a flap taken from the rectus sheath on one side which can be crossed anteriorly or wrapped around the bladder neck to compress the urethra. The technique is somewhat different between males and females, especially because in after-pubertal females a combined vaginal and abdominal approach is adopted [33]. Most of the authors report favorable outcomes of this procedure; however, considering that this approach is mostly applied in children with neurogenic disorders, the success rate is high, especially when the technique is combined with other surgeries aimed to improve bladder capacity. An important limit regarding this approach is represented by the absence of studies reporting long-term outcomes with >5 years of follow-up [34–36]. Gormely et al. in 1994 used a pubovaginal sling to treat incontinence in 15 female adolescents. The etiology of incontinence was spinal dysraphism in ten patients and prior trauma in three. Simultaneous bladder augmentation was performed in the remaining two patients for poor bladder compliance. Three patients required additional procedures including repeated slings in two and repeated augmentation in one. Out of 13 patients, followed for more than 6 months, 11 remained dry, 1 had a leakage of small amounts wearing 1 pad per day, and 1 did not achieve acceptable continence and was subsequently managed with bladder augmentation and a Mitrofanoff procedure. The authors reported satisfying outcomes regarding the upper urinary tract, which resulted normal in 13 patients during the follow-up. These authors concluded that the pubovaginal sling has proved to be safe and successful in these children, describing an overall continence rate of 92%. Larger experience with the application of pubovaginal sling by vaginal approach in 24 girls suffering from neurogenic bladder secondary to spina bifida has been reported by Dik et al. [36]. One of the possible applications of suburethral slings in children is represented by the incontinence in subjects suffering from bladder exstrophy. In fact, post-exstrophy incontinence is a challenge because continence is difficult to achieve and even more difficult to maintain. Wadie et al. described in 2016 the feasibility and outcomes of a bulbourethral sling to treat post-exstrophy incontinence [37]. In this study the authors applied a retropubic bulbourethral sling to male patients with incontinence post-exstrophy-epispadias repair. They enrolled children with total incontinence who underwent multiple previous anti-incontinence procedures, ranging from bladder neck injection to bladder neck reconstruction. The technique consisted in the implant of a polypropylene sling suspended by four pairs of nylon sutures to support the bulbar urethra within its covering muscles with the sutures tied on the rectus muscles. The cohort was comprehensive of 17 children with a median age of 8.7 years. After surgery, five children (29.27%) were dry, four micturated through the urethra, and one by catheterizing his cutaneous stoma every 3–4 h. In none patient the PVR exceeded 10% of expected bladder capacity; four children underwent re-tightening 1–4 weeks after removal of urethral catheter; perineal wound dehiscence occurred in 1, perineal/suprapubic pain in 7, and epididymo-orchitis in 1 child. Other experience with similar results have been reported in literature using intestinal submucosal slings and Gore-Tex combined with bladder augmentation, with the same study limits described for the fascial slings [38, 39]. Although these studies have been well performed, literature is still lacking of large, prospective, long-term randomized trials regarding the use, efficacy, and safety of slings in pediatric population with long-term outcomes.

31.5 Final Considerations

In 2012 the International Children's Continence Society's recommendations for therapeutic intervention in congenital neuropathic bladder and bowel dysfunction in children was published [40]. This was a report of a consensus from the members of the International Children's Continence Society on the therapeutic intervention in congenital neuropathic bladder and bowel dysfunction in children. Many statements emerging from Literature reviewed by the authors of this consensus has been reported in our chapter. However, a very important statement of the consensus is that the nonsurgical intervention is promoted before undertaking major surgery. Indicators for nonsurgical treatments depend on issues related to intravesical pressure, upper urinary tract status, prevalence of urinary tract infections, and the degree of incontinence. The optimal age for treatment should also be adequately and carefully planned. For these reasons it has to be strongly taken into consideration that, when surgery is needed, the mini-invasive approaches or endoscopic techniques like those described in this chapter have to be preferred as an initial choice. Another very important aspect is that there are many papers regarding children, but very few of them also focus the attention on adolescents. Nowadays, thanks to the high level of care in developed countries, large rate of children with congenital neurologic diseases, malformations, and consequences of obstetric trauma reach adulthood

(70% of subjects with CP and 80–90% with SB). Therefore, specific guidelines could result of crucial support for the clinicians who are going to take care of young adults with voiding dysfunctions and UI who were previously treated and followed by pediatricians or pediatric urologists. In fact, as strongly sustained by current literature, contrary to popular perception, young adults-ages are surprisingly unhealthy and need a specific care. The Institute of Medicine and National Research Council recently released a report titled "Investing in the Health and Well-Being of Young Adults" [41]. The report concludes that young adulthood is a critical developmental period, and it is recommended that young adults ages should be treated as a distinct subpopulation in policy, planning, programming, and research. The report also recommends actions to improve the transition from pediatric to adult medical and behavioral health care, to enhance preventive care for young adults, and to develop evidence-based practices. These recommendations should be adopted by all the sanitary systems to guarantee continuity of care for all patients during this delicate phase of their life. However, to support the achievement of these goals, clinicians should define precise protocols for transitional care in the different therapeutic fields.

References

1. Abrams P, Cardozo L, Khoury S, Wein A. Incontinence. Plymouth: Health Publications Ltd; 2013.
2. Karsenty G, Denys P, Amarenco G, De Seze M, Gamé X, Haab F, Kerdraon J, Perrouin-Verbe B, Ruffion A, Saussine C, Soler JM, Schurch B, Chartier-Kastler E. Botulinum toxin A (Botox) intradetrusor injections in adults with neurogenic detrusor overactivity/neurogenic overactive bladder: a systematic literature review. Eur Urol. 2008;53(2):275–87. Epub 2007 Oct 16. Review
3. Linsenmeyer TA. Use of botulinum toxin in individuals with neurogenic detrusor overactivity: state of the art review. J Spinal Cord Med. 2013;36(5):402–19.
4. European Association of Urology Guidelines 2016. Section: NeuroUrology. http://uroweb.org/guideline/neuro-urology/
5. Dmochwoski R, Sand PK. Botulinum toxin A in the overactive bladder: current status and future directions. BJU Int. 2007;99(2):247–62.
6. Mangera A, Apostolidis A, Andersson KE, Dasgupta P, Giannantoni A, Roehrborn C, Novara G, Chapple C. An updated systematic review and statistical comparison of standardised mean outcomes for the use of botulinum toxin in the management of lower urinary tract disorders. Eur Urol. 2014;65(5):981–90.
7. Kuo HC, Botulinum A. Toxin urethral injection for the treatment of lower urinary tract dysfunction. J Urol. 2003;170:1908–12.
8. Apostolidis A, Dasgupta P, Denys P, Elneil S, Fowler CJ, Giannantoni A, Karsenty G, Schulte-Baukloh H, Schurch B, Wyndaele JJ, European Consensus Panel. Recommendations on the use of botulinum toxin in the treatment of lower urinary tract disorders and pelvic floor dysfunctions: a European consensus report. Eur Urol. 2009;55:100–19.
9. Hoebeke P. The effect of botulinum a toxin in incontinent children with therapy resistant overactive detrusor. J Urol. 2006;176:328–30.
10. Kajbafzadeh AM, Ahmadi H, Montaser-Kouhsari L, Shariufi-Rad L, Nejat F, Bazargan-Hejazi S. Intravesical electromotive botulinum toxin type-A administration-part II: clinical application. Urology. 2011;77:439–45.
11. Radojicic ZI, Perovic SV, Milic NM. Is it reasonable to treat refractory voiding dysfunction in children with botulinum-A-toxin? J Urol. 2006;176:332–6.

12. Franco I, et al. The use of botulinum toxin A injection for the management of external sphincter dyssynergia in neurologically normal children. J Urol. 2007;178:1775–9.
13. Mokhless I, Zahran AR, Saad A, Yehia M, Youssif ME. Effect of Botox injection at the bladder neck in boys with bladder dysfunction after valve ablation. J Pediatr Urol. 2014;10(5):899–904. Epub 2014 Feb 6
14. Tran CN, Reichard CA, McMahon D, Rhee A. Anterior urethral valve associated with posterior urethral valves: report of 2 cases and review of the literature. Urology. 2014;84(2):469–71. https://doi.org/10.1016/j.urology.2014.04.034. Epub 2014 Jun 21
15. Keihani S, Kajbafzadeh AM. Concomitant anterior and posterior urethral valves: a comprehensive review of literature. Urology. 2015;86(1):151–7. https://doi.org/10.1016/j.urology.2015.02.019. Epub 2015 Apr 8
16. Gholdoian CG, Thayer K, Hald D, Rajpoot D, Shanberg AM. Applications of the KTP laser in the treatment of posterior urethral valves, ureteroceles, and urethral strictures in the pediatric patient. J Clin Laser Med Surg. 1998;16(1):39–43.
17. Shoukry AI, Abouela WN, ElSheemy MS, Shouman AM, Daw K, Hussein AA, Morsi H, Mohsen MA, Badawy H, Eissa M. Use of holmium laser for urethral strictures in pediatrics: a prospective study. J Pediatr Urol. 2016;12(1):42.e1–6. Epub 2015 Aug 11
18. Lopez PJ, Celis S, Reed F, Zubieta R. Vesicoureteral reflux: current management in children. Curr Urol Rep. 2014;15(10):447.
19. Kirsch AJ, Arlen AM. Evaluation of new Deflux administration techniques: intraureteric HIT and double HIT for the endoscopic correction of vesicoureteral reflux. Expert Rev Med Devices. 2014;11(5):439–46. https://doi.org/10.1586/17434440.2014.929491. Epub 2014 Jun 14
20. Kirsch AJ, Arlen AM, Lackgren G. Current trends in dextranomer hyaluronic acid copolymer (Deflux) injection technique for endoscopic treatment of vesicoureteral reflux. Urology. 2014;84(2):462–8. https://doi.org/10.1016/j.urology.2014.04.032. Epub 2014 Jun 26
21. Herbst KW, Corbett ST, Lendvay TS, Caldamone AA. Recent trends in the surgical management of primary vesicoureteral reflux in the era of dextranomer/hyaluronic acid. J Urol. 2014;191(5 Suppl):1628–33. Epub 2014 Mar 26
22. Cosentino M, Caffaratti J, Bujons A, Garat JM, Villavicencio H. Vesico-ureteral reflux, endoscopic management. Arch Argent Pediatr. 2013;111(4):349–52.
23. Vorstman B, Lokhart J, Kaufman MR, Politano V. Polytetrafluoroethylene injection for urinary incontinence in children. J Urol. 1985;133:248–50.
24. Malizia AA Jr, Reiman HM, Myers RP, Sandle JR, Bahrman SS, Benson RC Jr, Dewanjee MK, Utz WJ. Migration and granulomatous reaction after periurethral injection of polytef (Teflon). JAMA. 1984;251:3277–81.
25. Bomalski MD, Bloom DA, McGuire EJ, Panzi A. Glutaraldehyde cross linked collagen in the treatment of urinary incontinence in children. J Urol. 1996;155:699–702.
26. Chernoff A, Horowitz M, Combs A, Libretti D, Nitti V, Glassberg KL. Periurethral collagen injection for the treatment of urinary incontinence in children. J Urol. 1997;157:2303–5.
27. Capozza N, Caione P, De gennaro M, Nappo S, Patricola M. Endoscopic treatment of vesicoureteral reflux and urinary incontinence. Technical problems in the pediatric patient. Br J Urol. 1995;75:538–42.
28. Sundaram CP, Reinberg Y, Aliabadi HA. Failure to obtain durable results with collagen implantation in children with urinary incontinence. J Urol. 1997;157:2306–7.
29. Guys JM, Breaud J, Hery G, Camerlo A, Le Hors H, De Laguaise P. Endoscopic injection with polydimethylsiloxane for the treatment of pediatric urinary incontinence in the neurogenic bladder: long term results. J Urol. 2006;175(3 Pt 1):1106–10.
30. Dyer L, Franco I, Firlit CF, Reda EF, Levit SB, Palmer LS. Endoscopic injection of bulking agents in children with incontinence: dextranomer/hyaluronic acid copolymer versus polytetrafluoroethylene. J Urol. 2007;178(4 Pt 2):1628–31.
31. Lund L, Yeung CK. Periurethral injection therapy for urinary incontinence using a laparoscopic port. J Endourol. 2003;17(4):253.
32. Woodside JR, Borden TA. Pubovaginal sling procedure for the management of urinary incontinence in myelodysplastic girl. J Urol. 1986;78:808–9.

33. Kakizaki H, Shibata T, Kobayashi S, Matsumara K, Koyanagi T. Fascial sling for the management of incontinence due to sphincter incompetence. J Urol. 1995;153:644–7.
34. Elder JS. Periurethral and puboprostatic sling repair for incontinence in patients with myelodysplasia. J Urol. 1990;144:434–7.
35. Dik P, Klijn AJ, van Gool JD, de Jong TP. Transvaginal sling suspension of bladder neck in female patients with neurogenic sphincter incontinence. J Urol. 2003;170:580–1.
36. Gormley EA, Bloom DA, McGuire EJ, Ritchey ML. Pubovaginal slings for the management of urinary incontinence in female adolescents. J Urol. 1994 Aug;152(2 Pt 2):822–5.
37. Wadie BS, Helmy TE, Dawaba ME, Ghoneim MA. Retropubic bulbourethral sling in incontinence post-exstrophy repair: 2-year minimal follow up of a salvage procedure. Neurourol Urodyn. 2016;35(4):497–502.
38. Colvert JR 3rd, Kropp BP, Cheng EY, Pope JC, Brok JW 3rd, Adams MC, Austin P, Furness PD 3rd, Koyle MA. The use of small intestinal submucosa as an off-the-shelf urethral sling material for pediatric urinary incontinence. J Urol. 2002;168:1872–5.
39. Goodbole P, Mackinnon AE. Expanded PTFE bladder neck slings for incontinence in children: the long term outcome. BJU Int. 2004;93:139–41.
40. Rawashdeh YF, Austin P, Siggaard C, Bauer SB, Franco I, de Jong TP, Jorgensen TM, International Children's Continence Society. International Children's Continence Society's recommendations for therapeutic intervention in congenital neuropathic bladder and bowel dysfunction in children. Neurourol Urodyn. 2012;31(5):615–20.
41. Stroud C, Walker LR, Davis M, Irwin CE Jr. Investing in the health and well-being of young adults. J Adolesc Health. 2015;56(2):127–9.

Laparoscopic Procedures

32

Rafał Chrzan

32.1 Introduction

A variety of congenital and acquired anomalies of the lower urinary tract (LUT) can lead to urinary incontinence. Some patients require surgical treatment to increase bladder outlet resistance. The goals and the consequences of such an operation should be thoroughly explained to the patient and his/her parents (care providers). In this chapter, only laparoscopic bladder neck (BN) procedures in children are discussed. The indications and the general rules for bladder neck surgery are described elsewhere in this book (see Chap. 33).

Various terms (minimally invasive surgery [MIS], endoscopy, laparoscopy) are used in relation to procedures that are done under magnification and by means of instruments inserted via a trocar (cannula) into a body cavity. In this Chap. 32, uniform names are used: *laparoscopy* and *vesicoscopy*. The latter refers to surgery done inside the bladder, filled with CO_2.

32.2 Laparoscopic Surgery in Children

Laparoscopy has made remarkable progress during the last two decades and has established its place also in children [1–3]. Laparoscopy can be done safely regardless of the patient's age [4, 5]. For a number of urological procedures (laparoscopy for nonpalpable testis, nephrectomy, pyeloplasty), laparoscopy has become the gold standard [6, 7]. However, because of anatomical and physiological differences between adults and children, laparoscopy is challenging in children [8, 9]. The small operating

R. Chrzan
Department of Pediatric Urology, Children's University Hospital, Jagiellonian University Medical College, Krakow, Poland
e-mail: rafal.chrzan@uj.edu.pl

© Springer International Publishing AG, part of Springer Nature 2018
G. Mosiello et al. (eds.), *Clinical Urodynamics in Childhood and Adolescence*,
Urodynamics, Neurourology and Pelvic Floor Dysfunctions,
https://doi.org/10.1007/978-3-319-42193-3_32

field and very delicate structures require meticulous tissue handling to avoid unintentional injury to the surrounding organs. It must be kept in mind that children are more sensitive to CO_2 [10]. Hypercapnia and increased intra-abdominal pressure can lead to respiratory, cardiac, renal, and central nervous system impairment [11, 12]. These negative effects correlate with the height of the pressure and the duration of the procedure [13, 14]. On the other hand, laparoscopy is advantageous in terms of its cosmetic outcome and is associated with less postoperative pain and fewer intra-abdominal adhesions [15]. Laparoscopy provides a magnificent view of the operating field which, together with fine instruments, can result in superior precision [16].

The intravesical procedure in children was first described in 2001 by Gill et al., who performed ureteral reimplantation inside a bladder filled with glycine [17]. The camera was put in the urethra and additional ports were introduced percutaneously. Young et al. proposed to adopt CO_2 to maintain sufficient intravesical pressure during the surgery [18]. Although the results of vesicoscopic ureteral reimplantation are at least as good as those of the open procedure, there have been only a few reports on that topic [19, 20]. This is probably because of the technical challenges related to this technique. There is little room inside the bladder, which requires more experience from the operating surgeon. Port placement and fixation must be done properly to avoid displacement, because CO_2 leakage results in loss of the operating field. Vesicovaginal fistula repair and vesicoscopic diverticulectomy have also been reported [21, 22].

Robotic-assisted laparoscopy (RAL) has evolved enormously over the years [23, 24]. RAL offers a magnificent view and outstanding freedom of movement, which is very important in small operating fields. Moreover, the surgeon stays in a very ergonomic position during the whole procedure. RAL is mainly used in the adult population, and one of the reason why it has not become that popular in children is the size of the ports. The length of the incision matters in terms of postoperative pain and cosmetic outcome. The longer the wound, the higher the wound healing tension [15]. Furthermore, there is no evidence that RAL is superior to laparoscopy and open surgery, and it is still more expensive [25–28] Nevertheless, in pediatric urology, RAL is used for various indications: pyeloplasty, nephrectomy, and ureteral reimplantation [24, 29–32]. Also, complex RAL procedures such as reconstructive surgery in duplex system anomaly and bladder augmentation with appendicovesicostomy have been described [33, 34].

32.3 Laparoscopic Procedures of the Bladder Neck

32.3.1 Preperitoneal Approach

A laparoscopic sling procedure in a 13-year-old boy was reported by Mattioli et al. [35]. They proposed to put a fascia sling around the bladder neck, which was mobilized by a preperitoneal approach. The authors provided a comprehensive description of the procedure, with special attention to the technical challenges. The short-term outcome in this patient was satisfactory, but no larger experience from this center has been published to date.

Burch colposuspension has been proposed for the management of stress urinary incontinence (UI) in adults [36]. The European Association of Urology (EAU) recommends this procedure for patients who cannot be treated by means of midurethral slings [37]. The results of the laparoscopic technique are the same as of the open one, provided it is done by an experienced surgeon [37, 38]. In children, colposuspension can be offered to those with refractory UI based on congenital bladder neck insufficiency. The indications and preoperative work-up are described elswhere in this textbook. Since 2011 this procedure has also been done in our department, by means of laparoscopy. For this procedure the patient is in the lithotomy position. Cystoscopy is done first to evaluate the anatomy of the LUT. A balloon catheter is left in the bladder. A small incision is made under the umbilicus. Monopolar diathermy is used to open the anterior sheath of the right rectus muscle. This approach allows the prevesical space to be entered by means of a blunt tip obturator without injury to the peritoneum. The Retzius space is entered and the bladder is emptied. Two additional ports are put into the suprapubic region medially to the epigastric vessels (Fig. 32.1). Subsequently, the bladder neck and the vaginal wall are freed. The anterolateral wall is fixed to the Cooper's ligaments at the level of the bladder neck by means of 2.0 polyglactin sutures (Fig. 32.2). The bladder catheter is left for 2 days. We described the details of this technique and the primary results in 2014 [39]. We have already done 28 laparoscopic Burch colposuspensions in children aged 9–17 years (Figs. 32.3 and 32.4). Analysis of prospectively collected data on 18 procedures with follow-up of at least 1 year showed full responses in 8/18 and partial responses in 5/18. Six patients had a history of recurrent urinary tract infections (UTIs) and 4/6 were infection free after the procedure.

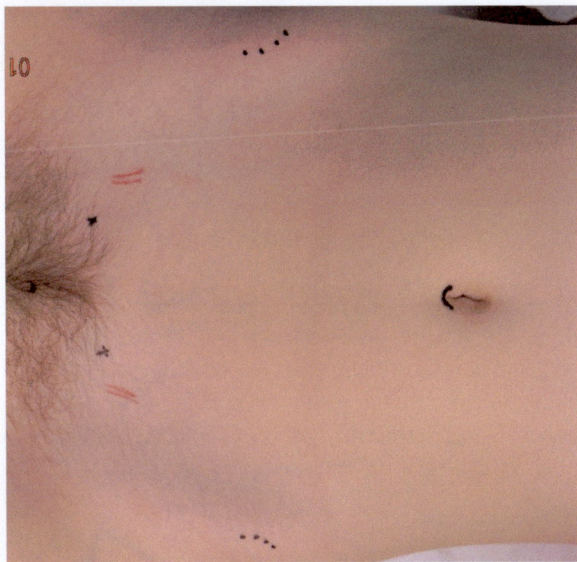

Fig. 32.1 Laparoscopic Burch colposuspension. The landmarks shown are the epigastric vessels (red line), skin incisions (cross), and anterior superior iliac spine (dotted line)

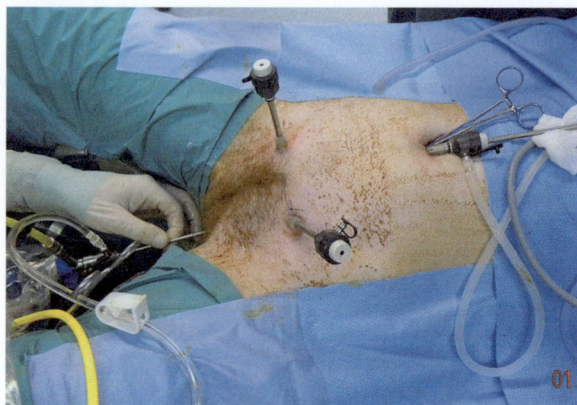

Fig. 32.2 Laparoscopic Burch colposuspension: cystoscopy and port placement

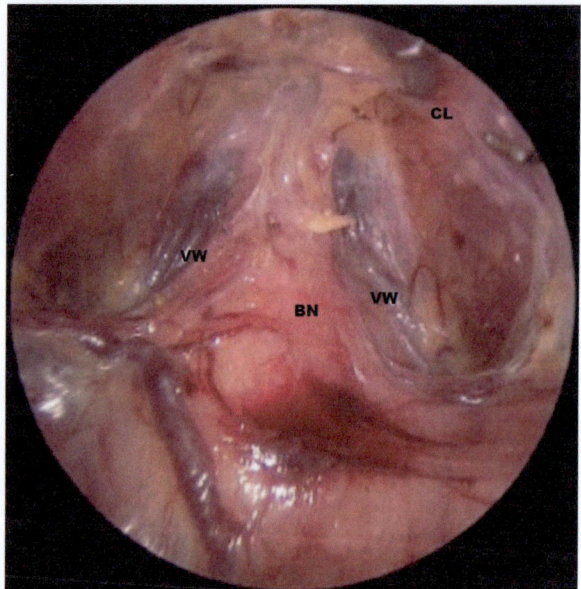

Fig. 32.3 Laparoscopic Burch colposuspension: intraoperative view before suspension. *BN* bladder neck, *CL* Cooper's ligament, *VW* vaginal wall

32.3.2 Transperitoneal Approach

Storm et al. described the first robotic-assisted laparoscopic sling procedure in children [40]. The bladder neck was approached transperitoneally, and then a circumferential dermal allograft was placed. This procedure was done in two girls and took about 3 h. The robotic system was found to be very helpful for working in the small pelvis. Gargollo recently published a series of 38 RAL Mitchell–Leadbetter bladder neck procedures in combination with a sling [41]. During a mean follow-up of

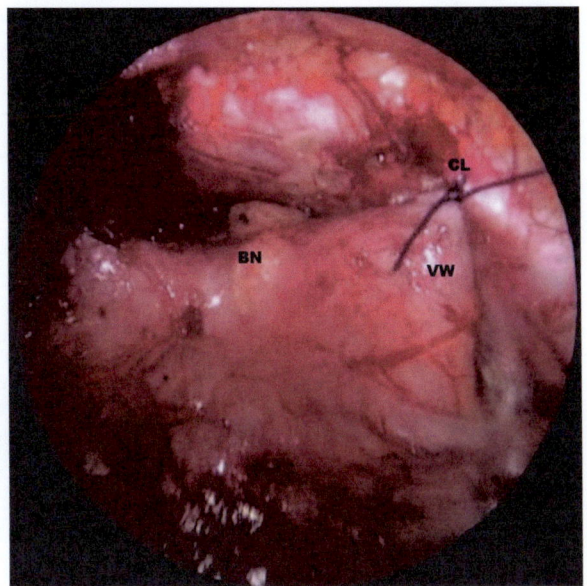

Fig. 32.4 Laparoscopic Burch colposuspension: intraoperative view after suspension. *BN* bladder neck, *CL* Cooper's ligament, *VW* vaginal wall

21 months, 82% of them were dry at 3 h intervals, and this result was comparable to that of the open approach. In 4/38, conversion was needed because of extensive adhesions. The author pointed out that RAL reconstruction took more time than the open procedure, and the operating surgeon should be aware of this. He also emphasized that during the RAL procedure, the same steps must be followed as during the open surgery.

32.4 Vesicoscopic Bladder Neck Procedure

This procedure is done in the lithotomy position (Fig. 32.5). A cystoscopy is done first to assess the LUT and to insert three 6 mm ports into the bladder under direct vision. A sharp-tip obturator should be used to enter the bladder smoothly (Figs. 32.6 and 32.7). The fluid is removed from the bladder, and insufflation with CO_2 begins at the same time, to reach a pressure of 10 mmHg (which correlates with approximately 14 cm H_2O). It is very important to prevent port displacement. The bladder wall can be fixed to the anterior abdominal wall percutaneously. Balloon trocars can be used optionally. A catheter is left in the urethra. A U-shaped incision is made with monopolar cautery around the bladder neck on the anterior wall (Fig. 32.8). A strip of the mucosa is freed and closed with interrupted sutures. The second layer is done over the first line and the suprapubic tube is left after the surger (Figs. 32.9 and 32.10).

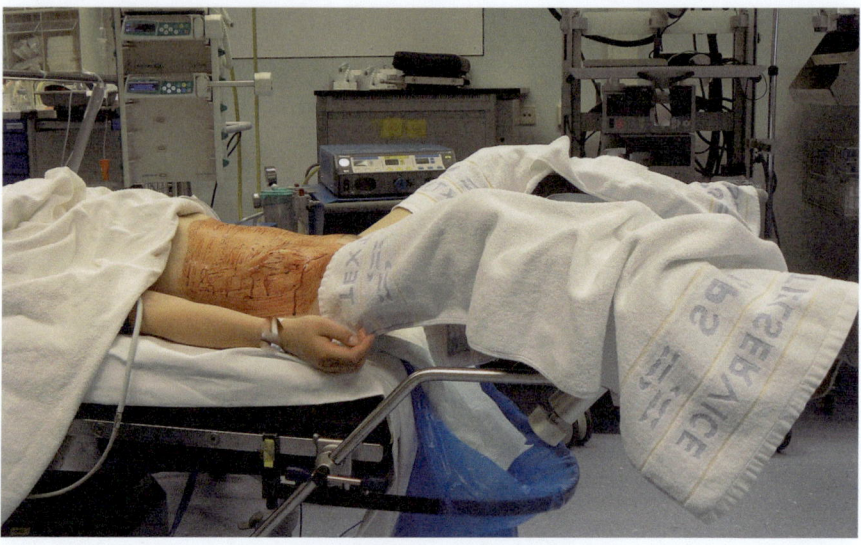

Fig. 32.5 Vesicoscopic bladder neck procedure: lithotomy position

Fig. 32.6 Vesicoscopic bladder neck procedure: port placement and fixation of the bladder wall

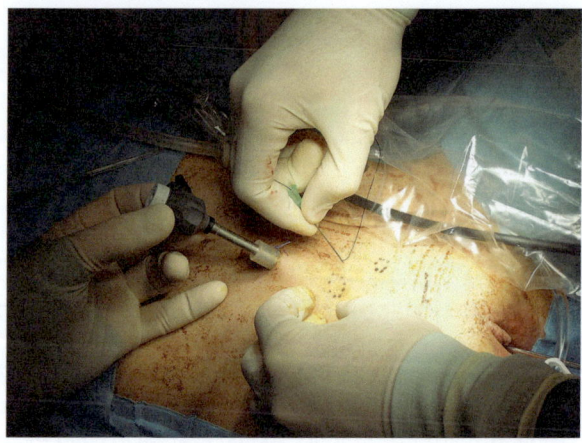

Our primary experience with this procedure was encouraging. In the short term, 4/8 patients were dry and 2/8 improved [42]. However the long-term results were rather disappointing, with a full response in only 2/18 and a partial response in only 6/18 [43]. It is worth mentioning that almost all of them failed a bladder neck procedure before and 50% had clean intermittent catheterization (CIC) via the urethra. We presume that the bladder neck plasty could be destroyed during catheterization. To the author's knowledge, there is no other literature on the vesicoscopic approach to the bladder neck in children.

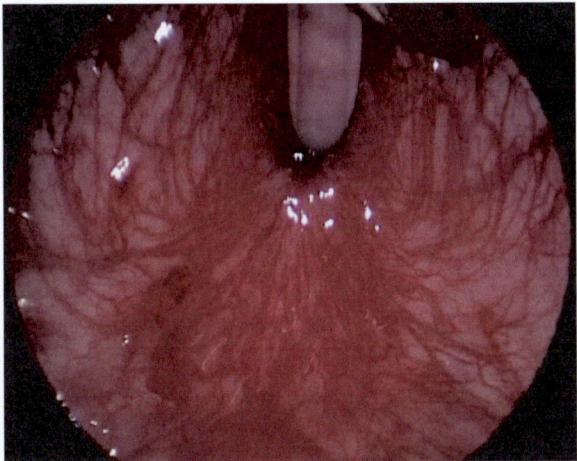

Fig. 32.7 Vesicoscopic bladder neck procedure: bladder neck and trigone

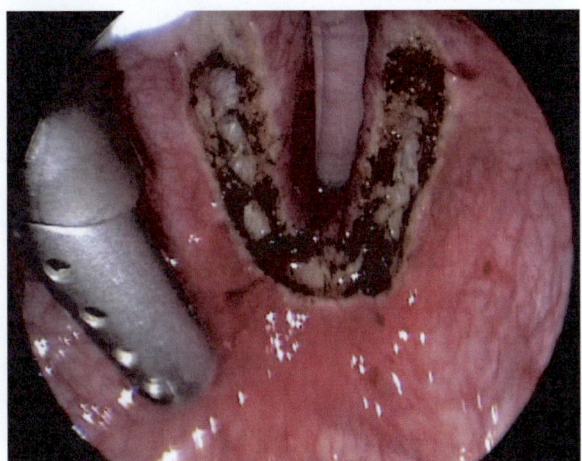

Fig. 32.8 Vesicoscopic bladder neck procedure: U incision on the anterior wall

32.5 Summary

Laparoscopy was introduced into pediatric surgery and urology in the early 1990s and over time it has become a part of routine surgical care. Laparoscopy means using technological findings to perform a procedure; still, one has to keep in mind that the general surgical rules should be followed [3]. Laparoscopy can bring new solutions and can help to optimize the results, together with minimizing the postoperative complication rate. On the other hand, its limitations should be taken into consideration. Not every procedure that is feasible for the laparoscopic surgeon is

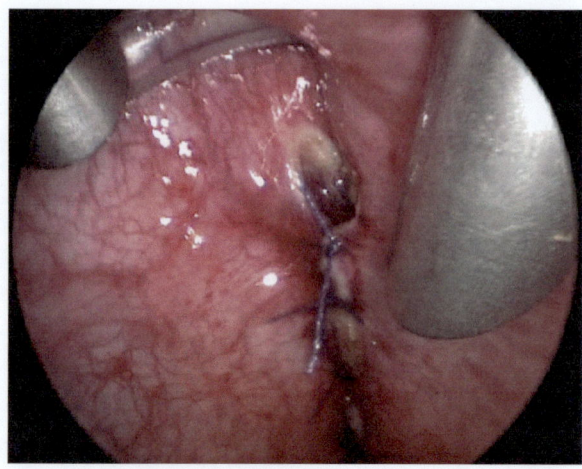

Fig. 32.9 Vesicoscopic bladder neck procedure: final result

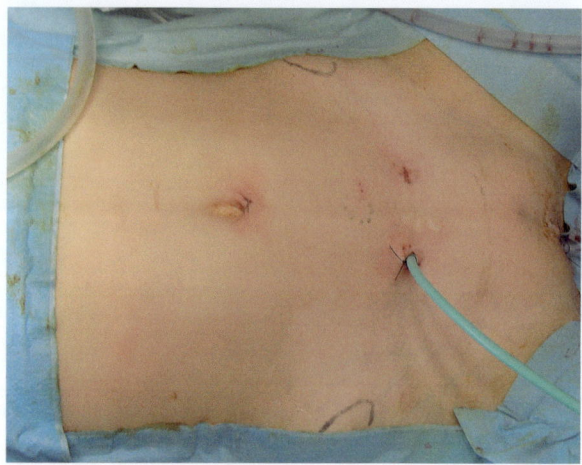

Fig. 32.10 Vesicoscopic bladder neck procedure: abdominal wall after surgery

advantageous for the patient. Technology can also contribute to improvement of ergonomics during the surgery, and RAL is the best example of that.

The success rate of surgical treatment of UI based on a bladder outlet incompetence event, even in the most experienced hands, usually does not exceed 70–80% [44, 45]. The weak point is that there is no uniform score system to compare the outcomes. It has already been shown that volume matters, and the complication rate decreases when the surgeon gains more experience [46]. Bladder neck procedures are not very common in the pediatric population, which means that the learning process can be quite long. Laparoscopic procedures require different skills and additional training can be needed [3, 47]. Putting those facts together, one can conclude that laparoscopic bladder neck surgery should be done by a well-prepared team at a center that is properly equipped and where the preoperative patient selection process is well established.

References

1. Peters CA. Laparoscopy in pediatric urology: challenge and opportunity. Semin Pediatr Surg. 1996;5(1):16–22. http://www.ncbi.nlm.nih.gov/pubmed/8988293. [cited 2015 Aug 14]
2. da Cruz JAS, Passerotti CC. Reconstructive laparoscopy in pediatric urology. Curr Opin Urol. 2010;20(4):330–5. http://www.ncbi.nlm.nih.gov/pubmed/20531199. [cited 2012 Mar 28]
3. Blinman TA. MIS-behavior: practical heuristics for precise pediatric minimally invasive surgery. Urol Clin North Am. 2015;42(1):131–40. http://www.ncbi.nlm.nih.gov/pubmed/25455179. [cited 2015 Mar 22]
4. Kuebler JF, Ure BM. Minimally invasive surgery in the neonate. Semin Fetal Neonatal Med. 2011;16(3):151–6. https://doi.org/10.1016/j.siny.2011.03.001. [cited 2012 Apr 5]
5. Lacher M, Kuebler JF, Dingemann J, Ure BM. Minimal invasive surgery in the newborn: current status and evidence. Semin Pediatr Surg. 2014;23(5):249–56. http://www.ncbi.nlm.nih.gov/pubmed/25459008. [cited 2015 Mar 22]
6. Blanc T, Muller C, Abdoul H, Peev S, Paye-Jaouen A, Peycelon M, et al. Retroperitoneal laparoscopic pyeloplasty in children: long-term outcome and critical analysis of 10-year experience in a teaching center. Eur Urol. 2013;63(3):565–72. http://www.ncbi.nlm.nih.gov/pubmed/22902039. [cited 2015 Nov 8]
7. Bowlin PR, Farhat WA. Laparoscopic nephrectomy and partial nephrectomy: intraperitoneal, retroperitoneal, single site. Urol Clin North Am. 2015;42(1):31–42. http://www.ncbi.nlm.nih.gov/pubmed/25455170. [cited 2015 Mar 22]
8. Gupta R, Singh S. Challenges in paediatric laparoscopic surgeries. Indian J Anaesth. 2009;53(5):560–6. http://www.pubmedcentral.nih.gov/articlerender.fcgi?artid=2900088&tool=pmcentrez&rendertype=abstract. [cited 2015 Mar 22]
9. Tomaszewski JJ, Casella DP, Turner RM, Casale P, Ost MC. Pediatric laparoscopic and robot-assisted laparoscopic surgery: technical considerations. J Endourol. 2012;26(6):602–13. http://www.ncbi.nlm.nih.gov/pubmed/22050504. [cited 2015 Mar 22]
10. McHoney M, Corizia L, Eaton S, Kiely EM, Drake DP, Tan HL, et al. Carbon dioxide elimination during laparoscopy in children is age dependent. J Pediatr Surg. 2003;38(1):105–10. discussion 105–10. http://www.ncbi.nlm.nih.gov/pubmed/12592630. [cited 2015 Mar 22]
11. Gómez Dammeier BH, Karanik E, Glüer S, Jesch NK, Kübler J, Latta K, et al. Anuria during pneumoperitoneum in infants and children: a prospective study. J Pediatr Surg. 2005;40(9):1454–8. http://www.ncbi.nlm.nih.gov/pubmed/16150348. [cited 2015 Mar 22]
12. Ure BM, Suempelmann R, Metzelder MM, Kuebler J. Physiological responses to endoscopic surgery in children. Semin Pediatr Surg. 2007;16(4):217–23. http://www.ncbi.nlm.nih.gov/pubmed/17933662. [cited 2015 Mar 22]
13. Sümpelmann R, Schuerholz T, Marx G, Härtel D, Hecker H, Ure BM, et al. Haemodynamic, acid-base and blood volume changes during prolonged low pressure pneumoperitoneum in rabbits. Br J Anaesth. 2006;96(5):563–8. http://www.ncbi.nlm.nih.gov/pubmed/16531448. [cited 2015 Mar 22]
14. Sümpelmann R, Schuerholz T, Marx G, Jesch NK, Osthaus WA, Ure BM. Hemodynamic changes during acute elevation of intra-abdominal pressure in rabbits. Paediatr Anaesth. 2006;16(12):1262–7. http://www.ncbi.nlm.nih.gov/pubmed/17121557. [cited 2015 Mar 22]
15. Blinman T, Ponsky T. Pediatric minimally invasive surgery: laparoscopy and thoracoscopy in infants and children. Pediatrics. 2012;130(3):539–49. http://pediatrics.aappublications.org/content/130/3/539.long. [cited 2015 Mar 22]
16. Turner RM, Fox JA, Ost MC. Advances in the surgical pediatric urologic armamentarium. Pediatr Clin N Am. 2012;59(4):927–41. http://www.ncbi.nlm.nih.gov/pubmed/22857839. [cited 2015 Mar 22]
17. Gill IS, Ponsky LEEE, Desai M, Kay R, Ross JH. Laparoscopic cross-trigonal Cohen ureteroneocystostomy: novel technique. J Urol. 2001;166(5):1811–4.
18. Yeung CK, Sihoe JDY, Borzi PA. Endoscopic cross-trigonal ureteral reimplantation under carbon dioxide bladder insufflation: a novel technique. J Endourol. 2005;19(3):295–9. http://www.ncbi.nlm.nih.gov/pubmed/15865516. [cited 2012 Apr 5]

19. Kutikov A, Guzzo TJ, Canter DJ, Casale P. Initial experience with laparoscopic transvesical ureteral reimplantation at the Children's Hospital of Philadelphia. J Urol. 2006;176(5):2222–5. discussion 2225–6. http://www.ncbi.nlm.nih.gov/pubmed/17070297. [cited 2015 Jul 12]
20. Valla JS, Steyaert H, Griffin SJ, Lauron J, Fragoso AC, Arnaud P, et al. Transvesicoscopic Cohen ureteric reimplantation for vesicoureteral reflux in children: a single-centre 5-year experience. J Pediatr Urol. 2009;5(6):466–71. http://www.ncbi.nlm.nih.gov/pubmed/19428305. [cited 2012 Apr 5]
21. Grange P, Giarenis I, Rouse P, Kouriefs C, Robinson D, Cardozo L. Combined vaginal and vesicoscopic collaborative repair of complex vesicovaginal fistulae. Urology. 2014;84(4): 950–4. http://www.ncbi.nlm.nih.gov/pubmed/25150182. [cited 2015 Nov 8]
22. Marte A, Cavaiuolo S, Esposito M, Pintozzi L. Vesicoscopic treatment of symptomatic congenital bladder diverticula in children: a 7-year experience. Eur J Pediatr Surg. 2016;26(3):240–4. http://www.ncbi.nlm.nih.gov/pubmed/25988747. [cited 2015 Nov 8]
23. Peters CA. Robotically assisted surgery in pediatric urology. Urol Clin North Am. 2004;31(4):743–52. http://www.ncbi.nlm.nih.gov/pubmed/15474601. [cited 2015 Jul 12]
24. El-Ghoneimi A. Robotic paediatric urology. BJU Int. 2012;110(1):13. http://www.ncbi.nlm.nih.gov/pubmed/22429862. [cited 2015 Jul 12]
25. Smith RP, Oliver JL, Peters CA. Pediatric robotic extravesical ureteral reimplantation: comparison with open surgery. J Urol. 2011;185(5):1876–81. http://www.ncbi.nlm.nih.gov/pubmed/21421231. [cited 2015 Jul 12]
26. Casella DP, Fox JA, Schneck FX, Cannon GM, Ost MC. Cost analysis of pediatric robot-assisted and laparoscopic pyeloplasty. J Urol. 2013;189(3):1083–6. http://www.ncbi.nlm.nih.gov/pubmed/23017518. [cited 2015 Nov 8]
27. Sukumar S, Roghmann F, Sood A, Abdo A, Menon M, Sammon JD, et al. Correction of ureteropelvic junction obstruction in children: national trends and comparative effectiveness in operative outcomes. J Endourol. 2014;28(5):592–8. http://online.liebertpub.com/doi/abs/10.1089/end.2013.0618. [cited 2015 Aug 14]
28. Chang S-J, Hsu C-K, Hsieh C-H, Yang SS-D. Comparing the efficacy and safety between robotic-assisted versus open pyeloplasty in children: a systemic review and meta-analysis. World J Urol. 2015;33(11):1855–65. http://www.ncbi.nlm.nih.gov/pubmed/25754944. [cited 2015 Aug 12]
29. Olsen LH, Rawashdeh YF, Jorgensen TM. Pediatric robot assisted retroperitoneoscopic pyeloplasty: a 5-year experience. J Urol. 2007;178(5):2137–41. discussion 2141. http://www.sciencedirect.com/science/article/pii/S0022534707017934. [cited 2015 Aug 14]
30. Autorino R, Eden C, El-Ghoneimi A, Guazzoni G, Buffi N, Peters CA, et al. Robot-assisted and laparoscopic repair of ureteropelvic junction obstruction: a systematic review and meta-analysis. Eur Urol. 2014;65(2):430–52. http://www.ncbi.nlm.nih.gov/pubmed/23856037. [cited 2015 Jul 12]
31. Schober MS, Jayanthi VR. Vesicoscopic ureteral reimplant: is there a role in the age of robotics? Urol Clin North Am. 2015;42(1):53–9. http://www.ncbi.nlm.nih.gov/pubmed/25455172. [cited 2015 Nov 8]
32. Weiss DA, Shukla AR. The robotic-assisted ureteral reimplantation: the evolution to a new standard. Urol Clin North Am. 2015;42(1):99–109. http://www.ncbi.nlm.nih.gov/pubmed/25455176. [cited 2015 Jul 12]
33. Kutikov A, Nguyen M, Guzzo T, Canter D, Casale P. Laparoscopic and robotic complex upper-tract reconstruction in children with a duplex collecting system. J Endourol. 2007;21(6): 621–4. http://online.liebertpub.com/doi/abs/10.1089/end.2006.0227. [cited 2015 Aug 14]
34. Gundeti MS, Acharya SS, Zagaja GP, Shalhav AL. Paediatric robotic-assisted laparoscopic augmentation ileocystoplasty and Mitrofanoff appendicovesicostomy (RALIMA): feasibility of and initial experience with the University of Chicago technique. BJU Int. 2011;107(6): 962–9. http://www.ncbi.nlm.nih.gov/pubmed/20942829. [cited 2015 Jul 12]
35. Mattioli G, Buffa P, Torre M, Pini-Prato A, Disma N, Avanzini S, et al. Preperitoneoscopic approach for bladder neck sling suspension in a boy: preliminary experience. J Laparoendosc Adv Surg Tech A. 2010;20(5):497–501. http://www.ncbi.nlm.nih.gov/pubmed/20367124. [cited 2015 Nov 8]

36. Burch JC. Urethrovaginal fixation to Cooper's ligament for correction of stress incontinence, cystocele, and prolapse. Am J Obstet Gynecol. 1961;81:281–90. http://www.ncbi.nlm.nih.gov/pubmed/13688914. [cited 2013 Mar 29]
37. Lucas MG, Bosch RJL, Burkhard FC, Cruz F, Madden TB, Nambiar AK, et al. EAU guidelines on surgical treatment of urinary incontinence. Eur Urol. 2012;62(6):1118–29. http://www.ncbi.nlm.nih.gov/pubmed/23040204. [cited 2013 Mar 20]
38. Reid F, Smith ARB. Laparoscopic versus open colposuspension: which one should we choose? Curr Opin Obstet Gynecol. 2007;19(4):345–9. http://www.ncbi.nlm.nih.gov/pubmed/17625416. [cited 2013 Mar 20]
39. Chrzan R, Klijn AJ, Kuijper CF, Dik P, de Jong TPVM. Laparoscopic burch colposuspension in children: technical challenges and primary results. J Laparoendosc Adv Surg Tech A. 2014;24(7):513–7. http://www.ncbi.nlm.nih.gov/pubmed/24844777. [cited 2015 Aug 12]
40. Storm DW, Fulmer BR, Sumfest JM. Robotic-assisted laparoscopic approach for posterior bladder neck dissection and placement of pediatric bladder neck sling: initial experience. Urology. 2008;72(5):1149–52. http://www.ncbi.nlm.nih.gov/pubmed/18805574. [cited 2012 Mar 20]
41. Gargollo PC. Robotic-assisted bladder neck repair: feasibility and outcomes. Urol Clin North Am. 2015;42(1):111–20. http://www.ncbi.nlm.nih.gov/pubmed/25455177. [cited 2015 Mar 22]
42. Chrzan R, Klijn AJ, Dik P, de Jong TPVM. U2B-dry: preliminary results of a new vesicoscopic technique for bladder neck repair in children. J Laparoendosc Adv Surg Tech A. 2010;20(3):293–6. http://www.ncbi.nlm.nih.gov/pubmed/19943779
43. Chrzan R, Dik P, Klijn AJ, Kuijper CF, van den Heijkant MMC, de Jong TPVM. Vesicoscopic bladder neck procedure in children: what we have learned from the first series. J Laparoendosc Adv Surg Tech A. 2013;23(9):803–7. http://online.liebertpub.com/doi/abs/10.1089/lap.2013.0016. [cited 2015 Aug 12]
44. Dave S, Salle JLP. Current status of bladder neck reconstruction. Curr Opin Urol. 2008;18(4):419–24. http://www.ncbi.nlm.nih.gov/pubmed/18520766
45. Grimsby GM, Menon V, Schlomer BJ, Baker LA, Adams R, Gargollo PC, et al. Long-term outcomes of bladder neck reconstruction without augmentation cystoplasty in children. J Urol. 2016;195(1):155–61. http://www.ncbi.nlm.nih.gov/pubmed/26173106. [cited 2015 Nov 8]
46. Sukumar S, Djahangirian O, Sood A, Sammon JD, Varda B, Janosek-Albright K, et al. Minimally invasive vs open pyeloplasty in children: the differential effect of procedure volume on operative outcomes. Urology. 2014;84(1):180–4. http://www.sciencedirect.com/science/article/pii/S0090429514001186. [cited 2015 Aug 14]
47. Passerotti CC, Franco F, Bissoli JCC, Tiseo B, Oliveira CM, Buchalla CAO, et al. Comparison of the learning curves and frustration level in performing laparoscopic and robotic training skills by experts and novices. Int Urol Nephrol. 2015;47(7):1075–84. http://www.ncbi.nlm.nih.gov/pubmed/25913053. [cited 2015 Aug 12]

Open Surgery for Incontinence

Tom P.V.M. de Jong and Aart J. Klijn

33.1 Surgical Treatment

33.1.1 Introduction

In children, indications for surgical treatment of urinary incontinence (UI) are predominantly related to neurogenic lower urinary tract dysfunction (LUTD). Also a number of congenital non-neurogenic urogenital anomalies can lead to involuntary leakage of urine and may require surgical intervention. In children who cannot void spontaneously dryness is probably a more appropriate term to describe the normal state (no leakage) but in this chapter a uniform term continence will be used regardless of the underlying pathology. Bladder and bladder outlet (BO) are equally important for continence and both must be thoroughly examined when surgical treatment is considered. However, for practical reasons they are discussed separately.

Significant increase in the intravesical pressure can result in incontinence and if necessary must be treated before of together with the bladder outlet. On the other hand, one has to keep in mind that any surgical procedure that increases the BO resistance can lead to the serious changes of the bladder function and finally deterioration of the upper urinary tract and kidney function. That means that all patients in whom BO procedure is considered require a very careful preoperative checkup and a close follow-up after surgery. Adequate bladder volume and proper compliance are needed to achieve continence. When the bladder is too small which is referred to

---

T.P.V.M. de Jong (✉) • A.J. Klijn
Department of Pediatric Urology, University Children's Hospitals UMC Utrecht and AMC Amsterdam, 85090, Utrecht, 3508AB, The Netherlands
e-mail: T.P.V.M.deJong@umcutrecht.nl

© Springer International Publishing AG, part of Springer Nature 2018
G. Mosiello et al. (eds.), *Clinical Urodynamics in Childhood and Adolescence*, Urodynamics, Neurourology and Pelvic Floor Dysfunctions, https://doi.org/10.1007/978-3-319-42193-3_33

the expected bladder capacity (EBX) and the compliance is poor (high end-filling pressure), then bladder augmentation should be chosen. In selected cases, with adequate volume and poor compliance, detrusorectomy can be done.

A wide variety of techniques are described to improve bladder outlet resistance. None of them are universal and many factors have influence on the decision which one should be used. Underlying pathology, general condition of the patient and the kidney function as well as the age and the social situation must be considered. The most important issues are as follows: (1) is patient expected to void, (2) is the patient able to empty the bladder on his own, and (3) does he/she need a stoma. The surgeon must bear in mind that the school-age children are dependent on their care providers and the clean intermittent catheterization (CIC) is usually done on time but during adolescence the well-established CIC schedule can be neglected by the child. Hence, the question is how tight the BO should be. Is there any pop-off mechanism needed? If not, then bladder neck closure can be the best definitive option. Furthermore, if the urethra is supposed to be used for a CIC, then the BO procedure should not get destroyed in time. Different techniques are used depending on the etiology of UI and the preferences/experience of the surgeon. Bladder neck and the urethra must be constructed in children with bladder/cloacal exstrophy. Girls with epispadias may require urethra lengthening with cranial repositioning of the bladder neck. In children with neurogenic LUTD a remodeling/plasty of the bladder neck can be done (Young-Dees, Koff, Mitchell-Leadbetter, Pippi-Sale, etc). A number of suspension techniques using allo- and autologous material can also be used in these patients.

Indication for a BO procedure is made on the base of the clinical symptoms, urodynamic study (UDS), and in some cases ultrasound of the pelvic floor. Stress urinary leakage usually indicates a poor bladder outlet resistance. A UDS is done to assess the bladder function: volume and compliance, to exclude detrusor overactivity and to assess the detrusor leak point pressure is measured. Strict reference point does not exist, but pressure >40 H_2O is considered high and dangerous for the upper tract. It is worth to remember that it is not always possible to reproduce the symptoms during the UDS. Ultrasound of the pelvic floor provides an additional information of its anatomy and function. Continuously open bladder neck and absence of the vesicourethral angle during filling phase in combination with hypermobility of this region during straining (cystocoele) can suggest a congenital bladder neck incompetence. Those girls can be cured by a (Burch) colposuspension procedure.

Children with a neurogenic bladder have a denervated, paralyzed sphincter and pelvic floor in approximately 40% of cases. They need surgery to become dry and CIC to empty the bladder after surgery.

The children with spinal dysraphism and an overactive pelvic floor run a high risk to end up needing bladder surgery because of the development of a contractile overactive bladder with risks for the upper urinary tract. The development of a hostile bladder can be prevented by starting antimuscarinic treatment immediately after birth, a treatment that will be needed lifelong.

When doing bladder outlet surgery, one should think about bladder surgery at the same moment to reduce subsequent risks for the upper tracts. A recent publication by Grimsby et al. is quite convincing that these risks are high and should be prevented as much as possible [1].

Bladder outlet surgery can be done in many ways. The most popular ways of lengthening the urethra cranially into the bladder are known under the names of

Young-Dees-Leadbetter, Kropp, Pippi Salle, and Mitchell and a simple lengthening of the urethra over the anterior surface of the bladder wall, a procedure that also can be done vesicoscopically. The basic principle of all these procedures is the creation of a 2.5–3 cm long channel into the bladder that is supposed to be leak-proof by way of flap valve, compression of surrounding tissues, and/or the fact that the proximal urethra is brought into the abdominal cavity in a way that increasing pressures in the abdomen are also transmitted onto the proximal urethra thus keeping it closed.

33.2 Bladder Neck Procedures

In a YDL procedure, the surgery starts by bilateral ureteric reimplantation to bring the ureters higher up in the bladder. A mucosal strip is created, 12 mm wide, from the bladder neck 2.5 cm long. The adjacent part of the bladder is denuded from mucosa, and these bare triangles of detrusor are incised from lateral up till the level of the proximal end of the mucosal strip. The mucosal strip is sutured into a tube over a 10 Fr catheter. The two triangles of detrusor are wrapped around the mucosal tube in a hand-over-vest fashion (Fig. 33.1). Bladder drainage is done by suprapubic

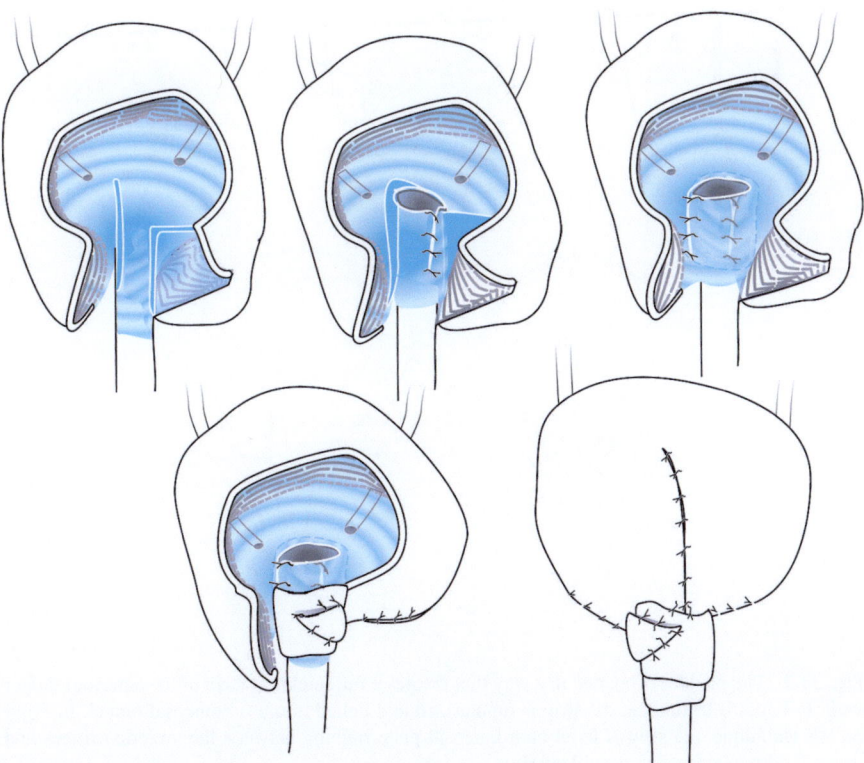

Fig. 33.1 Classical Young-Dees-Leadbetter technique for a bladder neck reconstruction

catheter, and a transurethral stent is left for 3 weeks. CIC is reinstituted after 3 weeks. The procedure costs approximately 30 mL of bladder volume [2].

In Kropp's tube the bladder is opened anteriorly, the last 3 cm up till the bladder neck in an inverted U fashion creating a 20-mm-wide full-thickness flap of the anterior wall. A mucosal incision is made around the bladder neck from 3-6-9 o'clock position, and the flap is sutured into a full-thickness tube. Starting at the mucosal incision, a 2.5 cm submucosal tunnel is created cranially between the ureteric orifices, and the tube is buried and fixed into this tunnel (Fig. 33.2). Again, after 3 weeks, CIC can be reinstituted. The advantage of the procedure is that it does not cost much volume. The disadvantage in male patients is that it may create an angle between prostatic urethra and proximal tube hampering CIC [3].

Pippi Salle's procedure has the same opening of the bladder as Kropp's, but now the incision is done to create a flap 15 mm wide. Starting at the bladder neck, a mucosal strip, 10–12 mm wide, is created, in general after bilateral ureteric reimplantation to bring the ureters in a more cranial position. The flap is sutured to the mucosal strip creating a flap valve. The constructed tube is covered by mucosa

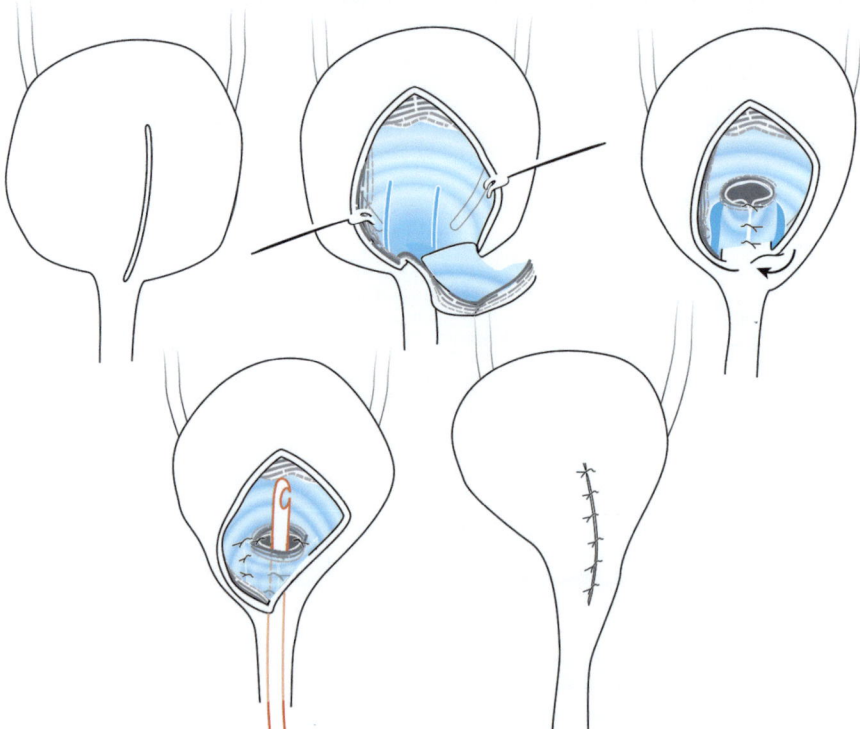

Fig. 33.2 The bladder is opened in a way that creates a full thickness strip of the anterior bladder wall. In Kropp's technique, the strip is tubularized and pulled into a submucosal tunnel. In Pippi Salle's technique, the strip is fixed on a mucosal plate running between the ureteric orifices and covered with mucosa, harvested laterally

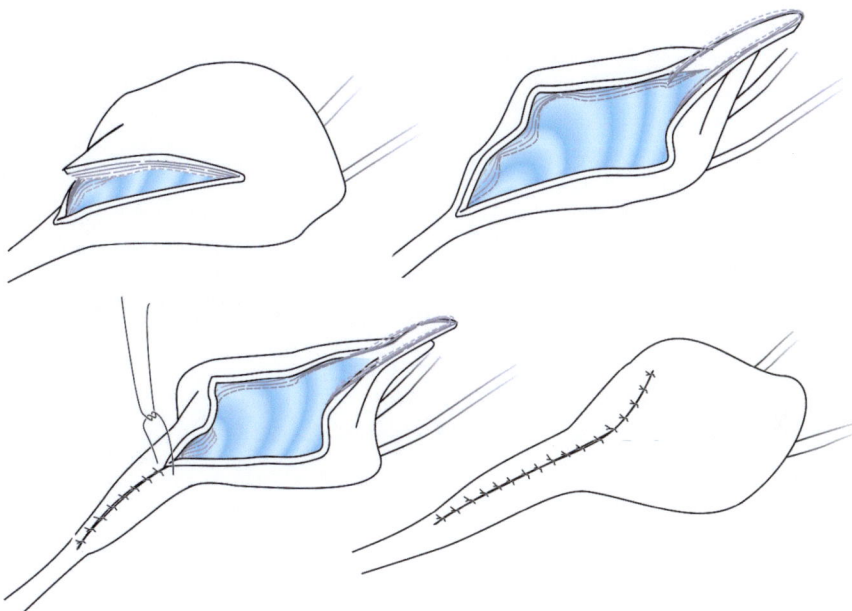

Fig. 33.3 Mitchel's technique of funneling the bladder neck

mobilized from left to right. Stenting and drainage are done for 3 weeks, and CIC should be restarted after 3 weeks. The procedure has the same advantages and disadvantages as Kropp's [4].

In Mitchell's procedure, the bladder is opened, starting at the level of the bladder neck, in a fashion that a 2-cm-wide and 2.5–3-cmlong strip of full-thickness bladder wall is left at the bottom of the bladder. In general, the ureters need to be taken up. The strip and the bladder are simply closed longitudinally creating a lengthening of the urethra into the abdominal cavity (Fig. 33.3). Again, drainage and splinting are done for 3 weeks before restarting CIC. Also this procedure, in males, may cause an angle in the urethra [5].

"Keeling" of the urethra. When lengthening the urethra over the anterior aspect of the bladder wall, the bladder is opened transversely or higher up longitudinally. A U-shaped incision is made around the bladder neck on the anterior aspect of the bladder. Best is to make it near full thickness. The strip is closed over a catheter, and the bladder is closed in a fashion that the created tube runs over the anterior aspect of the bladder (Fig. 33.4). The tube is covered with mucosa, mobilized from left to right. Drainage and stenting for 3 weeks are done before restarting CIC. The advantage of this procedure is that the tube follows the direction of the prostatic procedure with less problems in doing CIC afterward [6].

Of course many alternatives exist such as the creation of a tube from the bladder wall to replace the urethra as has been described by Tanagho or even the use of a distal ureter as the urethra.

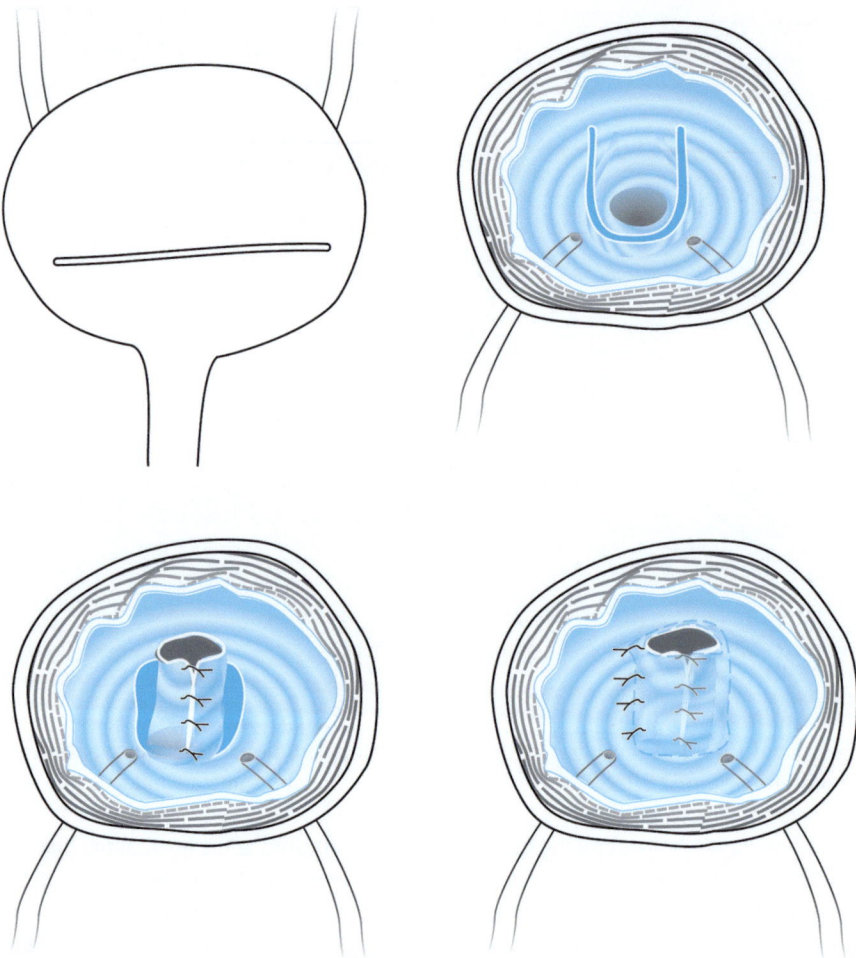

Fig. 33.4 Creation of a lengthening of the urethra on the anterior aspect of the bladder. This procedure can also be done vesicoscopically

33.2.1 Slings

A totally different approach is to create a closing mechanism by suspending and compressing the bladder neck with a sling. The advantage of sling procedures is that drainage and stenting can be done for a shorter period of time and that CIC can be reinstituted earlier, after 7–10 days [7, 8]. The disadvantage is that, in males, approximately 10–15% will develop problems with normal transurethral CIC afterward bringing the need for a secondary catheterizable stoma from the bladder to the abdominal skin. Another disadvantage is that finding the way around the bladder neck may result in a leak and subsequent failure of the procedure or erosion of the sling into the bladder neck. Also a vesicovaginal fistula may be created in female patients. All these complications may lead to the decision to do a bladder neck closure and create a catheterizable stoma. Several tips may help to prevent this complication. For the sling, mostly the rectus abdominis fascia is used, but some like to use artificial material [9–11]. This has the theoretic disadvantage, when done before puberty, that after the pubertal growth spurt, the sling may be too tight, but we have no experience with that. We do have the experience that a rectus abdominis fascia sling, when done at a young age, will stay good and dry when passing puberty without creating prostatic problems in male patients. Normally the sling is harvested in the midline. Sometimes the quality of the fascia is not good enough, or the patient may have had an earlier operation with transverse incision of the fascia. In those cases the sling may be harvested from a lateral side, a strip of fascia taken cranially from Poupart's ligament.

33.2.2 Puboprostatic Sling in Male Patients

Depending on the need for bladder surgery during the same procedure, the abdomen is opened by transverse lower abdominal incision with longitudinal opening of the rectus fascia up till the level of the umbilicus or by a longitudinal lower abdominal incision. The sling is harvested over a length of approximately 10–15 cm, 2 cm wide, not detached from the pubic bone. Most textbooks advise to find the way around the bladder neck by opening the urogenital diaphragm left and right of the bladder neck and going around the bladder neck through these openings with a right angle. Alternatively, Lottmann described a way by freeing the whole bladder from the peritoneum and putting the sling around the bladder neck caudally of the ureters [12]. In our experience, when combined with a ureteric reimplantation, this may reduce the blood supply to the bladder resulting in bladder fibrosis in one patient that had a detrusorectomy during the same procedure with a subsequent ileocystoplasty 6 months later.

We have chosen for a perineal approach to develop the plane between the bladder neck and the rectum (Fig. 33.5). With the patient in an exaggerated lithotomy position, an inverted-U incision is made in front of the anus, with the transverse part of the incision at the level of the caudal rim of the symphysis. With a gauze roll in the rectum, the plane can be felt easily. Following a transurethral catheter, the perineal body is opened sharply, and the plane between the rectum and the prostate is developed by blunt finger preparation. In the midline, sometimes sharp dissection of structures is needed. By pulling the balloon of the catheter to the bladder neck, one can feel when the right level has been reached. From this level, following the rami of the pubic bone closely with a fingertip, a hole is made left and right from the bladder neck in the urogenital diaphragm into the prevesical space by pushing the finger through. In some cases, the diaphragm can be so tight that a very strong finger is needed. A rubber band is brought from the perineal wound into the prevesical space. The sling is taken around the bladder neck, fixed to these rubber bands.

Many ways of putting the sling around the bladder neck exist. In general, we take the sling down through the left rectus abdominis muscle, take the sling around in a simple U shape, bring it up through the contralateral rectus muscle and fascia, and

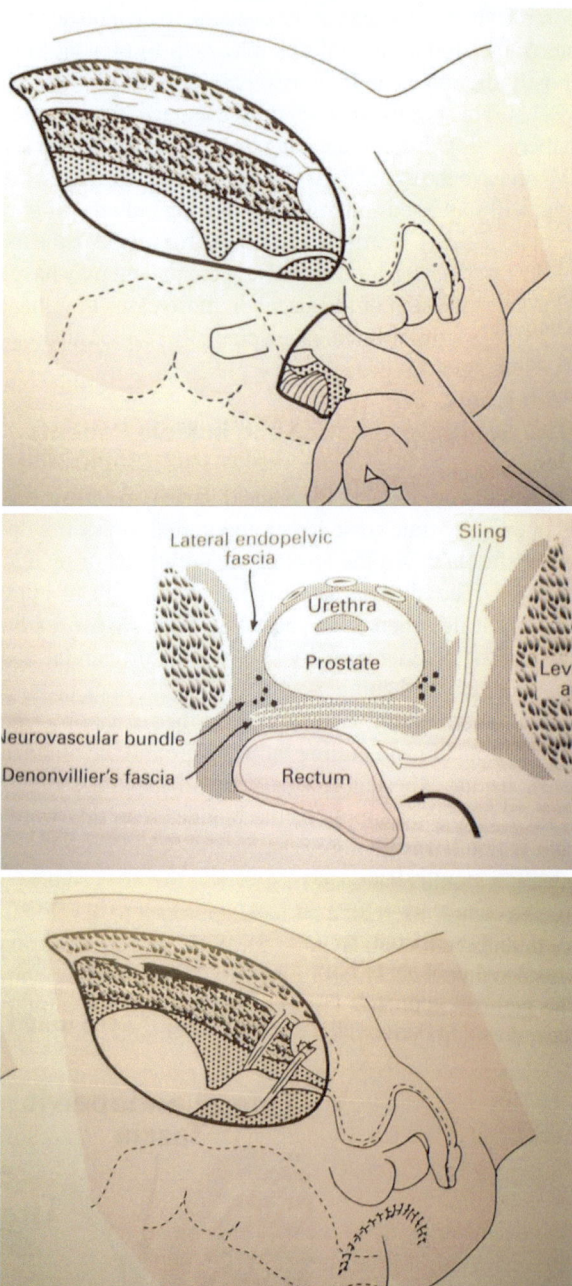

Fig. 33.5 Technique to create a puboprostatic sling in a male patient with perineal access to the plane between the bladder neck and the rectum

suture it to the fascia and pubic bone. In theory, by doing this, contraction of the rectus abdominis muscle tightens the sling. Whether if this is truly the case has not been proven. The tightness of the sling is dictated by the ability to pass a 12 Fr (prepubertal) or a 14–16 Fr catheter (after puberty) through the bladder neck. Several authors have published this sling making a full turn around the bladder neck and claim excellent result. In our hands, the few cases that we did this way were failures. In case the sling appears too short, it can be fixed to Cooper's ligament instead of the rectus fascia [13].

33.2.3 Rectus Abdominis Fascia Sling in Female Patients

In female patients, surgeons with limited experience have trouble to find the plane between the bladder neck and the vagina with a risk for damaging the bladder neck with subsequent erosion of the sling or even development of a vesicovaginal fistula. We have learned many years ago that this risk can be avoided by simply putting the sling through the vagina. After opening of the abdomen with longitudinal opening of the rectus abdominis fascia, the anterior vaginal wall, the urethra, and the bladder neck are exposed. Filling of the bladder and a catheter balloon with some traction allows to identify the bladder neck and the limit of the bladder connection to the anterior vaginal wall. One centimeter laterally of this limit, at the level of the bladder neck, a small hole is burnt into the vagina on a small sponge that pushes the vaginal wall up at the elected site left and right. Rubber bands are put through the holes and are used to pass the sling through the holes. The sling is passed through the contralateral rectus abdominis muscle and fascia and sutured at the fascia (Fig. 33.6). In case of a neurogenic bladder, the sling is tightened in such a way that one finger may pass between the symphysis and the bladder neck. In non-neurogenic cases that are expected to void spontaneously after the procedure, two fingers of space are left behind the symphysis. CIC can be started a few days after the procedure. By doing a sling this way, the procedure has become much easier, and the risk for erosion or fistulas has been dramatically reduced. Again, when the sling is too short, one may choose to fix it to Cooper's ligament [14].

33.2.4 Urethral Slings

Coming out of surgery for adult male incontinence after radical prostatectomy for prostatic cancer, a system has been developed to cure this by putting a sling of artificial material tightly to the bulbous urethra fixed to the pubic bones with bone anchors (Advance®). Few departments claim success by these slings, for example, for persistent incontinence in male patients with epispadias [9].

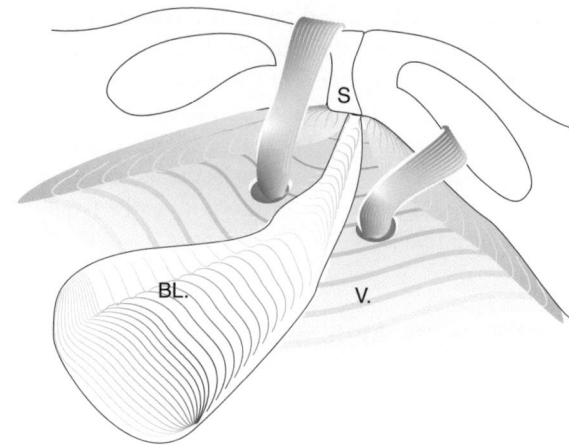

Fig. 33.6 Transvaginal rectus fascia sling in a female

33.2.5 Colposuspension Technique

Several types of colposuspension to cure bladder neck incompetence and congenital cystocele have been described. Colposuspension techniques that fix the anterior vaginal wall to the retropubic periosteum have been left because of the risk for developing overactive bladder complaints. Needle suspension techniques have been left because of disappointing results on the long term. In girls with therapy-resistant stress incontinence, mostly in combination with generalized hyperlaxity of joints, after failed conservative treatment that included good physical therapy of the pelvic floor with anal balloon biofeedback, one can reach the point that surgery is the only option left. Also girls with an open bladder neck resulting in overactive bladder complaints and recurrent urinary tract infections may, in rare cases that are refractory to conservative treatment, end up with an indication for colposuspension. The mechanism is that due to the open bladder neck, urine is always present in the proximal urethra. Urine in the proximal urethra triggers the micturition reflex resulting in OAB complaints counteracted by the pelvic floor that is responsible for dysfunctional voiding, insufficient emptying, and recurrent lower urinary tract infections.

The type of colposuspension that has best results is that described by Burch. Suspension is done of the anterior vaginal wall, left and right of the bladder neck, to Cooper's ligament. The operation is nice and easy in prepubertal girls and can be difficult in overweight postpubertal females. Because of that, it is a blessing that, nowadays, it can also be done by laparoscopy. When doing other types of surgery, for example, ureteric reimplantations, in a girl with a low standing open bladder neck or absent vesicourethral angle, we always combine the procedure with a few suspension sutures. In those cases the procedure takes only a few minutes extra OR time. No proof exists that it really produces extra benefit for the patient, but proof exists that it does no harm.

33.3 Technique

Transverse lower abdominal incision. Preferably the rectus fascia is opened in the midline to take into account the possible need for a later sling suspension in case of failure. The prevesical space is developed, the bladder neck, urethra, and anterior vaginal wall identified with a balloon catheter in the bladder and some filling of the bladder. Bladder margin at the anterior vaginal wall is identified. This can be tedious, especially when the bladder is completely empty. In left and right of the vagina, the optimal point is chosen with an instrument that lifts the vaginal wall unilaterally. Chosen point to put the suture is chosen approximately 1 cm lateral of the bladder neck and is marked by diathermia for better fixation afterward. This depends also on the suture material chosen. Polyglycolic acid sutures may dissolve without any tissue reaction, and some tissue reaction is required in cases where the anterior vaginal wall is suspended to keep the suspension intact. Suspension suture is taken at full thickness through the vaginal wall. The suture is then passed through the Cooper's ligament that is strongly developed in any subject. Sutures are tied in such a way that a good suspension exists. In most cases, it is not possible to get a complete junction between the anterior vaginal wall and Cooper's ligament, but apparently this does not matter. Looking into the literature, one may find many ways of suturing and types and number of suture material. In general, we use one strong polyglycolic acid suture on each side with approximately 60% good result at long-term follow-up [15]. In our hands, simple colposuspension was without any success in cases with a neurogenic bladder. Literature on this subject is inconsistent; some have reported reasonable success. Simple colposuspension has been proven to remain successful after later pregnancy and vaginal delivery [16].

33.3.1 Minimal Invasive Slings, TVT, and TOT

In pediatric urology, these are rarely used. Concerns exist about the lack of space for vaginal surgery in girls and concerns about possible problems in later pregnancy and vaginal delivery.

33.3.2 Artificial Sphincter Placement

Several reports exist on series of artificial sphincter placement for neurogenic incontinence. The technique, in males, is comparable to that needed for bladder neck sling suspension where the bladder neck is circled from above. We will not describe in detail the technique needed. Literature reports show that only a minority of the patients will not need CIC afterward and is able to void volitionally. For the majority of patients, an artificial sphincter is an expensive type of sling with a repeated need for reoperations.

33.4 Bladder Surgery

Bladder surgery at pediatric age is mostly needed in children with neurogenic bladder, sometimes in severe cases of posterior urethral valves, exstrophy of the bladder, and in oncologic cases. The use of cultured bladders is standing at the horizon for many years but still is not clinically available. Because of this the only possibilities that we have to come to a bigger bladder or a bladder with better compliance and lower pressures are introducing a piece of gastrointestinal tract into the bladder, megaureters when available, or removing a substantial part of the detrusor muscle to bring the pressure down. When bladder augment surgery is done, of course, this can be combined with any other procedure needed such as a sling, bladder neck repair, ureteric reimplantation, or construction of a catheterizable stoma [17, 18].

33.4.1 Bladder Augmentation by Enterocystoplasty

In the last decades, people have used different parts of the intestinal tract for bladder augmentation. Gastrocystoplasty has been popular, but most have abandoned this technique based on experiences with late complications. Colonic augments have been popular and are still being used in several pouch techniques, but most pediatric urologic surgeons, over the last 10 years, prefer the ileum as material for the bladder augmentation.

33.5 Technique for Ileocystoplasty

An ileocystoplasty can be done through a transverse lower abdominal incision, but a lower midline incision gives a better overview. The bladder needs to be opened extensively in the midline from the bladder neck anteriorly till between the ureteric orifices posteriorly to avoid a later hourglass bladder: a small retracted ring at the junction of the bowel and detrusor. An ileal segment is chosen to isolate and insert into the bladder. At least 25–30 cm is needed for redundant volume afterward. Preferably, the last 25 cm of the ileum is left in place to avoid vitamin B problems years after surgery. Vasculature of the chosen segment is controlled by looking at the vessels through the mesentery with a strong backlight. The segment is isolated, and the mesentery is opened and vessels clamped. Where in the past, I truly developed a vascular pedicle based on two vessels, nowadays I open the mesentery for not more than 5 cm. The segment is cut in between clamped ilea; ileal-ileal anastomosis is done. We prefer interrupted 4–5.0 polyglycolic acid sutures; many alternatives exist. Most pediatric urologists do too few of these procedures a year to be very dexterous with staplers. The isolated segment is opened antimesenterically. This is done by inserting a 30 Fr silicon drain in the segment and opening it by diathermia cutting on the tube. Depending on the length of the segment, this can be folded into a U or a W with a running 3.0 suture. The created patch is sutured into the bladder using several

3.0 running sutures. The bladder is closed with a 16 Fr suprapubic catheter left to avoid mucous problems in the days after surgery. It is questionable whether the neobladder should be put intraperitoneally or extraperitoneally. We try to bring the bladder extraperitoneally by closing the peritoneum as much as possible. In theory one should see less spontaneous perforations, and indeed, we very rarely have had one. But in contrast, also cycling of the bladder into a good volume may be hampered by doing so, and indeed, we have seen a few patients that took some time to develop adequate volume or even needed distension under anesthesia.

Cycling the bladder by clamping the catheter is started at day 3–4, and the patient is sent home when clamping can be done for 3 h. CIC can be started at day 7 in a normal child without nocturnal polyuria. For reasons of mucous, CIC should ideally be done with a 14 or 16 Fr catheter. Patients with mucous problems may have their bladder flushed once a day with a solution of acetylcysteine (expensive), 0, 9% NaCl, or water.

33.5.1 Alternative for Ileocystoplasty: Detrusorectomy or Autoaugmentation of the Bladder

In well-selected cases, detrusorectomy can be the ideal choice. Patients need to have a reasonable bladder volume, at least 75% of expected volume for age, and especially bad compliance of the bladder and severe dependency on anticholinergics are a strong indication to do a detrusorectomy. Many reports have been published about failed detrusorectomies. These were reports where the exposed bladder mucosa has been left uncovered or has been covered by peritoneum or omentum. Success has been reported in cases where the exposed bladder mucosa has been covered by demucolized sigmoid colon. We have chosen, with rather good success, to cover the exposed mucosa with the well-vascularized adventitional layers surrounding the bladder, the layers that make the bladder slide up and down unnoticed when filling and emptying. The procedure can be combined with any other surgery for bladder outlet and even intravesical surgery for ureteric reimplantations [19–22].

With the bladder exposed, meticulous removal of the adventitional layers from the detrusor muscle is done from the anterior and lateral aspects of the bladder. The adventitional layers are marked with a suture to be able to find them back later. Cranially of the urachus, the peritoneum is freed from the detrusor. The bladder is filled by indwelling catheter connected to an infusion bag with 5% saline or glucose at 30 cm water pressure. The top of the bladder is fixed with a clamp at the urachal remnant. Detrusorectomy, incising the detrusor up till the level of the mucosa, is started with a circumferential incision around the urachal remnant with a diameter of 2–3 cm using a blunt scissors. Enlarging the diverticulum is done in all directions after good exposure of the circumferential mucosa. When a good diverticulum has been realized, we have chosen to make one extra vertical incision cranially, two lateral incisions backward, and one in the direction of the bladder neck on the anterior surface. This latter anterior incision may be tedious because here, the detrusor tends to be more securely fixed to the mucosa. The idea of the cranial and lateral incisions is to fool Laplace's law making circular contractions of the detrusor impossible. Remnant detrusor strips are excised by diathermia. An occasional mucosal leak is closed using 7.0 monophilic suture with a small isolated patch of detrusor glued on with Tissue coll®. After this, the bladder is emptied, the adventitional layers are meticulously closed in the midline, and the abdomen is closed with fixation of the urachal patch as high as possible to the rectus abdominis muscle. We have the habit of leaving a low-pressure suction tube in front of the adventitional layers when closing the wound. One may doubt if this is needed.

Aftercare is of utmost importance; the bladder should be challenged immediately. We do this by instilling a pressure of 20 cm water in the first 24 h after surgery (by putting the catheter bag on that level) and 30 cm in the second 24 h and starting clamping the catheter after 2 days. Patients are sent home with a clamping regime at day 4 or 5 and readmitted after 7–10 days to restart CIC.

33.5.2 Bladder Augmentation by Megaureters

In case of large megaureters and a small bladder, one can think about using the megaureter for augmentation of the bladder. This may happen in boys with posterior urethral valves with a nonfunctioning kidney and a refluxing megaureter or in exstrophy cases with the typically refluxing fishhook configuration of the ureters. In case of a nonfunctioning kidney, nephrectomy is done and as much as possible if the ureter is used as an augment. When the patient had an earlier cutaneous ureterostomy, the kidney can be left in place and be removed later. Some even have reported using the dilated pyelum of a nonfunctioning kidney as well with success. In exstrophy cases, the dilated distal ureters can be used as augment; the proximal ureters are reimplanted into the bladder [23–26].

Technique: the bladder is opened transversally. Literature reports advise opening the bladder into the ureteric orifices. For safety of blood supply, we leave the last 3 mm to the orifice unopened. The ureter that is going to be used as an augment is opened, taking care to leave as many vessels as possible untouched. When sufficient length of the ureter exists, the ureter is folded into a U shape with a running 4.0 polyglycolic suture. In exstrophy cases, the two ureters will be sutured to the bladder wall and to themselves. The bladder is closed leaving a suprapubic catheter in place. Again, cycling of the bladder is of utmost importance and will be started at day 2 or 3 by clamping the catheter.

33.6 CIC Stoma

A continent stoma for CIC has many advantages for the wheelchair-bound patients, especially for girls that need a transfer from their wheelchair for CIC. Other indications may be parental preference because of the need to lift a

25 kg child out of the wheelchair several times a day, parental preferences considering privacy of their child: exposing the genitalia several times a day for CIC when at school, problems with dexterity of the child doing CIC per urethram, and problems performing CIC in a boy caused by false route. This may happen in 10% of boys after a sling procedure. A stoma is a good solution for many patients, but the complication rate, especially in the first few months after surgery, should not be underestimated.

33.7 Techniques

Many alternatives exist. Any tube that can be connected to the bladder or constructed from the bladder can be used. Ideally, a distal part of the ureter may be used, when present. This can both be a ureteric remnant after removal of a nonfunctioning kidney and a distal ureter that is left in place with reimplantation of the proximal ureter into the bladder. In these cases, reflux often exists, and the distal ureter may need an extravesical anti-reflux procedure (Lich-Gregoire technique). The appendix as a CIC stoma has been published as early as 1910 and popularized by Mitrofanoff [27, 28]. When bladder volume is sufficient, a strip of bladder wall may be constructed into a tube with intravesical lengthening by a mucosal tunnel. Some have used urachal remnants with success. Looking into the literature, the bladder tube comes with less complications than appendix when used as catheterizable stoma.

33.8 Aftercare

In the past, many used prolonged catheterization to prevent stomal stenosis. Special technique to construct the skin connection has been reported (V-Q-Z technique) to overcome stomal stenosis. By now, most have adopted the practice of routine use of a readily available silicon ACE stopper into the stoma during the first year after surgery. Ace stoppers of 12- or 14 Fr diameter, with a length between 4 and 6 cm, can be used. We have learned to postpone the start of CIC till 5 weeks after surgery to overcome CIC problems. Patients go home with an intubated stoma and a suprapubic catheter that is opened every 3–4 h to keep the bladder at an adequate volume.

The ureter: When a distal ureter is present, this is simply brought to the skin through muscle layers and fascia and sutured to the skin that has been opened by a V-shaped incision with 5.0 polyglycolic sutures. The ureter is left intubated for 2 weeks, and CIC can be started by then.

Appendix: One may try finding the appendix by transverse abdominal incision; many prefer a lower abdominal midline incision. The appendix is located, the mesentery meticulously left intact, cut at the level of the coecum with the stump simply ligated. When the appendix is very long, the coecal part may be used as an antegrade colonic enema stoma. The mesentery is freed in such a way that mobilization of the appendix is sufficient to connect one part with the bladder and the other part to the skin, in the umbilicus, or on the right lower abdominal wall. Ideally, peristalsis should be in the direction of the bladder, meaning that the top of the appendix is sutured to the skin. Connection of the appendix to the bladder is done in a similar way as an extravesical anti-reflux procedure. The detrusor muscle is opened over a length of 3 cm, leaving the mucosa intact. A small opening in the mucosa is made, and the appendix is sutured to the mucosa with four interrupted 5.0 sutures, of those two stay sutured to the detrusor as well. With the appendix intubated by a 10–12 Fr silicon drain, the detrusor muscle is closed over the appendix with 4.0 sutures. One has to decide where to bring the appendix into the bladder. Doing this on the posterior bladder wall can be done, but may be clumsy, the mesentery with the vessels are in the way. Taking the anterior wall of the bladder is easier, but the bladder should be fixed to the rectus muscle to avoid kinking of the appendix with subsequent catheterization problems. The appendix is fixed to the skin at the level of the umbilicus, mostly a simple subumbilical circumferential incision, leading to a V-shaped skin tag sutured to the spatulated appendix. The appendix can be taken out of the abdomen in between the rectus abdominis muscles or taken through one or even both rectus muscles to create an extra sphincter: when the rectus contracts, the appendix is closed. Different insights exist: some claim good results considering dryness by doing this, while some claim extra complications by CIC problems. Peritoneum is closed as good as possible without hampering the vascular supply.

Common daily practice has taught us to leave the appendix intubated for 5 weeks before starting CIC. Many extra CIC problems occurred when starting CIC after 2 or 3 weeks in the past.

33.9 Bladder Tube

When bladder volume is large for expected volume for age, a bladder tube for a catheterizable stoma is preferable. Textbooks show nice pictures of slender Boari-type bladder flaps. Be aware that such a flap shrinks when the bladder is emptied. Creation of a tube around a 12 Fr catheter needs a 3 cm-long flap, 3 cm wide at the base and 2.5 cm at the top. Depending on the level of the top of the bladder, one must decide if the catheterizable channel follows the posterior or the anterior bladder wall, coming from the umbilicus. Again, the posterior wall channel has some more risk for kinking. The detrusor strip is closed over a 12 Fr catheter using interrupted 4.0 sutures. By using diathermia, a 2 cm-wide strip of mucosa is created over 2.5–3 cm length, in continuation with the tube. The strip is closed into a tube. Laterally of the strip, bladder mucosa is undermined and pulled over the tube as a second layer of mucosa, avoiding kissing suture lines. The tube is fixed to the umbilicus in a similar way as the appendix. The bladder is closed and, in case of an anteriorly placed tube, fixed to the rectus muscle to avoid kinking (Fig. 33.7).

Again, intubation of the stoma for 4–5 weeks is advised.

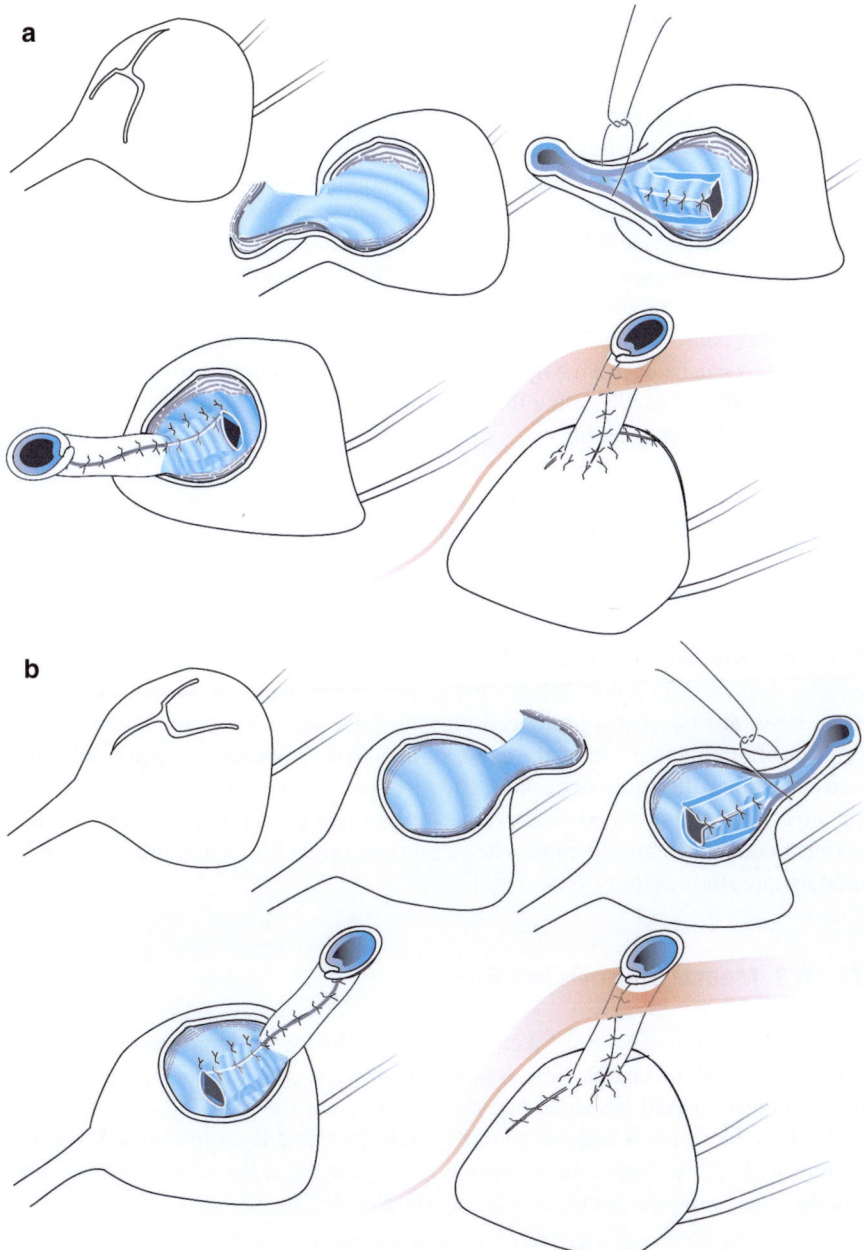

Fig. 33.7 (a) Upper picture shows the construction of a bladder tube with the tube running on the anterior aspect of the bladder. (b) Lower picture with the tube running into the dome of the bladder

33.9.1 Ileal Tubes: The Yang/Monti Procedure

Ileal tubes constructed by tapering an ileal segment are reported to come with many problems due to sacculation and CIC problems caused by the circumferential mucosal folds. To overcome this, a better catheterizable channel can be constructed by isolating a 2 cm segment of ileum, opening this antimesenterically and tubularizing this around a catheter [29]. In case that this is too short, two rings of ileum can be used, one opened at one side of the mesentery, the other at the contralateral side, and these can be connected into one long strip. The tube can be used similarly as an appendix between the bladder and the skin. The disadvantage is that sacculation and kinking may cause difficulties in performing CIC. When combined with an ileocystoplasty, this can be overcome by constructing the tube from two strips of ileum, cut from the split ileal patch. Doing this, the tube has enough support by the ileal mesentery to prevent sacculation.

33.10 Minor Surgery for Incontinent Children

33.10.1 Boys with Overactive Bladder Complaints

Every boy with urge incontinence based on overactive bladder complaints should also be suspected for a urethral narrowing as cause of the OAB. Sometimes, this is easy, when at first visit a prolonged plateau-shape uroflow points out the meatal stenosis after circumcision as the cause of the OAB. Stenoses in the proximal urethra can come with a normal uroflow, and many will not be detected by VCUG. One should consider, after failed conservative treatment of OAB complaints by antimuscarinic treatment and urotherapy, when a boy has a right for further investigation by urodynamic study and/or cystoscopy [30].

33.10.2 Meatal Stenosis in a Boy

The simple technique by doing a meatotomy and closing this transversely will have a recurrence risk of nearly 50%. It is better to avoid dilatation of the meatus and create a meatal-based V-shaped flap on the surface of the glans by using a cornea knife. This V incision is lengthened into the distal urethra. By suturing the V into the urethra with 7.0 polyglycolic sutures, a Y-V plasty is done with a considerably smaller chance for recurrence of the stenosis. Surgical loupes are needed.

33.11 Cystoscopy in a Boy, Suspected for Urethral Obstruction

The procedure is started with a cystoscope using a 25–30 grade optic. The bladder is inspected for trabeculation, the bladder neck observed with full and empty bladder. Prostatic urethra is inspected, and the top of the colliculus is sounded with a 3 Fr ureteral catheter. Normal depth of the utricular remnant is between 5 mm and 12 mm. In case of a utricular cyst, the catheter goes in much deeper. A membranous hood over the colliculus that may act as a cyst during voiding can, when present, easily be ruptured with the ureteral catheter. The sphincteric area is inspected for classical posterior urethral valves and for a possible syringocele. The whole length of the urethra is inspected meticulously for the possible presence of an anterior diverticulum.

Next, a resectoscope is inserted with a 0° optic and a diathermia hook. A very high and obstructive bladder neck may be incised at the 7 o'clock position over a depth of 2–3 mm. Classical posterior valves may be hooked and incised. One needs to feel the way around the corner in the sphincter area in the 12 o'clock position: a flap valve often cannot be seen but can be hooked and cut, when needed. A syringocele may be incised; the rim of an anterior diverticulum can be incised.

A 12 Fr cystoscope should pass the meatus in any boy over 10 months old without resistance. In case of distal urethral narrowing, an Otis urethrotomy needs to be done with a pediatric urethrotome till 14 Fr with a recurrence risk for narrowing of 25% within 1 year.

33.12 Girls with Dysfunctional Voiding, OAB, and Recurrent Urinary Tract Infections

When screening girls with LUTS in a third-line referral setting, we always look at hypermobility of joints. Hypermobility of the bladder neck is detected by asking them to cough with an ultrasound probe on the lower abdomen. When the bladder neck descends more than 2.5–3 cm, one may suspect a congenital cystocele. By doing perineal ultrasound, one can measure the length of the urethra. Urethral lengths under 20 mm may prevent the possibility of continence; under 15 mm needs bladder neck surgery to become dry. A congenital cystocele is detected by asking the patient to cough and strain. These are all rare anomalies.

Approximately 20% of girls with dysfunctional voiding and/or recurrent urinary tract infections have an anomaly of their meatus. The urinary stream is deflected anteriorly by a web that covers the meatus partially. They urinate against the toilet seat or against the clitoris. This can be seen at physical exam or detected by asking the girl and mother to inspect the stream during voiding with the legs at an angle of 90°. It is very useful to do this because treatment of this meatal anomaly will cure the LUTS in nearly 50% of cases, obviating the need for further urotherapy and medication [31, 32].

33.13 Meatal Correction in a Girl with Anterior Deflected Urinary Stream

In lithotomy position under general anesthesia, the stream is inspected by expression of the bladder. This can only be done when a caudal block has been given by the anesthesiologist.

The meatus is calibrated with olive catheters. When the olive catheter fits in tightly, a dorsal meatal incision is done on the olive catheter with a pointed knife. After this, the meatus is dilated to 24 Fr in girls over 5 years of age. An alternative is to pick up the dorsal meatus with two forceps and do a meatotomy using scissors. The incision may be closed by 2 or 3.6 or 7.0 sutures. Expression of the bladder should reveal normalization of the stream.

For practical reasons, this is combined with cystoscopy to look at patency of the bladder neck, vesicourethral angle, and urethral length and aspect.

Acknowledgment We thank Mrs. Ingrid Visser for drawing the pictures in this chapter.

References

1. Grimsby GM, Menon V, Schlomer BJ, Baker LA, Adams R, Gargollo PC, et al. Long-term outcomes of bladder neck reconstruction without augmentation cystoplasty in children. J Urol. 2016;195(1):155–61.
2. Ferrer FA, Tadros YE, Gearhart J. Modified Young-Dees-Leadbetter bladder neck reconstruction: new concepts about old ideas. Urology. 2001;58:791.
3. Belman AB, Kaplan GW. Experience with the Kropp anti-incontinence procedure. J Urol. 1989;141:1160.
4. Salle JL, McLorie GA, Bagli DJ, Khoury AE. Urethral lengthening with anterior bladder wall flap (Pippi Salle procedure): modifications and extended indications of the technique. J Urol. 1997;158:585.
5. Jones JA, Mitchell ME, Rink RC. Improved results using a modification of the Young-Dees-Leadbetter bladder neck repair. Br J Urol. 1993;71:555.
6. Chrzan R, Dik P, Klijn AJ, Kuijper CF, van den Heijkant MM, de Jong TP. Vesicoscopic bladder neck procedure in children: what we have learned from the first series. J Laparoendosc Adv Surg Tech A. 2013;23:803.
7. Elder JS. Periurethral and puboprostatic sling repair for incontinence in patients with myelodysplasia. J Urol. 1990;144:434.
8. Chrzan R, Dik P, Klijn AJ, de Jong TP. Sling suspension of the bladder neck for pediatric urinary incontinence. J Pediatr Urol. 2009;5:82.
9. Groen LA, Spinoit AF, Hoebeke P, Van LE, De TB, Everaert K. The AdVance male sling as a minimally invasive treatment for intrinsic sphincter deficiency in patients with neurogenic bladder sphincter dysfunction: a pilot study. Neurourol Urodyn. 2012;31:1284.
10. Garcia FA, Vagni R, Garcia AJ, Flores M, Sentagne L, Badiola F. Urethral mini-sling for the treatment of neurogenic sphincteric incompetence in pediatric and young adult patients. Arch Esp Urol. 2013;66:295.
11. Barbalias G, Liatsikos E, Barbalias D. Use of slings made of indigenous and allogenic material (Goretex) in type III urinary incontinence and comparison between them. Eur Urol. 1997;31:394.
12. Lottmann H, Traxer O, Aigrain Y, Melin Y. Posterior approach to the bladder for implantation of the 800 AMS artificial sphincter in children and adolescents: techniques and results in eight patients. Ann Urol (Paris). 1999;33:357.
13. Dik P, van Gool JD, de Jong TP. Urinary continence and erectile function after bladder neck sling suspension in male patients with spinal dysraphism. BJU Int. 1999;83:971.
14. Dik P, Klijn AJ, van Gool JD, de Jong TP. Transvaginal sling suspension of bladder neck in female patients with neurogenic sphincter incontinence. J Urol. 2003;170:580.
15. Burch JC. Urethrovaginal fixation to Cooper's ligament for correction of stress incontinence, cystocele, and prolapse. Am J Obstet Gynecol. 1961;81:281.

16. de Kort LM, Vijverberg MA, de Jong TP. Colposuspension in girls: clinical and urodynamic aspects. J Pediatr Urol. 2005;1:69.
17. Rawashdeh YF, Austin P, Siggaard C, Bauer SB, Franco I, de Jong TP, et al. International Children's Continence Society's recommendations for therapeutic intervention in congenital neuropathic bladder and bowel dysfunction in children. Neurourol Urodyn. 2012;31:615.
18. Veenboer PW, Nadorp S, de Jong TP, Dik P, van Asbeck FW, Bosch JL, et al. Enterocystoplasty vs detrusorectomy: outcome in the adult with spina bifida. J Urol. 2013;189:1066.
19. Chrzan R, Dik P, Klijn AJ, Kuijper CF, de Jong TP. Detrusorectomy reduces the need for augmentation and use of antimuscarinics in children with neuropathic bladders. J Pediatr Urol. 2013;9:193.
20. Djordjevic ML, Vukadinovic V, Stojanovic B, Bizic M, Radojicic Z, Djordjevic D, et al. Objective long-term evaluation after bladder autoaugmentation with rectus muscle backing. J Urol. 2015;193:1824.
21. Gurocak S, De Gier RP, Feitz W. Bladder augmentation without integration of intact bowel segments: critical review and future perspectives. J Urol. 2007;177:839.
22. Hansen EL, Hvistendahl GM, Rawashdeh YF, Olsen LH. Promising long-term outcome of bladder autoaugmentation in children with neurogenic bladder dysfunction. J Urol. 2013;190:1869.
23. Johal NS, Hamid R, Aslam Z, Carr B, Cuckow PM, Duffy PG. Ureterocystoplasty: long-term functional results. J Urol. 2008;179:2373.
24. Reinberg Y, Allen RC Jr, Vaughn M, McKenna PH. Nephrectomy combined with lower abdominal extraperitoneal ureteral bladder augmentation in the treatment of children with the vesicoureteral reflux dysplasia syndrome. J Urol. 1995;153:177.
25. Tekgul S, Oge O, Bal K, Erkan I, Bakkaloglu M. Ureterocystoplasty: an alternative reconstructive procedure to enterocystoplasty in suitable cases. J Pediatr Surg. 2000;35:577.
26. Kajbafzadeh AM, Farrokhi-Khajeh-Pasha Y, Ostovaneh MR, Nezami BG, Hojjat A. Teapot ureterocystoplasty and ureteral Mitrofanoff channel for bilateral megaureters: technical points and surgical results of neurogenic bladder. J Urol. 2010;183:1168.
27. Mitrofanoff P. Trans-appendicular continent cystostomy in the management of the neurogenic bladder. Chir Pediatr. 1980;21:297.
28. Makkas M. Zur behandlung der Blasenektopie. Umwandlung des ausgeschalteten Coecum zur Blase und der Appendix zur Urethra. Zentralbl Chir. 1910;37:1073.
29. Lemelle JL, Simo AK, Schmitt M. Comparative study of the Yang-Monti channel and appendix for continent diversion in the Mitrofanoff and Malone principles. J Urol. 2004;172:1907.
30. de Jong TP, Kuijper CF, Chrzan R, Dik P, Klijn AJ, Vijverberg MA. Efficacy and safety of urethral de-obstruction in boys with overactive bladder complaints. J Pediatr Urol. 2013;9:1072.
31. Hoebeke P, Van LE, Raes A, van Gool JD, Vande WJ. Anomalies of the external urethral meatus in girls with non-neurogenic bladder sphincter dysfunction. BJU Int. 1999;83:294.
32. Klijn AJ, Bochove-Overgaauw D, Winkler-Seinstra PL, Dik P, de Jong TP. Urethral meatus deformities in girls as a factor in dysfunctional voiding. Neurourol Urodyn. 2012;31:1161.

Index

A
Abdominal pain, 315
Abdominal pressure, 75, 79
Adventitional layers, 360
Aftercare, 360, 362, 363
Alfuzosin, 300
Alpha-adrenergic antagonists, 300
Alpha-blockers, 242, 244, 299
American Urological Association (AUA) guideline, 95, 291
Anal atresia, 309
Anatomic obstruction, 121
Anorectal physiology testing, 110
Antegrade colonic enema stoma (ACE), 132
Antibiotic prophylaxis, 284
Antibiotics, 130
Anticholinergics, 131, 297
Antimuscarinics, 148
Artificial sphincter placement, 358
Attention deficit hyperactivity disorder (ADHD), 170–172, 177
Autism, 169–170

B
BCR, see Bulbocavernous reflex (BCR)
BD, see Bladder diary (BD)
Bedwetting, 118–119
    alarm therapy, 191
    diary, 32
    features, 178
Behavioral problems, 180
Behavioral therapy, 262
Behavioural issues, 123
Beta-3 adrenergic receptor agonists, 301–302
BFB, see Biofeedback (BFB)

Biofeedback (BFB), 199, 277, 282, 283
    childhood, 279
    constipation, 291
    dysfunctional voiding, 284, 285
    OAB, 280
    pain, 291
    pelvic floor (see Pelvic floor rehabilitation)
    urinary tract infection, 290
    vesicoureteral reflux, 290
Bladder, 3
    Botox injection, 59
    capacity, 6–9
    diverticulum, 56, 57
    endoscopic evaluation of, 55
    injections into, 59
    normal and abnormal function, 265
    recovery, 237
    small bladder capacity, 271
    training, 263
    wall thickness, 38, 39
Bladder and bowel dysfunction (BBD), 303
Bladder augmentation, 331, 332
    enterocystoplasty, 359
    megaureters, 361
Bladder autoaugmentation, 360–361
Bladder bowel dysfunction (BBD), 313
Bladder contraction, 297
Bladder diary (BD), 29, 181
    example of, 31
    limitations of, 33
    in paediatric population, 32–33
    voiding and, 30–32
Bladder drainage, 350
Bladder dysfunction, 121, 242
    pharmacotherapy, 297
    and renal failure, 243

© Springer International Publishing AG, part of Springer Nature 2018
G. Mosiello et al. (eds.), *Clinical Urodynamics in Childhood and Adolescence*, Urodynamics, Neurourology and Pelvic Floor Dysfunctions,
https://doi.org/10.1007/978-3-319-42193-3

Bladder exstrophy, 225
    anatomy of, 225–226
    complete primary repair of bladder exstrophy, 231
    embryology of, 225
    epispadias, 232–236
    presentation of, 226–228
    radical soft tissue mobilisation, 230
    staged approaches, 229–230
    surgical techniques, 228–229
    urodynamics and outcomes, 231–232
Bladder emptying, functional disturbances of, 120–121
Bladder exstrophy-epispadias complex (BEEC), 225
Bladder leak point pressure (BLPP), 85
Bladder neck (BN)
    colposuspension, 357
    injections into, 59
    laparoscopy, 338, 340
    Mitchel's technique, 352
    preperitoneal approach, 338
    procedures, 350–352, 354–357
    puboprostatic sling, 354
    rectus abdominis fascia sling, 356
    with slings, 352–354
    transperitoneal approach, 340
    urethral sling, 357
    vesicoscopy, 341–344
    Young-Dees-Leadbetter technique, 350
Bladder neck incision (BNI), 242
Bladder outlet obstruction (BOO), 66, 68, 209, 243
Bladder overactivity, 176
Bladder sensation, 83
Bladder stone, 59
Bladder surgery, 358, 359
Bladder tube, 363, 364
Bladder tumor, 58, 59
Bladder voiding, 313
Bladder/bowel dysfunction (BBD), 24, 25, 205, 208
Bladder–brain dialogue, 177
Bladderscan, 38
Botox®, 131, 244
Botulinum toxin (BTX), 131, 148, 200, 201, 328
Bowel diary, 182
Bowel dysfunction, 121, 313
    management, 315
    measures, 24
Bristol Stool Form Scale (BSFS), 24, 190, 314–316

Bulbocavernous reflex (BCR), 106–107
Bulbourethral sling, 332
Bulking agent, 330, 331
Burch colposuspension, 339–341

C
Campylobacter jejuni, 158
Cantwell-Ransley repair, 234
Catheterization, 281
Cauda equina syndrome, 106
Cerebral palsy (CP), , , –, 18, 153, 169, 170
    detrusor overactivity, 155
    detrusor underactivity, 155
    incontinence, 154
    management, 155–156
    pathogenesis, 155
    specific recommendations, 156–157
    symptomatology, 154
Child Behaviour Checklist (CBCL), 23, 264
Childhood, 308
    biofeedback, 279
    bowel dysfunction management, 315–317
    pelvic floor rehabilitation, 279
    SNM (*see* Sacral neuromodulation (SNM))
    survival strategies, 265
Chronic constipation, 315, 316
Classical conditioning, 262
Clean intermittent catheterization (CIC), 81, 127, 129, 132, 241, 242, 342, 350–352, 356, 361, 362
Cognitive therapy, 261–262
    overactive bladder, 200
Colonic transit times, 112
Colposuspension, 339, 357
Comorbidities, 196
Complete primary repair of bladder exstrophy (CPRE), 231
Congenital defect, 251
Congenital neuropathic bladder, 332
Constipation, 120, 122, 123, 172, 180, 264, 301, 304, 308, 313–315, 317
    chronic (*see* Chronic constipation)
    functional (*see* Functional constipation)
    intractable, 317
    and overactive bladder, 195
    probiotics, 316
    rehabilitation and, 291
    treatment, 315
Continence, 165–169
Continuous incontinence, 117
Cultured bladders, 358
Cystography, 307

Index

Cystometrogram, 103
Cystometry, 73, 76, 77, 283
   detrusor compliance, 83
   flowmetry and ultrasound PVR measurement, 77
   Fr double-lumen catheter, 78
   indication for, 74–75
   leakage, 81
   procedures, 77
   quality control, 81–82
   recording, 80
   retrograde filling, 80
   setting of, 76
   slow filling rate, 80
   storage phase, interpretation, 82–85
   triple-lumen catheter, 79
   voiding, 81
Cystoscopy, 339, 365, 366

D

Daytime diary, 31
Daytime incontinence, 118, 119
Daytime lower urinary tract dysfunction
   BBD, 208
   bladder neck dysfunction, 210
   bladder outlet obstruction, 209
   diagnostic investigations, 206
   dysfunctional voiding, 208
   etiology and clinical presentation, 205
   giggle incontinence, 209
   overactive bladder, 207
   prevalence of, 205
   reference point for, 206
   storage dysfunction, 207
   toilet-trained children, 210
   underactive bladder, 207
   vaginal reflux, 208–209
   valve-bladder syndrome, 210
   voiding postponement, 207–208
   voiding/emptying phase dysfunction, 208
Defecation disorders
   anorectal physiology tests, 110–111
   colonic transit times, 112
   diagnostic tests for, 109
   digital rectal examination, 110
   patient history, 109–110
   physical examination, 110
   rectal biomechanics, 111
   rectal biopsy, 111
   rectal examination, 111–112
Demography, 238
Demucolized sigmoid colon, 360

Des-ethyl-oxybutynin (DEOB), 131
Desmopressin, 184, 191
Detrusor activity, 84
Detrusor compliance, 83
Detrusor leak point pressure (DLPP), 85
Detrusor muscle, 362
Detrusor overactivity (DO), 84, 287, 330
Detrusor pressure, 78, 82
Detrusor sphincter dyssynergia (DSD), 67, 84, 102, 103, 160
Detrusor underactivity, 86, 90, 118, 120
Detrusor underutilization disorder, 104
Detrusorectomy, 132, 354, 360
Dextranomer, 216
Diabetes insipidus, 180
Diabetes mellitus, 180
Digital rectal examination, defecation disorders, 110
Dilation of rectum, 315
Disruptive Behaviour Disorders Rating Scale, 23
Diurnal enuresis, 118
Down's syndrome, 121, 170–172
Doxazosin, 300
Dry mouth, 299, 301
Duckett's classification, 251, 252
Duplay technique, 256
Dysfunction voiding, 103
Dysfunctional elimination syndrome, 289, 290
Dysfunctional voiding (DV), 67, 118, 120, 171, 208, 274, 277, 327, 328
   doxazosin for, 300
   girls with, 366
   PTNS, 319, 323
   rehabilitation in, 284
Dysfunctional voiding scoring system (DVSS), 14, 22, 64, 299

E

Ectopic ureter
   clinical presentation, 214–215
   diagnosis, 215
   embryology, 213–214
   intervention, 216–217
   ultrasound of, 215
   VCUG, 216
Ectopic ureteric orifice, 18
Electrodes, 79
Electromyographic studies, 85
Electromyography (EMG), 101–104, 279, 280, 285, 286, 300
Encopresis, 280, 287

Endoscopy, 329–335
Enterocystoplasty, bladder augmentation, 359
Enuresis, 118, 283
    classification, 175
    family history, 181 (*see also* Monosymptomatic enuresis (MNE))
    pregnancy, labor, and birth history, 181
    psychosocial impact of, 177
    rehabilitation in, 280
Epispadias
    female epispadias, 234–236
    male epispadias, 232–234
Erectile dysfunction, 253
Estimated bladder capacity (EBC), 8
European Association of Urology (EAU), 339
European Bladder Dysfunction Study (EBDS), 286
European Society for Paediatric Gastroenterology Hepatology and Nutrition (ESPGHAN), 315
Expected bladder capacity (EBC), 30, 118
Exstrophy, 361

F

Faecal incontinence, 304, 313, 315, 316
Fascia sling, 331, 338
Fecal incontinence, 180
Female epispadias, 234
Fertility, sexual function and, 247
Flap valve, 351
Flowmeter, 269
Flowmetry index (FI), 66
Food and Drug Administration (FDA), 303
Frequency volume chart (FVC), 29, 96
Functional bladder capacity, 308
Functional constipation, 309, 314, 315

G

Gastrocystoplasty, 359
Giggle incontinence, 12, 119, 209, 281
Guillain-Barré syndrome, 309

H

Headache, 301
Health-related quality of life (HRQoL), 253
High voiding detrusor pressures, 87
Hinman bladder, 121
Hinman syndrome, 32, 277
Hinman-Allen syndrome, 208
Hirschsprung' s disease, 111

Holding manoeuvres, 118
Holmium/\yttrium aluminum garnet (Ho\:YAG) laser \urethrotomy (HLU), 330
Hyaluronic acid, 216
Hydrodistention implantation technique (HIT), 330
Hyperfiltration injury, 247
Hypospadias, 251
    critical process of, 251
    detrusor overactivity, 255
    diagnosis, 251
    Duckett's classification, 251, 252
    etiology, 251
    mictional cystography, 256
    neourethral stricture, 255–257
    with proximal meatus, 252
    psychosexual development, 253
    psychosocial features, 253
    scars, 257
    self-image, 253–254
    urinary flow, 255
    urodynamics in patients with, 254–255
Hypothermia, 46
Hypoxic ischemic encephalopathy (HIE), 158

I

ICCS, *see* International children continence society (ICCS)
Ileal tubes, 363
Ileocystoplasty, 132, 359–361, 363
Incompetent closure mechanism, 89
Incontinence, 85, 117, 154
Increased arousal threshold, 176
Institute of Medicine and National Research Council, 333
Intermittent catheterization, 147
Intermittent incontinence, 118
Intermittent self-catheterization, 275
International Children's Continence Society (ICCS), 29, 31, 33, 73, 277, 278, 313, 332
International Consultation on Incontinence (ICI), 327
International Continence Society (ICS), 29, 73
Intractable constipation, 317
Intravesical procedure, 338
Invasive urodynamics, monosymptomatic enuresis, 182

K
Kegel exercises, 277, 281
Kidney disease, 180
Kropp's tube, 350

L
Labial adhesions, 17
Laparoscopy, 331, 337, 338, 357
    bladder neck, 338–340
    Burch colposuspension, 339–341
Lazy bladder, 292
Loop ureterostomy, 241
Lower urinary tract dysfunction
    (LUTD), 280, 304, 308
    clinical care outcome, 25
    clinical patterns of, 11
    conditions affecting, 18–19
    definitions, 117
    gynaecologic examination, 17–18
    history taking, 13–14
    incontinence, 117
    labial adhesions, 17
    limitations of, 22
    measurement tool, 22–24
    musculoskeletal examination, 15
    neurologic causes of, 12
    neurological examination, 15–16
    non-neurogenic, 305
    pediatric urologist, 12–13
    pelvic floor rehabilitation
        (*see* Pelvic floor rehabilitation)
    physical examination, 15
    pitfalls, 22
    Rome III diagnostic criteria, 25
    routine intervention, 21
    in school-aged child, 11
    urogenital sinus anomalies, 17
    urological examination, 16–17
    warning signs, 122
Lower urinary tract symptoms
    (LUTS), 63, 179, 313
    standardization, 176
LUTD, *see* Lower urinary tract dysfunction
    (LUTD)
LUTS, *see* Lower urinary tract symptoms
    (LUTS)

M
Male epispadias, 232
Malone Anterograde Continence Enemas
    (MACE), 316
Maximum bladder capacity, 83
Maximum cystometric capacity
    (MCC), 86
Maximum voiding detrusor pressure, 87
Meatal stenosis, 365
Mechanism of action, PTNS, 322
Megaureters, bladder augmentation, 361
Mini-invasive approach, 328–330, 332
Minimal invasive sling, 358
Mirabegron, 301
Mitchell's procedure, 351, 352
Mitrofanoff procedure, 331
MNE, *see* Monosymptomatic enuresis
    (MNE)
Modern staged repair of bladder exstrophy
    (MSRE), 230
Monopolar diathermy, 339
Monosymptomatic enuresis
    (MNE), 280
    active treatment, 183
    alarm, 183–184
    bladder diary, 181–182
    blood tests, 182
    bowel diary, 182
    clinical assessment, 178–181
    definitions, 175
    desmopressin, 184
    enuresis, 177–178
    epidemiology, 176
    first-line treatment, 185
    general measures, 183
    invasive urodynamics, 182
    pathology, 176–177
    ultrasound, 182
    warning findings, 179
    X-rays, 182
MRI, 40–43
Mucopolysaccharidosis type 3 (MPS3),
    168–169
Mucosal strip, 350, 351
Mucosal tunnel, 362
Mullerian-inhibiting substance (MIS)
    deficiency, 52

N
Neourethral stricture, 255
Nephrectomy, 361
Nerve stimulation, *see specific nerve*
    stimulation
Neurogenic bladder (NB), 58, 121, 300, 304
Neurogenic bladder dysfunction (NBD),
    157, 158, 304, 305, 308–310

Neurogenic detrusor overactivity
 (NDO), 328
Neurogenic lower urinary tract dysfunction
 (NLUTD), 145
Neuromodulation, 199
 exclusion criteria, 305
 modalities of, 303
 sacral, 303–304
  evidence of, 307
  external pulse generator, 307
  implant, 306, 309
  indications, 304–305
  intraoperative test phase, 307
  neurogenic bladder dysfunction, 308
  patients selection, 305
  surgical technique, 306–308
Neuropathic bladder dysfunction, 161
Neurophysiological testing
 bulbocavernous reflex, 106
 cystometrogram, 103
 electromyography, 101
 noninvasive urodynamic study, 102
 somatosensory evoked potential, 104–106
Neurorehabilitation, 278
NMNE, *see* Nonmonosymptomatic nocturnal
 enuresis (NMNE)
Nocturnal polyuria, 30, 176, 182
Noninvasive rehabilitation program, 281
Nonmonosymptomatic nocturnal enuresis
 (NMNE), 33, 175
 epidemiology, 189
 pathophysiology, 190
 pretreatment patient examination, 190
 treatment, 191
Non-neurogenic bladder, 121, 300
Non-neurogenic vesical–sphincter
 dyssynergia, 284
Nonobstructive urinary retention
 (NOUR), 304
Nonrandomized controlled trials (NRCT),
 319, 322, 323

O

OAB, *see* overactive bladder (OAB)
Obesity, overactive bladder and, 197
Occult spina bifida, 105
Onabotulinum toxin A, 60, 328, 329
Onabotulinumtoxina (Botox®), 131
Operant conditioning, 262
Orifices, endoscopic evaluation of, 55
Otis urethrotomy, 366

Overactive bladder (OAB),
 67, 118, 119, 193, 274, 279
 anticholinergic agents, 298
 biofeedback therapy, 199
 botulinum toxin A, 200–201
 clinical presentation, 196
 cognitive therapy, 200
 comorbidities, 196–197
 complaints, 365
 conservative management, 198
 constipation, 195–196
 daytime LUTD, 207
 diagnosis, 197
 epidemiology, 194
 etiology, 194
 girls with, 366
 history, 197
 mirabegron, 301
 neuromodulation, 199–200
 and obesity, 197
 pathophysiology, 195
 peripheral nerve stimulation, 200
 pharmacologic treatment, 199
 physical examination, 198
 prognosis, 198
 psychotherapy, 200
 PTNS, 319, 322–324
 randomized controlled trials, 324
 refractory, 319
 rehabilitation in, 280
 sacral nerve modulation, 200
Overnight bladder drainage, 241
Oxybutynin, 244, 298, 299

P

Paediatric enuresis module to assess quality
 of life (PEMQOL), 24
Paediatric incontinence quality of life
 (PinQ), 24
Paediatric urology, 11
Pain, rehabilitation and, 291
Partial urogenital mobilization (PUM), 222
Pathogenesis, 121
Pediatric Penile Perception Score
 (PPPS), 253
Pediatric urinary incontinence quality of
 life score (PIN-Q), 64
Pediatric urologic endoscopy, 45
 advantages, 47
 anterior urethral valve, 51–52
 bladder, 55

bladder diverticulum, 56
bladder stone, 59
bladder tumors, 58
components of, 47
contraindications, 50
foreign objects, 59
indications, 50
injection, 59–60
neurogenic bladder, 58
posterior urethral valve, 53–55
preparation, 45–46
syringocele, 51
technique, 48–49
tools, 47–48
ureterocele, 57
urethral polyp, 53
urethral stricture, 50–51
utricular cyst, 52
VUR/STI, 55–56
Pediatric urologist, 12
Pelvic floor, 4
Pelvic floor muscles (PFMs), 65, 278
Pelvic floor rehabilitation, 277
in childhood, 279
constipation, 291
dysfunctional voiding, 284–290
monosymptomatic enuresis, 280
OAB, 280
pain, 291
posterior urethral valve ablation, 292
underactive bladder, 292
urinary tract infection, 290
vesicoureteral reflux, 290–291
Percutaneous tibial nerve stimulation (PTNS), 319
LUTD, 322
mechanism of action, 322
techniques of, 320–322
Perineal contraction, 278, 281, 282
Peripheral nerve stimulation, 200
PFS, *see* Pressure flow study (PFS)
Pharmacological therapy, 288, 297
alpha-blockers, 299–300
anticholinergics, 297–299
beta-3 adrenergic receptor agonists, 301
Pharmacotherapy, 244
Physiotherapy, 269
Pippi Salle's procedure, 351
Polyethylene glycol (PEG), 316
Polyglycolic acid suture, 358
Polypropylene sling, 332

Polyuria, 237, 246
Posterior urethral valve (PUV), 53, 121, 237, 329
antenatal diagnosis, 238
bladder dysfunction, 242–243
cystogram of, 243
demography, 238
diagnosis, 239
early diversion in, 241
endoscopic valve ablation, 239–240
endoscopic view of, 53
endoscopy for, 241
end-stage renal failure, 246–247
incision of, 54
isotope scans, 239
long-term outcome, 241
neonatal management, 239
newborn with, 240
pharmacotherapy, 244–245
postneonatal follow-up, 242
prenatal interventions, 239
prenatal ultrasound scanning, 238
reflux in, 245
rehabilitation, 292
transitional care, 247
urinary continence, 245–246
urodynamics in, 243–244
YAG laser, 239
Post-exstrophy incontinence, 332
Post-void residual (PVR), 33, 66, 74, 96, 243, 288
Preperitoneal approach, bladder neck, 338
Pressure flow study (PFS), 73
acontractile detrusor, 86
detrusor underactivity, 86
indication for, 74
normal voiding, 86
possible pathological findings, 88
procedures, 77–81, 86
voiding phase, 86–88
Primary monosymptomatic nocturnal enuresis, 324
Probiotics, 316
Prolonged lag time, 300
Psychiatry, 123–124
Psychosocial problems, 180
Psychotherapy, overactive bladder, 200
PTNS, *see* Percutaneous tibial nerve stimulation (PTNS)
Puboprostatic sling, 354, 355
Pubovaginal sling, 331

Q
Qmax, 66, 67, 69
Quality of life (QoL), 23, 315

R
Radical soft tissue mobilisation (RSTM), 230
Randomized controlled trials (RCT), 286, 319, 320, 323
    OAB, 324
    underactive bladder, 292
Rectal biomechanics, 111
Rectal biopsy, defecation disorders, 111
Rectus abdominis fascia sling, 353, 356
Reflux, in PUV boys, 245
Rehabilitation, 279
    pelvic floor (*see* Pelvic floor rehabilitation)
Renal failure, bladder dysfunction and, 243
Renal transplant, 246–247
Resectoscope, 48
Robotic-assisted laparoscopy (RAL), 338, 340, 341, 344
Rome III diagnostic criteria, 25, 190

S
Sacral agenesis, 12
Sacral nerve stimulation (SNS), 106
Sacral neuromodulation (SNM), 200, 303
    evidence of, 307
    external pulse generator, 307
    implant of, 306, 309
    indications, 304
    intraoperative test phase, 307
    with NBD, 308
    patients selection, 305–306
    surgical technique, 306
Sacral spinal cord lesions, 145
Sanfilippo disease, 168, 169
Sexual function, and fertility, 247
Short screening instrument for psychological problems in enuresis (SSIPPE), 23, 64
Sleep fragmentation, 177
Slings, 132, 331, 332, 352, 354
Small bladder capacity, 271
SNM, *see* Sacral neuromodulation (SNM)
Somatosensory evoked potential (SSEP), 104
Sphincter, 4
Sphincteric incompetence, 330
Spina bifida, 105, 308
    adolescents, 130
    antibiotics, 130–131
    anticholinergic medication, 131

    bladder, 128
    botulin toxin, 131–132
    bowel, 128
    combinations of medication, 131
    complications and solutions, 132–133
    early after birth, 129
    first years of life, 129
    history of, 127–128
    intravesical therapy, 131
    kidneys, 128
    laboratory tests, 130
    low pressures, 128
    overtreatment, 133–134
    school age, 129
    sexuality, 136–138
    surgical options, 132
    tomax, 138
    urodynamic study, 135–136
Spinal cord injury (SCI), 143
    botulinum toxin, 149
    epidemiology, 143–144
    intermittent catheterization, 147–148
    neurological bladder dysfunction, 146
    patient evaluation, 145
    pharmacotherapy, 148
    rehabilitation and treatment, 147
    sacral spinal cord lesions, 145
    suprasacral SCI, 144–145
    surgical treatment, 149
    treatment, 147
Spinal dysraphism, 135, 136, 299, 331
Staccato voiding curve, 67
STI, 55
STING procedure, 56
Stress urinary incontinence (SUI), 330
    management, 339
    neurogenic, 331
    suburethral slings, 331
Suburethral slings, SUI, 331
Suprapubic technique, 320
Suprasacral SCI, 144
Syringocele, 51, 365

T
Tamsulosin, 300
TENS, *see* Transcutaneous electrical nerve stimulation (TENS)
Tethered cord syndrome, 12, 105
Tissue coll®, 360
Tolterodine, 299
Total urogenital mobilization (TUM), 222
Transabdominal ultrasound, PFM, 278
Transanal irrigation, 316

Index

Transcutaneous electrical nerve stimulation (TENS), 319, 320
  advantages, 321
  LUTD, 322–324
  in physiological changes, 322
Transcutaneous posterior tibial nerve stimulation (TPTNS), 321, 323
Transperitoneal approach, bladder neck, 340–341
Transvaginal rectus fascia sling, 356
Transverse abdominal incision, 362
Transverse lower abdominal incision, 357
Transverse myelitis, 158–161
Trigon, endoscopic evaluation of, 55

U

UDS, *see* Urodynamic studies (UDS)
Ultrasound, 38–40
  antenatal diagnosis, 238
  bladder volume by, 38
  measurements of the rectal diameter, 40
  monosymptomatic enuresis, 182
  PFM, 278
Underactive bladder (UB), 118, 120, 292
UPP, *see* Urethral pressure profile (UPP)
Upper airway obstruction, 180
Upper urinary tract (UUT), 95
Ureteral ectopia, 122
Ureterocele, 57, 329
  clinical presentation, 217
  diagnosis, 217–219
  embryology, 217
  intervention, 219
  intravesical ureteroceles, 218
  VCUG, 218
Urethra, 4
Urethral diverticulum, 42, 51
Urethral meatus position, 254
Urethral obstruction, 365
Urethral overactivity, 91
Urethral polyp, 53
Urethral pressure profile (UPP), 73–74
  in children, 90
  filling phase, 90
  incompetent closure mechanism, 89
  indication for, 75
  pressure-recording catheter, 89
  procedures, 88, 89
  simultaneous bladder and, 89
  static measurement, 88
  terminology and clinical significance, 89–91
  urethral sphincter, 88
  voiding phase, 87
Urethral sling, 357
Urethral sphincter, 59, 88, 328, 331
Urethral stricture, 50, 51
Urethral valve (UV), 51, 329
Urethrocystoscopy, 47
Urethrotome, 48
Urethrovaginal fistula, 42
Urge incontinence, 118, 283, 303, 365
Urge syndrome, 280–283
Urge Visual Analogue Scale, 23
Urgency, 118
Urinalysis, 46
Urinary continence, 245
Urinary cystography, 307
Urinary flowmetry, 65–70
Urinary incontinence (UI), 305, 327, 337
  daytime, 279–281, 283, 284, 286, 288, 289
  minor surgery for, 365
  treatment algorithm, 298
Urinary tract infection (UTI), 64
  recurrent, 279, 366
  rehabilitation in, 290
Urine storage, functional disturbances of, 118–120
Urodynamic instrumented investigations, 63
Urodynamics, 12, 63, 95, 129, 277, 279, 284, 305
  equipment, 68
  evaluation, 63, 67, 305
  investigation, 68
  neurologic examination, 64
  noninvasive, 64, 244
  in non-neurogenic conditions, 97
  parameter, 309
  in patients with hypospadias, 254
  pitfalls of, 135
  physical examination, 64
  in PUV, 243
  Qmax, 66, 67
  question, 64
  spina bifida, 135
  surface electromyography, 66
  test, 307
  urinary flowmetry, 65
  variable, 308
  video, 305
  voiding diary, 64
  weekly bowel diary, 64

Uroflowmetry, 280, 284, 285
Urogenital sinus
  anomalies, 17
  clinical presentation, 220
  diagnosis of, 220–221
  embryology, 219–220
  treatment, 221–222
Urologic issues, 297
Urologists, 297
Urotherapist, 286
Urotherapy, 262
  biofeedback, 268
  bladder training, 263
  children for, 263–264
  drawbacks, 274–275
  ending the therapy, 272–273
  fluid intake, 266
  frequency of urinations, 270
  group training, 271–272
  instructions on proper toilet, 268
  intensive approach, 271
  intermittent self-catheterization, 275
  learning element, 268–271
  parents role, 273–274
  psycho-education, 264–268
  relaxed toilet position, 266
  relearning process, 268
  results, 274
  rewards and support, 272
  signal to urinate, 268
  small bladder capacity, 271
  standard treatment, 264–267
  tacking, 267
  therapist role, 273
  timed voiding, 271
  urinary frequency, 266
  urinary tract infections, 264
  voiding diary, 263, 268
  voiding history, 263

U-shaped incision, 341, 352
Utricular cyst, 52

V

Vaginal discharge, 18
Vaginal reflux, 119, 208
Vaginal voiding, 208
Valsalva's manoeuver, 17
Valve-bladder syndrome, 210
Vesical catheterization, 282
Vesicoscopy, bladder neck procedure, 341–344
Vesicoureteral reflux (VUR), 55, 245, 290, 330
Vesicovaginal fistula, 356
Video urodynamic (VUD), 305
  initial assessment and technique, 96
  neurological abnormalities, 98–99
  procedure, 97
  setting, 96
  UDS general considerations, 97–98
Video-urodynamic study (VUDS), 129, 135
Voided volume, 118
Voiding cystourethrogram (VCUG), 239
Voiding diaries, 30
Voiding dysfunction, *see* Dysfunctional voiding (DV)
Voiding function, 4–8
Voiding postponement, 118, 120
Voiding school (VS), 290
Voiding/emptying phase dysfunction, 208

Y

Yang/Monti procedure, 363
Young-Dees-Leadbetter (YDL) technique, 350
Y-V plasty, 365

MIX
Papier aus verantwortungsvollen Quellen
Paper from responsible sources
FSC® C105338

If you have any concerns about our products, you can contact us on
ProductSafety@springernature.com

In case Publisher is established outside the EU, the EU authorized representative is:
**Springer Nature Customer Service Center GmbH
Europaplatz 3, 69115 Heidelberg, Germany**

Printed by Libri Plureos GmbH
in Hamburg, Germany